PHARMACOTHERAPIES FOR THE TREATMENT OF OPIOID DEPENDENCE

PHARMACOTHERAPIES FOR THE TREATMENT OF OPIOID DEPENDENCE

Efficacy, Cost-Effectiveness, and Implementation Guidelines

Edited by

Richard P. Mattick
University of New South Wales
Sydney, Australia

Robert Ali
University of Adelaide
Adelaide, Australia

Nicholas Lintzeris
University of Sydney
Sydney, Australia

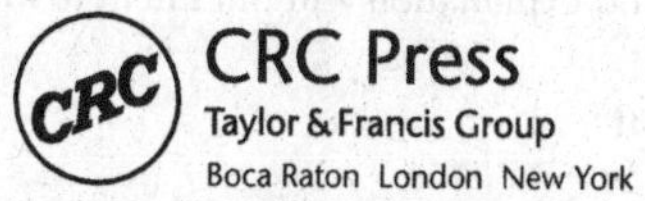

CRC Press is an imprint of the
Taylor & Francis Group, an **informa** business

First published in 2009 by Informa Healthcare

CRC Press
Taylor & Francis Group
6000 Broken Sound Parkway NW, Suite
300 Boca Raton, FL 33487-2742

© 2009 by Taylor & Francis Group, LLC
CRC Press is an imprint of Taylor & Francis Group, an Informa business

No claim to original U.S. Government works

ISBN-13: 978-1-84184-400-8 (pbk)

This book contains information obtained from authentic and highly regarded sources. While all reasonable efforts have been made to publish reliable data and information, neither the author[s] nor the publisher can accept any legal respon- sibility or liability for any errors or omissions that may be made. The publishers wish to make clear that any views or opinions expressed in this book by individual editors, authors or contributors are personal to them and do not neces- sarily reflect the views/opinions of the publishers. The information or guidance contained in this book is intended for use by medical, scientific or health-care professionals and is provided strictly as a supplement to the medical or other professional's own judgement, their knowledge of the patient's medical history, relevant manufacturer's instructions and the appropriate best practice guidelines. Because of the rapid advances in medical science, any information or advice on dosages, procedures or diagnoses should be independently verified. The reader is strongly urged to consult the relevant national drug formulary and the drug companies' and device or material manufacturers' printed instructions, and their websites, before administering or utilizing any of the drugs, devices or materials mentioned in this book. This book does not indicate whether a particular treatment is appropriate or suitable for a particular individual. Ultimately it is the sole responsibility of the medical professional to make his or her own professional judgements, so as to advise and treat patients appropriately. The authors and publishers have also attempted to trace the copyright holders of all mate- rial reproduced in this publication and apologize to copyright holders if permission to publish in this form has not been obtained. If any copyright material has not been acknowledged please write and let us know so we may rectify in any future reprint.

Except as permitted under U.S. Copyright Law, no part of this book may be reprinted, reproduced, transmitted, or uti- lized in any form by any electronic, mechanical, or other means, now known or hereafter invented, including photocopy- ing, microfilming, and recording, or in any information storage or retrieval system, without written permission from the publishers.

For permission to photocopy or use material electronically from this work, please access www.copyright.com (http:// www.copyright.com/) or contact the Copyright Clearance Center, Inc. (CCC), 222 Rosewood Drive, Danvers, MA 01923, 978-750-8400. CCC is a not-for-profit organization that provides licenses and registration for a variety of users. For organizations that have been granted a photocopy license by the CCC, a separate system of payment has been arranged.

Trademark Notice: Product or corporate names may be trademarks or registered trademarks, and are used only for identification and explanation without intent to infringe.

Visit the Taylor & Francis Web site at
http://www.taylorandfrancis.com

and the CRC Press Web site at
http://www.crcpress.com

A CIP record for this book is available from the British Library.

Library of Congress Cataloging-in-Publication Data available on application

Contents

Contributors

Robert Ali
WHO Collaborating Centre for the Treatment of Drug and Alcohol Problems
School of Medical Sciences
The University of Adelaide
Australia

Gabriele Bammer
National Centre for Epidemiology and Population Health
The Australian National University
Canberra
Australia

James Bell
The Langton Centre
Surry Hills
Australia

Rodger Brough
General Practitioner
Warnambool
Victoria
and Member, Drug and Alcohol Committee of the Royal Australian College of General Practitioners
Australia

Courtney Breen
National Drug and Alcohol Research Centre
University of New South Wales
Sydney
Australia

Tracey Burrell
Southside Health
Hurstville
Australia

Nicolas Clark
Mental Health and Substance Abuse
WHO
Geneva
Switzerland

Louisa Degenhardt
National Drug and Alcohol Research Centre
University of New South Wales
Sydney
Australia

Adrian Dunlop
Drug and Alcohol Clinical Services
Hunter New England Area Health Service and University of Newcastle
Newcastle
Australia

Amy Gibson
National Drug and Alcohol Research Centre
University of New South Wales
Sydney
Australia

Alan Gijsbers
Drug and Alcohol Liaison Unit
Royal Melbourne Hospital and Substance Withdrawal Unit
The Melbourne Clinic
Australia

Andrea L Gordon
Discipline of Pharmacology
School of Medical Sciences
The University of Adelaide
Adelaide
Australia

Linda Gowing
DASSA Evidence Based Practice Unit
Department of Clinical and Experimental Pharmacology
The University of Adelaide
Australia

Wayne Hall
School of Population Health
University of Queensland
Herston
Australia

Lynn Hawkin
DASSA Evidence Based Practice Unit
Department of Clinical and Experimental Pharmacology
The University of Adelaide
Australia

Sue Henry-Edwards
Principal Advisor
Alcohol and Other Drugs and Health Promotion
New South Wales Department of Corrective Services
Sydney
Australia

Mark R Hutchinson
Discipline of Pharmacology
School of Medical Sciences
The University of Adelaide
Adelaide
Australia

Katie Khoo
Monash University
Melbourne
Australia

Jo Kimber
Centre for Research on Drugs and Health Behaviour
London School of Hygiene and Tropical Medicine
London
UK

Sophie F La Vincente
Centre for International Child Health
Murdoch Children's Research Institute
and University of Melbourne
Department of Paediatrics
Royal Children's Hospital
Parkville, Victoria
Australia

Nicholas Lintzeris
Department of Addiction Medicine
University of Sydney
and Head of Department
Liverpool and Fairfield Hospitals
Drug Health Services
Sydney South West Area Health Service
Australia

Dolly Marope
Hunter New England Area Health Service
Newcastle
Australia

Richard P Mattick
Director
National Drug and Alcohol Research Centre
University of New South Wales
Sydney
Australia

Tim B Mitchell
Scientific Leader
Purple Hat Communications Ltd
London
UK

Benny Monheit
Alfred Hospital
Melbourne
Australia

Glynn A Morrish
Discipline of Pharmacology
School of Medical Sciences
The University of Adelaide
Australia

Peter Muhleisen
Department of Pharmacy
St Vincent's Hospital
Melbourne
Australia

David A Newcombe
Lecturer, Alcohol and Drug Studies
Social and Community Health
School of Population Health
University of Auckland
Auckland
New Zealand

Irvin Newton
Harm Minimization Committee
Drug of Dependence Advisory Committee
Kensington
Australia

David Osborn
Department of Neonatal Medicine
Royal Prince Alfred Hospital
Camperdown
Australia

Dimitra Petroulias
Turning Point Alcohol and Drug Centre
Fitzroy
Australia

Allan Quigley
Next Step Specialists Drug and Alcohol Services
East Perth
Australia

Alison Ritter
Drug Policy Modelling Program
National Drug and Alcohol Research Centre
University of New South Wales
Sydney
Australia

Marian Shanahan
Drug Policy Modelling Program
National Drug and Alcohol Research Centre
University of New South Wales
Sydney
Australia

Andrew A Somogyi
Discipline of Pharmacology
School of Medical Sciences
The University of Adelaide
Adelaide
Australia

Jeff Ward
School of Psychology
Australian National University
Canberra
Australia

Sue Whicker
Royal Australian College of General Practitioners
Australia

Jason M White
Discipline of Pharmacology
School of Medical Sciences
The University of Adelaide
Adelaide
Australia

Foreword

Pharmacotherapies for the treatment of heroin addiction matter – they matter greatly. Not only does it matter that they exist, but it also matters how they are provided. Provide the treatment well, and great public good can be achieved. Provide the treatment poorly, and some lesser level of public good may be achieved, but also opportunities will have been wasted. Fail to provide the treatment, and an opportunity to deliver individual and public good has been squandered. These observations are not obvious – there are plenty of examples where the manner of provision of treatment is not so important, provided the treatment is delivered. But in the field of pharmacotherapies for the treatment of opiate dependence, the organization of the provision of this treatment, and the quality of the treatment provided, have a great influence on the amount of individual and public good which is then achieved.

Providing treatment to individuals caught up in opioid dependence remains a controversial subject. Maintenance treatment programs are now a major component of treatment in many countries around the world, but are provided only in secret or are completely prohibited in many other countries. It is as if practitioners and policy makers have not been able to break out of the straitjacket of moral arguments and challenges about whether they do, or do not, "believe" in methadone maintenance (and similarly, but usually less passionately, with other maintenance treatments). Science needs to come to the fore, to encourage more objective consideration of the evidence, and to enable more rational planning of appropriate health care.

A long time ago, nearly 20 years ago, in the foreword to a predecessor of this book, I wrote that the world seemed split into three camps – those who know methadone maintenance to be good and efficacious, those who know it to be bad and ineffective, and a minority who are still receptive to new data and analyses of benefit and cost. I am sure that we all expected these matters to have been resolved in the intervening years, but sadly that observation remains true today. The good news is that the proportion of the world who are now receptive to consideration of new data and analyses has increased substantially, but progress is still hampered by unhealthy distractions and unreasoned attacks from both sides by those who believe, with the passion of religious zealots, that presentation and consideration of new data is in some way subversive. All three of these groups can benefit from this book with its clear presentations of the increasingly large and robust amounts of evidence about the benefits and harms that may result from provision (or nonprovision) of treatments for opioid dependence.

How much do we really know about the effects of maintenance treatment? What is the long-term outcome? What are the costs? How sure are we about the quality of the studies that have been done? These are questions that are repeatedly asked – and reasonably asked – but it is important for us all to move beyond merely repeatedly asking the questions. We must also be willing to listen to, and study, the answers that are provided. This new book edited by Richard P Mattick is an excellent source of answers to many of these questions, and it will stand many of us in better stead if we study and consider the issues laid out in clear format in this book, before we venture forth again into public debate. Not all the questions have been fully answered, and some of the initial conclusions are found to be less robust than others. But we need to know about the answers, and the quality of these answers, so that future debate, future commissioning of services, and future provision of treatment can be improved.

This new book provides an excellent and comprehensive review of this area. There are now several different pharmacotherapies to be considered, and these are each addressed in separate chapters and sections. There are also other aspects to treatment which are enormously important and relate to the organization and provision of the treatment programs themselves (i.e., there are important qualities which are not contained within the medicine bottle), and the findings from scientific study of these factors are usefully laid out for the reader.

So where does that leave us? With the planning of provision of pharmacotherapies for treatment of opioid dependence, there are ways of doing it well, and ways of doing it badly. With the actual direct clinical treatment of individuals afflicted by opioid dependence, there are ways of doing it well and ways of doing it badly. Without guidance from the extensive policy and clinical research literature, the planner and the practitioner are reliant on their instinct and intuition. They may get it right – but they may get it wrong, with disastrous consequences. Meaning well is just not good enough. Today, with access to the extensive literature on this form of treatment, decision making can be properly informed. But it is still often difficult to find balanced presentations of the large amount of data and opinions which are already out there in the public domain. This new book will be an invaluable resource for the reader looking for a balanced consideration of this extensive area, and particularly for balanced consideration of the relative merits of the different available and emerging pharmacotherapies which can be considered, alongside each other, in this most important area of healthcare planning and provision.

Professor John Strang
Director, National Addiction Centre
(Institute of Psychiatry, King's College London;
and South London and Maudsley NHS Foundation Trust)
London, UK

January 2009

Acknowledgments

The editors acknowledge the contribution of all the authors for their expertise in writing their chapters, and also Courtney Breen and Eva Congreve for their extensive and expert work in providing literature searches for many of the chapters of this book, and to Kati Haworth, for her work in co-ordinating between publishers and authors of chapters to ensure that this book reached publication.

Thanks go also to Professor John Strang, Director of the National Addiction Centre, Institute of Psychiatry, London, for writing the Foreword to this book, and for providing his overview on the research and understanding of pharmacotherapy treatments in the management of opioid dependence.

This work was supported by the authors institutions, and also partly by funding from the Australian Government Department of Health and Ageing, and the National Drug and Alcohol Research Centre at the University of New South Wales, Sydney, Australia.

—RPM, RA, NL
January 2009

PHARMACOTHERAPIES FOR THE TREATMENT OF OPIOID DEPENDENCE

chapter 1

Opioid dependence and management

Louisa Degenhardt, Richard P Mattick, and Amy Gibson

Illicit opioid use, typically involving the use of heroin, is a significant health problem internationally. In many developed countries, dependent heroin users are typically daily, or near daily, injectors of heroin, and of other opioid and sedative drugs when heroin is not available. They continue to use heroin despite the significant social and health problems that it causes them, such as, being arrested for drug or property crimes, with subsequent imprisonment, exposure to blood-borne viruses and increased potential for contracting infectious diseases, and opioid overdose often requiring resuscitation.

Research in the UK and the US indicates that dependent heroin users, who seek treatment or come to attention through the legal system, may continue to use heroin for decades.[1,2] In this population, daily heroin use is punctuated by periods of abstinence, drug treatment, and imprisonment. In the year after any episode of drug treatment, the majority of users relapse to heroin use.[3] When periods of voluntary and involuntary abstinence during treatment or imprisonment are included, it has been estimated that dependent heroin users use heroin daily for 40% to 60% of their 20-year addiction careers.[4,5] It is this long-term dependence on the drug that has focused the minds of clinicians and researchers on the best methods of management of these individuals to minimize the extent of the adverse social and health consequences.

Epidemiology of use and dependence

The prevalence of opioid use is relatively low in comparison with other illicit drugs, such as cannabis which is widely used. Annual estimates between 2001 and 2003 have found that just over 15 million people had used opioids in the previous year, including heroin, morphine, opium, and synthetic opioids. This number corresponds to approximately 0.4% of the global population aged between 15 and 64 years. Of these 15 million people, just over 9 million are believed to use heroin, equivalent to approximately 0.23% of the global population aged between 15 and 64 years.[6]

In considering these estimates, a number of cautions are warranted, as they most likely underestimate the true extent of the use of heroin and other illicit opioids. Since illicit opioid use is a stigmatized, covert activity, data on the level or nature of use are limited and prone to wide margins of error. When local opioid use data are extrapolated to national estimates, the error is amplified. The above estimates were sourced from the latest United Nations Office on Drugs and Crime (UNODC) annual World Drug Report.[7] The main limitation of these reports is that they primarily rely on the completeness of the data captured by annual reports questionnaires (ARQs) by various member states and submitted to the UNODC. Not all member states submit ARQs and some of those that do may not have adequate monitoring systems in place to provide reliable, internationally comparable data.[8]

There are substantial technical difficulties in estimating the number of heroin users. In most developed societies, heroin use is illegal and a stigmatized activity that is practiced in private by consenting adults who prefer others not to know about their behavior. There is no one widely accepted 'gold standard' method for producing credible estimates of the number of people who make up the 'hidden population' of dependent heroin users.[9]

The preferred strategy is to look for convergence in estimates produced by a variety of different methods of estimation.[10,11] These methods can be classified into two broad types: direct estimation methods that attempt to estimate the number of heroin users in representative samples of the population, and indirect methods which attempt to use information from known populations of heroin users (such as those who have died of opioid overdoses, and those who are in treatment or the criminal justice system) to estimate the size of the hidden population of heroin users.

Nearly 8 million of the world's 15 million opioid users are found in the Asian countries surrounding Afghanistan and Myanmar, the two biggest opium-cultivating countries. Some 4 million opioid users are in Europe, mostly in Eastern Europe, driven by a high prevalence of use in the Russian Federation. North and South America combined account for about 2.5 million opioid users, and Oceania has approximately 0.1 million users. Both Europe and Oceania have a prevalence of opioid use higher than the global average: 0.75% and 0.5% of the population aged 15 to 64, respectively.[6] That these estimates are imprecise should be unsurprising. That there is a significant international problem with illicit opioid use is equally obvious. The trends over time attest to the growth of this problem over the past decades.

Trends in opioid use

Over the past 30 years, there has been increased use of illicit opioids. For example, rising opioid overdose death rates indicate that the prevalence of dependent heroin use has increased in Australia since the late 1960s.[12] Increased overdose deaths and increased visibility of heroin use in major cities led to an increase in public and political concern about the impact of dependent heroin use on public health and public order in Australia. Similar concerns have been prominent in US and European cities, and more recently in Asia.

The trends shown by the birth cohort data mentioned above in proportional opioid overdose mortality are also consistent with historical data on post-war illicit heroin use, using Australia as an example.[13,14] These historical data suggest that illicit heroin use first came to police attention in major capital cities in the late 1960s after Australia began to host 'rest and recreation' visits by US servicemen who were on active service in Vietnam. US servicemen in Vietnam were subsequently shown to have high rates of exposure to heroin in Vietnam, where the drug was cheap, pure, and freely available.[15]

Dependent heroin use had become sufficiently widespread by the beginning of the 1970s to prompt the funding of treatment services for heroin-dependent persons. Methadone maintenance treatment was first developed in the USA in the 1960s and introduced into other countries in the 1970s,[16] and the first therapeutic communities were established around the same time.[17] The young adults who initiated heroin use in the late 1960s and early 1970s were members of the birth cohorts born between 1950–54 and 1955–59, (assuming an age of initiation between 15 and 25 years). The proportion of deaths attributable to opioid overdose began to increase in the late 1970s, in the case of the 1950–54 cohort, and in the early 1980s for the 1955–59 birth cohort.

Since the early development of the use of heroin, there has been stabilization of the extent of use, at least in some countries. Using the World Drug Reports, it is possible to consider yearly trends in drug use. In the most recent reports, heroin use in Western Europe is reported to be on a stable to declining trend, as evidenced by a fall in opioid overdose deaths. Stable or declining trends were also reported from most countries in East and South East Asia, Pakistan, and some Central Asian countries. However, China continues to report increases in opioid use, with the number of registered "addicts" reaching 1 million in 2003, a 15-fold increase since 1990. The strongest decrease in opioid use was recorded from Oceania, largely as a result of the 2001 Australian heroin shortage. In the United States, opioid use was stable, but increased in some countries in South America.

Risk factors for opioid use and dependence

Very few studies have examined the risk factors and life pathways that lead young people to use and become dependent on heroin, so that strong statements about the precursors of illicit opioid use are difficult. There is, however, a large literature on risk factors for early use of alcohol and cannabis which indicates that young people who are the earliest initiators and heaviest users of alcohol and cannabis are those who are most likely to use heroin.[18–20]

Two aspects of the family environment are associated with increased rates of licit and illicit drug use among children and adolescents. The first is the extent to which the child is exposed to a disadvantaged home environment, with parental conflict and poor discipline and supervision.[21] The second is the extent to which the child's parents and siblings use alcohol and other drugs.[21]

Children who perform poorly in school, those with impulsive or problem behavior in childhood, and those who are early users of alcohol and other drugs are most likely to use drugs like heroin.[21,22] The nature of the relationship between peer affiliations and adolescent substance use remains controversial, but affiliation with drug-using peers is an important risk factor for drug use, which operates independently of individual and family risk factors.[18]

Exposure to these risk factors is highly correlated. Young people who initiate substance use at an early age have often been exposed to multiple social and family disadvantages. They also tend to be impulsive, have performed poorly at school, to come from families with problems and a history of parental substance use, and to affiliate with delinquent peers.[18,20,21] However, simply being repeatedly exposed to use of opioids is probably sufficient to generate dependence.

Treatment

Of all the illicit drugs, worldwide treatment demand for opioids is the highest. Between 1998 and 2002, treatment demand for opioids accounted for 67% of drug treatment demand in Asia (including 33 Asian countries), 61% of drug treatment demand in Europe (32 European countries), and 47% of drug treatment demand in Oceania (Australia and New Zealand).[8] It is the exploration of these treatments for opioid dependence, and especially the available medications, which is the subject matter of this book.

Treatment ideologies

While illicit opioid dependence or addiction, as for alcohol, was sometimes viewed as a moral or a personality disorder, in the case of heroin dependence it has frequently been managed as a medical disorder. Although early attempts to achieve abstinence were prominent, the recognition that opioid dependence is a chronic relapsing disorder led to a focus on methods that would address the issue of relapse and especially that would draw dependent users into a pharmacologic intervention using medications to maintain the person in treatment and minimize their relapse to illicit opioid use.

Even so, in the past, most treatment services for opioid dependence in many countries (e.g., the US), other than methadone maintenance clinics, were largely non-medically orientated and had focused on abstinence as a treatment goal. In recognition of this issue, it was suggested that the recent registration of buprenorphine for use in general practice would mark a shift from ideologically driven treatment to a science-based treatment system.[23] It has, however, been the pharmacotherapies that have been and remain the mainstays of effective management of opioid dependence.

Management of opioid withdrawal

In opioid-dependent patients, management of opioid withdrawal alone does not constitute a treatment in and of itself, since relapse to opioid use is common following medication cessation.[24] Medications such as methadone, clonidine, naltrexone, and more recently buprenorphine, have been prominent in the management of withdrawal.

Opioid maintenance treatments

Methadone

The real breakthrough in the treatment of opioid dependence was the development of opioid agonists used for maintenance treatment. Methadone was the first of these agonist drugs, introduced by Dole and Nyswander in the early 1960s in New York. Their model of methadone maintenance treatment (MMT) used high or 'blockade' oral methadone doses at stabilization levels of between 50 and 150 mg/day.[25] Methadone treatment was administered as a component of a long-term supporting program with maintenance rather than opioid abstinence as the original treatment goal.[26] Unfortunately, the treatment was sometimes altered by those who wanted it to be abstinence oriented, and who then lowered methadone doses and punished patients for failure by expelling them from treatment. As MMT became the most common form of drug replacement treatment in the US, the goals of treatment changed from maintenance to achieving abstinence from opioids (including methadone) in lower dose and time-limited treatment programs.[26] This trend has still not been fully reversed and doses of methadone are still not adequate in many settings, including those countries where the treatment has been present for many decades. Treatment of opioid dependence in America for the most part remained confined to methadone clinics and remained outside of mainstream medicine.[24]

The most effective methadone programs are those that follow the original Dole and Nyswander model.[26] There have been only a small number of randomized controlled trials on the efficacy of MMT in comparison to control conditions, but they all have shown that methadone maintenance was more effective than detoxification, no treatment, or placebo at retaining subjects in treatment and in reducing opioid use. To confirm these findings, similar efficacy has been noted in observational studies, with the additional finding that MMT subjects have reduced participation in criminal activity.[26]

With the spread of HIV/AIDS in the 1980s, methadone treatment received additional support and funding in countries around the world as there were increased public health attempts to slow the spread of the virus among the population of injecting drug users. There is reasonable evidence that MMT is effective at this goal, providing it is given at adequate dose levels and patients remain in treatment.[27] Its efficacy in helping to reduce the prevalence of established blood-borne epidemics such as hepatitis C and B was, and remains, less clear.[27] Partly in recognition of its role in reducing the spread of HIV, methadone was included in the World Health Organization model list of essential medicines in 2005.[28]

LAAM

The full opioid agonist levo-alpha-acetylmethadol (LAAM) has been investigated since the 1970s as an alternative to methadone. It was approved for use in the treatment of opioid dependence in the United States in 1993,[29] while it is not approved for use in some other countries on the basis of concerns about some of its side-effects.

Buprenorphine

The partial opioid agonist buprenorphine was developed in the 1970s as an analgesic and was soon after investigated for the treatment of opioid dependence. In France, the country went from having no registered opioid maintenance treatments to registering both methadone and buprenorphine in 1995. By the following year, all registered doctors in France were able to prescribe buprenorphine without any additional training or licensing, while the number of places in methadone treatment remained limited.[30] This has resulted in approximately 65,000 patients per year being treated with buprenorphine, ten times the number treated with methadone in that country.[31] While other countries have not adopted France's liberal buprenorphine prescribing policies, it has been registered for use in the maintenance treatment of opioid dependence in Australia since 2001 and the US since 2002, and is registered in many European countries for the treatment of opioid dependence. In Australia, medical practitioners have to be registered as buprenorphine prescribers in a similar accreditation process to methadone prescribing. In the US, buprenorphine is less strictly regulated than methadone. Doctors are trained for 8 hours and registered with the Drug Enforcement Agency, but so far physician adoption of the treatment has been slower than expected.[32] Buprenorphine joined methadone on the World Health Organization model list of essential medicines in 2005.[28]

Heroin (diacetylmorphine)

The use of diacetylmorphine (heroin) as a maintenance treatment was investigated decades ago, and more recently again. Unfortunately, the symbolism associated with heroin reduces reasoned debate about its utility as a maintenance agent. Its use as a therapeutic agent is limited by its illicit status in many countries, but some countries have adopted the use of heroin as a maintenance agent for heroin dependence.

Naltrexone maintenance

Naltrexone is an opioid antagonist which acts to block opioid receptor sites. Naltrexone maintenance treatment was developed in the US and approved for use in the treatment of opioid dependence. The drug is not widely used, as it is unattractive to the target population. The drug only appears suitable for a small subset of highly motivated opioid-dependent people, as the efficacy is hampered by high early drop-out rates and lack of compliance with the medication.[29]

Factors affecting treatment effectiveness

There is a complex set of factors that influence the effectiveness of treatment for opioid dependence. These have been loosely categorized as factors originating in the treatment itself and recipient-based factors.

Treatment-based factors

Level of treatment provided

Higher methadone doses are associated with improved outcomes – especially reduced heroin use – and the concurrent provision of additional medical services may improve patient functioning.[33] Similarly, flexible dosing policies instead of dose restrictions are associated with better retention, and the length of time in treatment is associated with enhanced outcomes.

Ancillary services include services such as counseling and primary health care provided in addition to the core opioid replacement treatment. There is some evidence to show that the provision of ancillary services makes a positive contribution to the outcomes of methadone treatment.[33]

Accessibility and cost

While methadone treatment is effective whether delivered in the public or private sector,[32] the demand for treatment places in many cases is greater than the supply. Publicly funded treatment places are free to the patient and in greatest demand. In Australia, private methadone treatment generally involves a daily dispensing fee to a pharmacist, private methadone clinic, or medical practitioner.[33]

In accordance with harm minimization policy, methadone treatment in Australia is considered 'low threshold' treatment. For patients, this means no restrictions on the length of time in treatment, less intensive or absent urine testing, and drug use while on the program does not necessarily result in expulsion from treatment.[33] Pregnant, indigenous, HIV-positive opioid users, or opioid users recently released from prison, all receive priority for entry into public methadone treatment programs. Although low threshold treatment programs may offer less intensive services than more restricted treatment programs, the aim is to make a greater public health impact by providing some treatment to the greatest number of opioid users.

The difference in uptake of buprenorphine and methadone in France can be seen as an illustration of the impact of treatment accessibility.[31] Methadone is dispensed daily from registered clinics with compulsory urine testing, whereas buprenorphine is prescribed by general practitioners with no urine testing and take-away doses permitted. Buprenorphine recipients outnumber methadone recipients by nearly eight times.[31]

Culture and rules of treatment

The unattractiveness of methadone to many opioid users can be a barrier to entering treatment, whether this arises from 'street myths' surrounding methadone or the actual requirements of the treatment program.[29] Methadone requires daily attendance at a dispensing clinic or pharmacy, which limits patients' movements and their ability to work full time in some positions, especially if extended travel is involved. Some treatment services may also require regular supervised urine samples and high levels of security at the clinic, contributing to the treatment's unattractiveness and emphasizing the difference in power between clinicians and clients.

Recipient-based factors

Client's choice of treatment

Patient choice in the mode of treatment for their opioid dependence is an important factor in compliance with treatment and hence the outcomes achieved.[29] Patients often have clear ideas about which treatment they want and dissatisfaction in being allocated an unwanted treatment is one common reason for early drop-out of randomized controlled trials. For this reason it is important that a range of treatment options be available and that patients be informed about these options.

Drug use other than heroin

Polydrug use among injecting drug users is the rule rather than the exception.[34] Polydrug use is associated with riskier drug use behaviors such as sharing injection equipment and poorer psychosocial functioning, particularly in the case of drugs such as benzodiazepines.[35] It has been estimated that 37% of Australian MMT patients used benzodiazepine in the previous months,[36] and 28% of British injecting drug users in northern England were using temazepam.[34]

Use of cocaine by opioid users is widespread in the US and some parts of Europe. Concomitant cocaine and heroin use has also been associated with higher levels of HIV risk-taking behavior, whether the cocaine is injected or smoked.[35] The true impact of polydrug use on treatment effectiveness is unclear, as there is little research addressing the issue.

Comorbid mental health issues

The prevalence of many types of psychopathology including depression, anxiety, and antisocial personality disorder (ASPD) is high in injecting drug users. In a sample of 222 Australian MMT recipients, 73% of subjects had some degree of current depression, 51% of subjects scored higher than one standard deviation above the mean for anxiety symptoms, and 61% of subjects had a lifetime diagnosis of ASPD.[37] These trends are observed elsewhere and the management of comorbid disorders remains a significant issue for the general management of opioid dependence.

Summary

There is evidence of extensive illicit opioid use over the past decades, with increasing rates of use and harm occurring internationally. There is also now a range of treatments that are available to deal with this dependence on opioids. The rest of this book is focused on the analysis of the data related to the efficacy of these treatments, their clinical delivery, and to the evidence on the economic aspects of treatment choice.

Chapter 2 presents an overview of the pharmacology of opioid agonists and antagonists, followed by a review of the various methods of treatment for opioid withdrawal in Chapter 3. The following five chapters each discuss a pharmacotherapy used in the maintenance treatment of opioid dependence: methadone in Chapter 4, LAAM in Chapter 5, buprenorphine in Chapter 6, diamorphine (heroin) in Chapter 7, and naltrexone in Chapter 8.

Chapter 9 discusses the use of pharmacotherapies in the pregnant opioid-dependent person and Chapter 10 details the political issues surrounding policy development and research into the treatment of heroin addiction.

The Australian treatment guidelines for methadone, buprenorphine, and naltrexone are included in Chapters 11, 12, and 13, respectively. Chapter 14 concludes this book with a discussion on how health economics plays a role in informing treatment decisions and future directions of pharmacotherapies for the treatment of opioid dependence.

References

1. Goldstein A, Herrera J. Heroin addicts and methadone treatment in Albuquerque: A 22 year follow-up. Drug Alcohol Depen 1995; 40: 139–50.
2. Hser YI, Hoffman V, Grella CE, Anglin MD. A 33-year follow-up of narcotics addicts. Arch Gen Psychiatry 2001; 58(5): 503–8.
3. Gerstein DR, Harwood H. Treating Drug Problems Volume 1: A Study of Effectiveness and Financing of Public and Private Drug Treatment Systems. Washington: National Academy Press, 1990.
4. Maddux J, Desmond D. Methadone maintenance and recovery from opioid dependence. Am J Drug Alcohol Ab 1992; 18: 63–74.
5. Ball J, Shaffer J, Nurco D. The day-to-day criminality of heroin addicts in Baltimore – a study in the continuity of offence rates. Drug Alcohol Depen 1983; 12: 119–42.
6. United Nations Office on Drugs and Crime, World Drug Report 2006. 2007, United Nations: Vienna.
7. United Nations Office on Drugs and Crime, World Drug Report 2008. 2008, United Nations: Vienna.
8. United Nations Office on Drugs and Crime, 2004 World Drug Report. 2004, United Nations: Geneva.
9. Hartnoll R. Cross-validating at local level. In: European Monitoring Centre for Drugs and Drug Addiction, ed. Estimating the Prevalence of Problem Drug Use in Europe. Luxembourg: Office for Official Publications of the European Communities, 1997: 247–61.
10. European Monitoring Centre for Drugs and Drug Addiction, Estimating the Prevalence of Problem Drug Use in Europe. EMCDDA Scientific Monograph No. 1. 1997, Office for Official Publications of the European Communities: Luxembourg.
11. European Monitoring Centre for Drugs and Drug Addiction, Study to obtain comparable estimates of problem drug use prevalence for all EU Member States. 1999, EMCDDA: Lisbon.
12. Darke S, Hall W, Weatherburn D, Lind B. Fluctuations in heroin purity and the incidence of fatal heroin overdose. Drug Alcohol Depen 1999; 54: 155–61.
13. Manderson D. From Mr Sin to Mr Big: A History of Australian Drug Laws. 1993, Melbourne: Oxford University Press.
14. McCoy A. Drug Traffic: Narcotics and Organised Crime in Australia. 1980, Sydney: Harper & Row.
15. Robins LN, Helzer JE, Davis DH. Narcotic use in Southeast Asia and afterward: an interview study of 898 Vietnam returnees. Arch Gen Psychiat 1975; 32: 955–61.

16. Ward J, et al. Methadone maintenance and the human immunodeficiency virus: Current issues in treatment and research. Brit J Addict 1992; 87(3): 447–53.
17. Mattick RP, Hall W. Treatment Outline for Approaches to Opioid Dependence: Quality Assurance Project. 1993, Australian Government Publishing Service: Canberra.
18. Fergusson DM, Horwood LJ. Early onset cannabis use and psychosocial adjustment in young adults. Addiction 1997; 92(3): 279–96.
19. Chen K, Kandel DB. The natural history of drug use from adolescence to the mid-thirties in a general population sample [see comments]. Am J Public Health 1995; 85(1): 41–7.
20. Fergusson DM, Horwood LJ. Does cannabis use encourage other forms of illicit drug use? Addiction 2000; 95(4): 505–20.
21. Hawkins J, Catalano R, Miller J. Risk and protective factors for alcohol and other drug problems in adolescence and early adulthood: implications for substance abuse prevention. Psychol Bull 1992; 112: 64–105.
22. Hawkins J, et al. Exploring the effects of age of alcohol use initiation and psychosocial risk factors on subsequent alcohol misuse. J Stud Alcohol 1997; 58: 280–90.
23. Coffey C, et al. Cannabis dependence in young adults: an Australian population study. Addiction 2002; 97(2): 187–94.
24. Ling W, Smith D. Buprenorphine: blending practice and research. J Subst Abuse Treat 2002; 23: 87–92.
25. Dole V, Nyswander M. A medical treatment for diacetylmorphine (heroin) addiction. JAMA 1965; 193: 80–4.
26. Hall W, Ward J, Mattick RP. The effectiveness of methadone maintenance treatment 1: Heroin use and crime. In: Ward J, Mattick RP, Hall W, Eds. Methadone Maintenance Treatment and Other Opioid Replacement Therapies. 1998, Harwood Academic Publishers: Amsterdam.
27. Ward J, Mattick RP, Hall W. The effectiveness of methadone maintenance treatment 2: HIV and infectious hepatitis. In: Ward J, Mattick RP, Hall W, Eds. Methadone Maintenance Treatment and Other Opioid Replacement Therapies. 1998, Harwood Academic Publishers: Australia.
28. World Health Organization. WHO Model List of Essential Medicines. 2005. 14th Edition [Available from: http://www.who.int/medicines/organization/par/edl/expcom14/EML14_en.pdf.]
29. Mattick RP, et al. The effectiveness of other opioid replacement therapies: LAAM, heroin, buprenorphine, naltrexone and injectable maintenance. In: Ward J, Mattick RP, Hall W, Eds. Methadone Maintenance Treatment and Other Opioid Replacement Therapies. 1998, Harwood Academic Publishers: Australia.
30. Thirion X, et al. Buprenorphine prescription by general practitioners in a French region. Drug Alcohol Depen 2002; 65: 197–204.
31. Auriacombe M, et al. French field experience with buprenorphine. Am J Addict 2004; 13: S17–S28.
32. Vastag B. In-office opiate treatment 'not a panacea': physicians slow to embrace therapeutic option. J Am Med Assn 2003; 290(6): 731–5.

33. Ward J. Factors influencing the effectiveness of methadone maintenance treatment: change and innovation in New South Wales, Australia 1985–1995, in Faculty of Medicine. 1995, University of New South Wales: Sydney.
34. Klee H, Fluagier J, Hayes C, Boulton T, Morris J. AIDS related risk behaviour, polydrug use and temazepam. Brit J Addict 1990; 85: 1125–32.
35. Darke S. The effectiveness of methadone maintenance treatment 3: moderators of treatment outcome. In: Ward J, Mattick RP, Hall W, Eds. Methadone Maintenance Treatment and Other Opioid Replacement Therapies. 1998, Harwood Academic Publishers: Australia.
36. Darke S, et al. Benzodiazepine use and HIV risk-taking behaviour among injecting drug users. Drug Alcohol Depen 1992; 31(1): 31–6.
37. Darke S, Swift W, Hall W. Prevalence, severity and correlates of psychological morbidity among methadone maintenance clients. Addiction, 1994; 89: 211–17.

chapter 2

Pharmacology of opioid agonists and antagonists

Andrea L Gordon, Mark R Hutchinson, Sophie F La Vincente, Tim B Mitchell, Glynn A Morrish, David A Newcombe, Andrew A Somogyi, and Jason M White

This chapter reviews the pharmacology of the five major maintenance drugs discussed in later chapters: methadone, levo-alpha-acetylmethadol (LAAM), morphine, buprenorphine, and naltrexone. The first section covers the general pharmacology of opioids followed by consideration of each individual maintenance drug.

Opiates and opioids

The term 'opiate' refers to compounds that are derived from the opium poppy (*Papaver somniferum*), such as morphine, codeine, and their synthetic analogs, whilst the term 'opioid' refers to all compounds, both natural and synthetic, that have morphine-like actions. Opioids produce a variety of effects, the most notable being relief from pain, alterations in mood (e.g. euphoria), respiratory depression, sedation, miosis, decreased gastro-intestinal motility (constipation), nausea, and vomiting.[1] The first account of the use of opium to relieve pain and diarrhea can be found in the writing of Theophrastus in the 3rd century BC.[2] However, it is almost certain that the analgesic effects of an extract of poppy seeds were known long before then, since opium was imported from Cyprus to Egypt between 1551 and 1436 BC. One could safely assume that, because of its powerful euphoric effects, the non-analgesic use of opium has undoubtedly been known for at least 4000 years.

In 1806, Friedrich Wilhelm Adam Sertürner started work on isolating the major active constituent of opium and named it morphine (after Morpheus, Ovid's god of dreams, the son of sleep). However, the chemical structure of morphine was not elucidated until early last century.[3] Since then, many structural modifications have been made to morphine, producing semi-synthetic and fully synthetic compounds that are more potent, longer acting, more effective in the management of pain, and which have fewer side-effects. This has given rise to numerous other compound classes, such as morphinans (e.g. levorphanol), 4-phenylpiperidines (e.g. pethidine), 4-anilinopiperidines (e.g. fentanyl), and 3,3-diphenylpropylamines (e.g. methadone).

Endogenous opioids

The body is also able to synthesize its own compounds which act as opioids. The first evidence for endogenous opioids was reported in 1975, whereby isolated peptides were found to compete with morphine for binding at brain receptors.[4] These peptides, which have opioid-like actions, are encoded on three distinct genes. The products of these genes are known as preproopiomelanocortin (POMC), preproenkephalin, and preprodynorphin. Adrenocorticotropic hormone (ACTH), melanocyte-stimulating hormone, and β-endorphin are derived from POMC. All of these opioid peptides have the N-terminal amino acid sequence in common as this is required for binding to opioid receptors in the brain. The expression of these precursor peptides varies greatly throughout the body: POMC is located centrally in the pituitary and the hypothalamus, whilst the products of POMC are found centrally, peripherally, and in organs such as the adrenal medulla. The immune system is also capable of expressing these peptides in an active form.[5–7] More recently, smaller endogenous peptides called endomorphins have been discovered. Endomorphins have been shown to have the highest affinity and selectivity for the μ opioid receptor of all the known endogenous opioids.[8]

Opioid receptors

Evidence for the presence of specific receptors for endogenous opioid agonists came from binding studies using brain and nervous tissue.[9–11]

Martin et al[12] proposed the existence of three types of opioid receptors which were named after the drugs used in their study, μ: morphine, κ: ketocyclazocine, and σ: *N*-allylnormetazocine (SKF10047). The σ receptor was later shown to be non-opioid. However, Kosterlitz et al[13] determined the existence of a third opioid receptor type, delta (δ for deferens).[14] Each of these opioid receptor types has been cloned, with binding and functional properties confirmed,[15,16] and recently renamed,[17] with δ, κ, and μ opioid receptors recommended to be called OP_1, OP_2 and OP_3, respectively. The 'OP' nomenclature is for opioid, and the number a reflection of the order in which they were cloned. However, this naming system has not been generally accepted, and for simplicity the receptors will be referred to by their previous names throughout the chapter.

There have been recent reports of other receptors through which specific opioids may produce pharmacodynamic responses. For example, Brown et al[18] found two binding sites in brain membranes that had novel opioid ligand selectivity and antagonism. Specifically, the analgesia caused by a metabolite of morphine (morphine-6-glucuronide) and by diacetylmorphine (heroin) was antagonized by 3-methoxynaltrexone without interfering with μ, δ, or κ opioid receptor-mediated responses.[19] Moreover, an antisense clone of the μ opioid receptor blocked morphine, but not morphine-6-glucuronide analgesia.[19] Addition of antisense oligonucleotides of different G-proteins blocked the effect of morphine-6-glucuronide but not morphine.[20] This led to the conclusion that diacetylmorphine and morphine-6-glucuronide were acting not only at the μ opioid receptor, but also via a specific 3-methoxynaltrexone-sensitive binding site.[19,20] It has been suggested that alternative splicing of the μ opioid receptor produces various receptors of differing affinity, including the morphine-6-glucuronide receptor.[21] Since these discoveries, several other splice variants have been discovered[22] and functionally characterized,[23] many of which have altered ligand affinity and downstream signaling.

Opioid binding sites are located on both spinal cord pain transmission neurons and on the primary afferents that transmit pain messages to them. They are expressed both pre- (μ, κ, and δ) and post-synaptically (μ)[16] in many brain regions, some tissues in the periphery, and on the descending inhibitory pathway. Although the primary effects of opioids are mediated by the central nervous system, opioid receptors exhibit a wider anatomic distribution throughout peripheral cells and tissues that give rise to hormonal, immunologic, and some analgesic effects.[24]

Opioid receptors belong to the family of G-protein coupled receptors, specifically the inhibitory G_o and G_i subtypes. They reduce neuronal activity through inhibition of adenylate cyclase and voltage-gated calcium channels, and through increases in potassium conductance causing hyperpolarization and the inhibition of neurotransmitter release.[16,25–28] Although the primary effects of opioids are inhibitory, excitatory effects can occur on various neural pathways by preventing the release of inhibitory neurotransmitters.[28]

Opioid pharmacodynamics

For opioid ligands to produce a response, the ligand must occupy the binding site of an opioid receptor, and activate it. Receptor ligands with this ability are agonists. Agonists have varying efficacy, thus some agonists produce greater responses than others. Full agonists produce the maximal response possible from the tissue through activation of the relevant receptor types, whilst partial agonists only produce a submaximal response through the same receptor type. Ligands that bind to the active sites of receptors and block the binding of agonists are called antagonists and do not produce any response.

Opioid tolerance

When an opioid is administered repeatedly, tolerance develops and is typified by a reduction in the intensity and shortened duration of some but not all effects of the opioids, including analgesia, euphoria, sedation, and respiratory depression.[29] Tolerance does not develop to miosis or constipation. Tolerance to one opioid agonist often causes tolerance to other drugs of the same class; this is known as cross-tolerance.[30] There are a number of different forms of tolerance which include innate tolerance, acquired tolerance (pharmacokinetic and pharmacodynamic), and learned tolerances (behavioral and conditioned).[31] All of these forms of tolerance can modulate the efficacy of clinically prescribed or abused opioids. Innate tolerance refers to the genetically predetermined sensitivity to a drug that is evident upon first exposure. Acquired tolerance is obtained following repeated administration of a drug. Pharmacokinetic tolerance refers to altered metabolism and clearance (often increased) resulting in reduced concentrations of the drug. Pharmacodynamic tolerance is when there is a change in the organism that results in a reduced response to a given concentration of the drug, for example reduced receptor density. Learned tolerance results from compensatory mechanisms that cause a reduction in the observed drug effects in drug-associated environments.

While the mechanisms underpinning pharmacodynamic tolerance have yet to be fully elucidated, many pieces of the puzzle are now falling into place. Functional de-coupling of the opioid receptor from the G-protein and receptor internalization have also been postulated.[28] Others have suggested the downregulation of endogenous opioids, the downregulation of receptors, or the involvement of the *N*-methyl-D-asparate (NMDA) receptor.[32] Moreover, upregulation of cAMP pathways[33] and changes in nitric oxide and nitric oxide synthase levels have also been implicated in the development of tolerance.[34–38]

Opioid dependence and withdrawal (abstinence syndrome)

Physical dependence on opioids is revealed when opioid agonist administration is abruptly discontinued or when an opioid antagonist, such as naloxone, is administered and withdrawal is precipitated. Withdrawal is typically evident as anxiety, irritability, chills and hot flashes, joint pain, lacrimation, rhinorrhea, diaphoresis, nausea, vomiting, abdominal cramps, and diarrhea. These symptoms are often the opposite of those experienced when using the opioid. The mildest form of withdrawal is similar to viral 'flu-like' syndromes. For opioids with short half-lives, the onset of withdrawal symptoms can occur within 6 to 12 hours and peak at 24 to 72 hours after discontinuation of the opioid.[1] For opioids with longer half-lives, the onset of withdrawal may be delayed for 24 hours or more after drug discontinuation and may be of milder intensity but of longer duration.[1]

Methadone

Methadone (6-dimethylamino-4-4-diphenyl-3-heptone) is highly lipid soluble and contains a chiral carbon atom, giving rise to two stereo-isomeric forms, the levorotatory R-(–)-methadone and the dextrorotatory S-(+)-methadone.[39] Methadone is commonly administered as a 50:50 racemic mixture of the two enantiomers, with the (R)-enantiomer responsible for the majority of opioid effects.

Absorption and metabolism

Methadone is generally administered orally as a liquid or tablet preparation, with little variation in the extent of absorption of different preparations.[40] It is readily absorbed from the gastrointestinal tract, resulting in a high bioavailability of between 79 and 95%, although there is a large degree of variability between individuals.[41–43] Nilsson and coworkers showed a small but significant decrease in bioavailability at days 1 and 25 of methadone maintenance treatment.[43] Peak plasma concentration (and therefore maximal suppression of withdrawal and respiratory depression) occurs 2–4 hours after oral administration.[44–47]

Methadone is extensively metabolized in the body by the hepatic cytochrome P450 (CYP) enzyme family. The primary metabolic pathway of methadone is *N*-demethylation to the pharmacologically inactive primary metabolite 2-ethylidene-1,5-dimethyl-3,3-diphenylpyrrolidine (EDDP).[48] Methadone may also undergo minor metabolism to [α,β]-(±)methadol or hydroxylation to parahydroxymethadone, however little is known about these metabolites.

The main enzyme involved in methadone metabolism is CYP3A4. CYP2B6, 2C8, 2C18, 2C19, and 2D6 have also been shown to metabolize methadone, although there is controversy with regard to the degree of contribution of these isoforms,[49–53] which is likely to be small. Variation in the functional regulation and activity of these enzymes, particularly CYP3A4, may explain in part the large variation in dose, pharmacokinetics, and treatment outcomes for individuals on methadone maintenance treatment as reported by Dyer and White.[54] Shinderman et al[55] have shown that effective methadone dose is related to CPY3A4 activity. Inhibitors of CYP450 enzymes such as fluconazole, ketoconazole, fluoxetine, paroxetine, sertraline, ciprofloxacin, and fluvoxamine have been shown to increase plasma methadone concentrations (reviewed by Eap et al[56] and Davis and Walsh[57]). Likewise, St John's wort,[58] rifampin, phenobarbital, amylobarbitone, phenytoin, carbamazepine, spironolactone, fusidic acid, nevirapine, efavirenz, amprenavir, nelfinavir, and ritonavir decrease methadone plasma concentrations by inducing CYP450 enzymes (reviewed by Eap et al,[56] Davis and Walsh,[57] and Weschules and Bain[59]). A decrease in trough methadone concentrations during late pregnancy has been reported,[60,61] and is likely to be due to auto-induction of CYP450 enzymes.

Methadone inhibits CYP3A4 activity in vitro[62] and in vivo[63] after a single dose. Thus, increasing methadone dose during induction should be carefully monitored as clearance may be reduced, resulting in greater than expected toxicity. There is also evidence suggesting that chronic methadone exposure may induce CYP450 activity,[43,64,65] although this remains controversial. Methadone has also been shown to inhibit CYP2D6 activity in vitro[66] and in vivo, resulting in a change from extensive metabolism to poor metabolism phenocopying in methadone maintenance treatment (MMT) patients.[67]

Neuropharmacology

Displacement studies show that racemic methadone primarily binds to the μ opioid receptor, although it also has weak affinity for the δ and κ opioid receptors.[68,69] (R)-methadone has an approximately 20-fold higher affinity for the μ receptor compared with (S)-methadone,[68,70] and thus it is the (R)-enantiomer that contributes to the majority of opioid effects. Methadone demonstrates non-opioid properties, including acting as a non-competitive antagonist for the NMDA receptor[71] and stereoselective inhibition of norepinephrine and 5-HT (serotonin) re-uptake,[70,72,73] although the clinical significance of these actions is unknown.

Pharmacokinetics

Racemic methadone pharmacokinetics have been investigated during single and chronic dosing and in various treatment groups including normal healthy volunteers, methadone-maintained patients, and pain patients. There appear to be no substantial differences between these groups.

Methadone exhibits considerable tissue distribution and binding, with a volume of distribution between 2 and 6 l/kg.[42,43,46,74] High tissue binding of methadone contributes to the prolonged withdrawal after cessation of chronic dosing compared with the cessation of heroin or morphine.

Methadone is also highly and stereoselectively bound to plasma proteins with a mean racemic methadone free fraction of 12% reported in healthy volunteers.[75] Methadone is primarily bound to α1-acid glycoprotein (AAG). AAG shows variability between individuals and concentration alters with health status. A significant correlation between racemic methadone binding ratio and AAG concentration,[75] suggesting variations in free fraction of methadone up to 6-fold,[76] may be in part due to variation in AAG levels.

Methadone is primarily cleared via the hepatic metabolism as previously discussed. Renal clearance of methadone at normal urine pH is low,[43] but acidifying the urine increases renal clearance up to 35% of total body clearance and alkalizing the urine reduces renal clearance.[45] Low hepatic extraction and minimal renal excretion results in a relatively low total body clearance of between 100 and 180 ml/min.[42,43,45,46,77,78]

This low systemic clearance of methadone results in a relatively long terminal elimination half-life of between 22 and 52 hours.[42,44–46,77–83] A half-life greater than 24 hours allows once-daily dosing of methadone to be effective in preventing symptoms of withdrawal.

Pharmacokinetic studies of the individual methadone enantiomers are scarce. Foster et al[83] have investigated this in a large population pharmacokinetic study with 59 MMT subjects. They found marked stereoselective differences in methadone disposition (70–80% greater values for volume of distribution parameters for (R)-methadone vs (S)-methadone) and terminal half-life (51 vs 31 hours for (R)- and (S)-methadone, respectively) but similar values for mean apparent oral clearance (145 vs 138 ml/min for (R)- and (S)-methadone, respectively), although the individual clearance values were highly variable, ranging between 50 and 420 ml/min. These differences result in an increased time for (R)-methadone to reach steady-state during induction and reduced (R)-methadone peak plasma concentration, compared with (S)-methadone. These stereoselective differences should be considered when interpreting racemic data.

Pharmacodynamics

The majority of methadone's pharmacodynamic effects are due to the (R)-enantiomer.

In humans, (R)-methadone is approximately 50 times more potent than the (S)-enantiomer in producing analgesia,[84] and is effective in preventing opioid withdrawal whereas (S)-methadone is ineffective.[85] Although it contributes little to the opioid effects of racemic methadone, animal studies have shown that (S)-methadone may attenuate the development of tolerance to opioids.[86]

The major symptoms of complaint in patients chronically administered methadone include constipation (to which tolerance is incomplete), excessive sweating, insomnia, and reduced libido.[54,87–89] Prolongation of the QT interval by methadone resulting in *torsades de pointes* has also been reported.[90,91]

Changes in pharmacodynamic response over the 24-hour dosing interval, consistent with changes in plasma methadone concentration, have been observed in MMT. Opioid effects, including miosis and respiratory depression, correlate with plasma methadone concentration, with maximal opioid effects occurring approximately 2–4 hours after methadone ingestion.[92] Withdrawal symptoms display an effect–time course inversely related to methadone plasma concentration,[92] with small changes in plasma concentrations resulting in significant mood change.[93]

Levo-alpha-acetymethadol

Levo-alpha-acetymethadol, a long-acting synthetic congener of methadone, is an agonist at the μ opioid receptor and so has qualitatively similar actions to both morphine and methadone. However, unlike methadone it is metabolized to nor-LAAM and dinor-LAAM that are more active than LAAM.

Neuropharmacology

To date, the affinity of LAAM for all three opioid receptor subtypes (μ, δ, and κ) has been examined in rat[70] and monkey brain.[94] In these studies LAAM was shown to be 20 to 70 times more selective for μ than δ receptors, and 100 times more selective for μ than κ receptors.[70,94] Nor-LAAM has between 10 and 30 times, and dinor-LAAM between 10 and 15 times greater affinity for the μ opioid receptor than LAAM.[95–97] Functional assays demonstrated that LAAM was approximately 15,[98] and 30 times,[99] less potent than its nor-metabolites. However, the latter studies and in vivo animal studies have shown that LAAM itself has some intrinsic activity.[98,100–102] Therefore, it is likely that it is the combined activity of LAAM, nor-LAAM, and dinor-LAAM that contributes to the overall opioid effect seen following LAAM administration.

Absorption and metabolism

Following oral administration LAAM is rapidly absorbed from the gastrointestinal tract and LAAM and its metabolites appear in plasma within 30 minutes of ingestion.[103] The plasma concentrations of LAAM reach a peak about 2 to 4 hours after ingestion, and for nor-LAAM and dinor-LAAM about 2 to 4 hours later, with considerable inter-individual variability.[103,104] LAAM undergoes first-pass metabolism and is sequentially *N*-demethylated to noracetylmethadol (nor-LAAM) and then to dinoracetylmethadol (dinor-LAAM).[103–106] Studies evaluating the CYP isoforms contributing to the metabolism of LAAM have revealed the primary role of CYP3A4,[50,107] with minor contributions from 2D6 and 2E1,[50] and 2B6 and 2C18.[108] Similar to methadone, therapeutically important drugs are likely to alter LAAM pharmacokinetics. The inhibition of CYP3A4-mediated LAAM metabolism, with changes in plasma LAAM and metabolite concentrations, has been demonstrated following the administration of the antifungal agent ketoconazole,[109] and the antiviral drug delavirdine,[110] while induction of CYP3A4-mediated LAAM metabolism has been demonstrated following nevirapine administration.[111] Few other drug–drug interactions have been reported for LAAM. Thus, this could be an important future research concern, as variability in LAAM disposition will significantly affect the clinical effectiveness of LAAM.

Pharmacokinetics

Relatively few studies have investigated the pharmacokinetics of LAAM and its metabolites in human plasma,[103–105,112,113] and all have reported considerable interindividual variability. Following chronic LAAM treatment there is substantial accumulation of nor-LAAM and especially dinor-LAAM, with maximum concentrations between 3- and 10-fold greater than following a single dose.[103] The temporal variation in the active metabolites across the interdosing interval is less than for LAAM.[113]

Following chronic oral dosing LAAM has an elimination half-life estimated to range from 35 to 47 hours, while the half-lives of nor-LAAM and dinor-LAAM are estimated to range up to 47 hours and 175 hours, respectively.[103,104] It is the long terminal half-lives and the relatively flat plasma concentration versus time profiles for the two active metabolites that provide stability of opioid effect and hence adequate suppression of withdrawal across the inter-dosing interval for LAAM.[113,114]

Excretion

Following oral dosing in humans, less than 25% of the total dose is excreted via urine, although predictably there are large interindividual differences in the proportion excreted.[103,104] In a recent study in maintenance subjects, unchanged LAAM comprised relatively little of the recovered dose in urine (mean±SD: 1.6±1.0% dose, % coefficient of variation (CV)=60), in comparison to nor-LAAM (7.0±5.7% dose, % CV=82), and dinor-LAAM (14.8±6.0% dose, % CV=41) (Newcombe, unpublished data). Furthermore, although biliary excretion is a major route of elimination of LAAM and its nor-metabolites in animals, this has yet to be verified in humans.[104,115]

Pharmacodynamics

Acute dosing

Fraser and Isbell[116] demonstrated that, following administration of a single oral dose of LAAM (30–40 mg), objective opioid effects (miosis and euphoria) were observed within 90 minutes and peaked by 4 hours, but following parenteral administration (10–30 mg), obvious drug effects were delayed up to 4 to 6 hours, and tended to be less intense. Opioid effects persisted for up to 72 hours following both routes of administration. Walsh and coworkers[117] demonstrated that noticeable opioid effects (e.g. miosis and euphoria) occur soon after intravenous administration of LAAM, at a time when the parent drug was present in plasma, but the metabolites were below the level of detection, and concluded that LAAM itself has significant opioid activity.

Chronic dosing

Early clinical studies demonstrated the potential for cumulative toxicity (respiratory depression, severe nausea and vomiting, mental confusion, and even coma) when LAAM is dosed on a more frequent dosing regimen of twice daily than the 3 times a week or alternate daily dosing schedule that is typically used in maintenance treatment.[116,118] Only a few published papers have investigated the time course of opioid effects following repeat dosing in the context of maintenance treatment.[106,113] Newcombe and colleagues[113] demonstrated that miosis and respiratory depression were at a maximum 4 to 6 hours following dosing, and returned to pre-dosing levels by about 12 hours post dosing. Kaiko and Inturrisi[106] showed that the time course of miosis was more closely correlated to the underlying plasma concentration–time profile of nor-LAAM than LAAM. This would be consistent with in vitro findings of the greater potency of nor-LAAM compared to dinor-LAAM and LAAM.

Fraser and Isbell[116] demonstrated LAAM's capacity to substitute for morphine in morphine-dependent individuals and to suppress opioid withdrawal symptoms for up to 72 hours following 60 mg oral LAAM. When the interdosing interval was increased to 96 hours, all patients complained of mild symptoms at 84 hours, and significant, but mild withdrawal symptoms prior to their next dose. Later studies demonstrated the ability of 75 to 80 mg LAAM 3 times a week to effectively suppress withdrawal for up to 72 hours after dosing,[119,120] while doses in the range 50 to 70 mg resulted in only mild withdrawal.[121] The long duration of action of LAAM is due in part to the long half-lives of nor- and dinor-LAAM. Moreover, LAAM (75 mg) has been shown to confer cross-tolerance to the effects of co-administered opioids such as intravenous heroin 25 mg, hydromorphone 6 mg or 12 mg administered at 72 hours post-LAAM.[121,122]

Side-effects and toxicity

LAAM produces similar opioid side-effects to methadone, including constipation, excessive sweating, insomnia, impotence, nervousness, and feelings of discomfort.[120,123–125] In addition, there have been reports of a biphasic action of LAAM, with excessive stimulation (hyperactivity, irritability, anxiety, and nervousness) occurring on the day of dosing and relative sedation the day after.[105,119,120,126]

Following the reporting to the FDA of 10 cases of serious cardiac arrhythmia, regulatory authorities have recommend restricting the use of LAAM[127] or switching to alternative treatments.[128] LAAM has been reported to cause a delay in cardiac repolarization, leading to prolongation of the QT interval and to life-threatening cardiac rhythm disorders, such as *torsades des pointes*,[129] particularly in patients taking other drugs known to prolong the QT interval, such as fluoxetine and iv cocaine.[129] In 2003 the distributors of LAAM announced that they would cease its distribution in the US.

Slow-release oral morphine

Morphine is a μ opioid receptor agonist characterized by a short duration of action (4 to 6 hours)[130] that has traditionally limited its value as a substitution treatment for opioid dependence. Although experience with injectable and oral morphine maintenance dating back to the 1920s indicates that it can be used effectively to stabilize opioid dependence,[131–136] the inconvenience and costs associated with frequent dosing have traditionally made morphine an unfavorable option given the availability of longer-acting opioids such as methadone, LAAM, and buprenorphine. However, with the advent of slow-release oral morphine (SROM) formulations, particularly those permissive of once-daily dosing, the potential for morphine to be used as an opioid substitution treatment has been greatly enhanced.

Absorption and metabolism

Morphine is characterized by low oral bioavailability (estimates range from 19 to 47%)[137] due to extensive hepatic first-pass metabolism, and a short and variable half-life (approximately 2 hours).[138,139] Metabolism occurs mainly in the liver, primarily involving conjugation with uridine diphosphate glucuronic acid to form morphine-3-glucuronide (M3G) (about 50% of the dose) and morphine-6-glucuronide (M6G) (about 10% of the dose), with the majority of the dose excreted as these and other metabolites in urine.[140] M6G and M3G are up to 9 and 56 times more abundant than morphine in plasma after oral dosing, respectively.[137] Binding of morphine to plasma proteins is negligible, with an unbound fraction of about 0.75.[140]

Neuropharmacology

Morphine is an opioid agonist highly selective for the μ opioid receptor.[70] In animals, the intrinsic efficacy of morphine at the μ opioid receptor is less than for methadone.[140,141] M6G and M3G both show significant passage across the blood–brain barrier[142,143] and have been associated with pharmacologic effects, although the clinical significance of these is unclear.[137] M6G shows high affinity for μ opioid receptors, but may work through a μ receptor variant, and produces significant analgesic effects in both humans[145–147] and animals.[148,149] M3G has negligible affinity for opioid receptors, but in some studies has been found to act as a functional antagonist of morphine and M6G,[150,151] probably due to its excitatory effects. In humans, high plasma concentrations of M3G are associated with hyperalgesia, allodynia, myoclonus, and delirium.[137,152]

Pharmacokinetics and pharmacodynamics

Morphine exhibits a pharmacodynamic profile typical of μ opioid receptor agonists, such that it suppresses opioid withdrawal, but can also cause unwanted and adverse effects (e.g, euphoria, nausea, drowsiness, respiratory depression, constipation). Slow-release oral morphine is differentiated from other maintenance pharmacotherapies by the wide range of formulations commercially available, usually intended for either once- or twice-daily dosing, for which different pharmacokinetic and pharmacodynamic profiles apply.[153,154] The SROM formulations of greatest relevance to the present review are those permissive of once-daily dosing, as these require no alteration to the orthodox once-daily supervised dosing practice that normally applies for methadone. Slow-release oral morphine sulfate capsules are currently available in Australia as Kapanol® and Kadian®, available in 10, 20, 50, and 100 mg capsules, and MS Mono®, available in 30, 60, 90, and 120 mg capsules. Of these, formal pharmacokinetic and pharmacodynamic assessments have been reported only for Kapanol®, and only once in an opioid substitution setting. Tradenames for other once-daily SROM capsule formulations marketed elsewhere in the world include Reliadol®, MXL®, Avinza®, and Morphelan®.

Acute dosing

Four reports have described the single-dose pharmacokinetics and pharmacodynamics of SROM administered as Kapanol® to healthy volunteers.[155–158] These studies have shown that, in comparison to oral morphine solution,

Kapanol® is characterized by equivalent bioavailability, but with a more stable and prolonged plasma morphine concentration–time profile following dosing. This is evidenced by an approximate 5- to 8-fold reduction in maximum plasma morphine concentrations (Cmax) and 8-fold increase in the time to achieve Cmax (Tmax: means ranged from 7.4 to 11.6 hours). The most common side-effects reported in these studies involved the central nervous system, including nausea, drowsiness, and headache, and the gastrointestinal tract, including constipation and stomach discomfort, and were predictable in opioid-naïve subjects.

Chronic dosing

Only one formal investigation of the steady-state pharmacokinetics and pharmacodynamics of SROM has been conducted in an opioid substitution treatment setting. Mitchell and colleagues[159] transferred methadone maintenance patients reporting either adequate or inadequate withdrawal suppression between doses from methadone (mean dose 78 mg) to SROM (mean dose 349 mg) for an evaluation period of approximately 6 weeks. Indices of opioid effects and plasma concentrations for (R)-methadone and morphine were measured over a single 24-hour interdosing interval during methadone and SROM maintenance. Slow-release oral morphine was at least as effective as methadone in suppressing opioid withdrawal. Opioid effects such as withdrawal suppression, miosis, and respiratory depression were of a similar magnitude for each drug and showed an inverse relationship with plasma drug concentrations, which peaked later in the dosing interval for morphine in comparison to (R)-methadone (6.5 vs 2.5 hours). Although the plasma morphine concentration–time profile was relatively flat, the peak to trough plasma concentration ratio of 3.23 ± 1.81 was significantly greater and more variable than for methadone (1.83 ± 0.35). Most subjects stated a preference for SROM over methadone in this study. Consistent with these findings, other reports describing the use of SROM for opioid substitution treatment have generally supported its clinical efficacy and tolerability.[160–166]

Further evaluation of SROM is needed to address issues such as how patient response is affected by the choice of formulation and morphine's metabolites (particularly M6G) and also to overcome obstacles which may impede effective clinical implementation of SROM maintenance.

Obstacles include problems relating to the low oral bioavailability of morphine (which gives patients access to several times the desired therapeutic dose if injected intravenously), preventing dose chewing, which may compromise slow-release characteristics, and detecting illicit heroin use (since urinary detection of morphine cannot be used).

Buprenorphine

Buprenorphine [21-cyclopropyl-7α-[(*S*)-1-hydroxy-1,2,2-trimethylpropyl]-6, 14-*endo*-ethano-6,7,8,14-tetrahydrooripavine] is a derivative of the morphine alkaloid thebaine[167,168] and was introduced into medical practice in 1978 as an intramuscular analgesic and then in 1981 as a sublingual tablet.[169] Buprenorphine is up to 25–50% more potent and longer acting as an analgesic than morphine.[168,170]

Absorption and metabolism

Buprenorphine has a low oral bioavailability of approximately 6.5%[171] due to extensive first-pass metabolism.[172] For this and other reasons, it is, for the purposes of opioid maintenance therapy, administered as a sublingual tablet, either alone or in combination with naloxone. Buprenorphine as a sublingual tablet under acute dosing conditions has an absolute bioavailability of approximately 15%[171,172] compared to buprenorphine sublingual liquid preparations, that have an absolute bioavailability of between 28 and 51% (the relative bioavailability of tablet to liquid lies between 49 and 58%).[171,173–175] However, under chronic dosing conditions the relative bioavailability of the tablet to the solution increases to between 64 and 71%.[176,177] The time taken to reach peak plasma buprenorphine concentrations is between 0.5 and 3 hours.[176–184]

Buprenorphine is metabolized by a combination of phase I and phase II enzymes. The major metabolic pathway involved is *N*-dealkylation to form the pharmacologically active, major metabolite norbuprenorphine.[185,186] CYP3A4 and 3A5 are responsible for up to 75% of norbuprenorphine formation with CYP2C8 also significantly contributing.[187,188] The possibility of the formation of up to five other phase I metabolites has recently been observed with CYPs 3A4, 3A5, 3A7, and 2C8 contributing to their formation.[187,188]

Buprenorphine also undergoes glucuronidation to buprenorphine-3-glucuronide and about 75% of buprenorphine glucuronide formation is due to uridine diphosphate glucuronyltransferase (UGT) 1A1,[189] with UGT1A3 playing a minor role.[190]

The most common mechanism by which drug interactions occur with buprenorphine is by induction or inhibition of CYP3A4, whereby buprenorphine metabolism is inhibited or induced by other drugs or where buprenorphine causes inhibition or induction of metabolism of other drugs, and may lead to serious adverse events.[191] In opiate-dependent patients, buprenorphine is often administered in conjunction with other drugs such as benzodiazepines.[191–193] Buprenorphine itself has been shown to inhibit CYP3A4, which also metabolizes many benzodiazepines, therefore resulting in the potential for enhanced plasma concentrations of benzodiazepines and observed increases in sedation.[191–194] Several deaths have also been reported due to benzodiazepine misuse in conjunction with high-dose buprenorphine.[195] Interactions with buprenorphine and antiretroviral drugs have been noted and may result in a risk of buprenorphine overdose due to increased plasma concentrations as a result of inhibition of CYP3A4.[196–198] Other drugs that induce or inhibit CYP3A4 are barbiturates, rifampicin, antidepressants, St John's wort, and oral contraceptives, thus co-administration with buprenorphine could result in adverse effects.

Neuropharmacology

Buprenorphine is a potent partial agonist at the μ opioid receptor with high affinity (binds tightly to the receptor) and low intrinsic activity, thus it does not activate the receptor to the same extent as a full μ opioid agonist (K_i=0.08 nM).[170,186,199] Buprenorphine is also a partial agonist at κ opioid receptors with low efficacy, but shows potent antagonist activity (K_i=0.11 nM).[186] Buprenorphine has high affinity at δ opioid receptors (K_i=0.42 nM), displaying no agonistic activity, but acts as a competitive antagonist at this receptor.[186]

Nor-buprenorphine exhibits high affinities for μ, δ, and κ opioid receptors (K_I values of 0.07 nM, 3.14 nM, and 0.91 nM, respectively). Earlier research suggested that, similarly to buprenorphine, norbuprenorphine is also a partial agonist at μ and κ opioid receptors, however it acts as a full agonist at δ opioid receptors. More recent research observing the acute toxicity and respiratory effects of norbuprenorphine in rats, however, has suggested that it may also be a full agonist at μ opioid receptors.[200] Nor-buprenorphine has also been shown to be a relatively potent analgesic.[186]

An inverse correlation between lipophilicity and the rate of dissociation from opioid binding sites has previously been reported. Considering buprenorphine's high lipophilicity (octanol/water partition coefficient: 1943±50), it dissociates exceedingly slowly from opioid receptor binding sites. This is thought to be a major contributing factor to the drug's long duration of action and its relative resistance to challenge with antagonists.[201]

By displacing a full agonist from the receptor, a partial agonist can reduce the effect of a full agonist and therefore behave as an antagonist. For this reason, when beginning buprenorphine treatment, caution must be taken and an appropriate time period allocated between the last opioid administration and the first buprenorphine dose in order to prevent precipitated withdrawal. The probability of precipitated withdrawal due to buprenorphine administration is dependent on the type and dose of opioid previously administered, the length of time it was administered, and the dose of buprenorphine to be administered.[202–204]

Pharmacokinetics

The terminal half-life of buprenorphine when administered sublingually is highly variable (approximately 26 hours, range 9 to 69 hours).[183] However, reports have shown that when administered sublingually its duration of action is at least as long as that of methadone, if not longer (24 to 69 hours).[178,205] This may be due to the slow dissociation of buprenorphine from its binding sites[206] or the contribution from norbuprenorphine.[186] Buprenorphine is highly bound to plasma proteins (approximately 96%), predominantly α- and β-globulin fractions,[207] and has a large volume of distribution (90–190 l/kg).[208,209] The clearance of buprenorphine has been found to be between 900 and 1300 ml/min when administered intravenously.[180,208]

Buprenorphine is primarily excreted via feces (about 40% of dose mainly as unconjugated buprenorphine), with less than 10% recovered in urine mainly as buprenorphine conjugates. Norbuprenorphine is also excreted via feces (about 20% of the dose), with total urinary recovery of norbuprenorphine low (about 10% of the dose) over the course of 4 days.[185]

Pharmacodynamics

Reported subjective responses and physiologic actions produced by buprenorphine resemble those of morphine and methadone and include sedation, euphoria, miosis, and respiratory depression.[184,210] As a partial agonist, it has ceiling effects and for some actions there appears to be an inverted U-shaped dose–response curve. That is, there are dose-related increases in efficacy and opioid effect in the lower dose range, with higher doses producing no greater or even decreased effects.[170,178,184] During chronic dosing in maintenance subjects, physiologic and subjective changes over the dosing interval are relatively small.[211]

In subjects with experience with opioids, but who were not physically dependent, sublingual doses of 32 mg of buprenorphine have been shown to cause a decrease in respiratory rate of 4 breaths per minute. Relative to doses used to produce analgesia, a dose of 32 mg of buprenorphine is equivalent to 530 mg of intramuscular morphine and 1060 mg of oral methadone.[178] While these doses of morphine and methadone are in the lethal range, the equivalent dose of buprenorphine only shows marginal effects on respiratory function relative to other opioid agonists.[178,212] Chronic daily dosing with 16 mg of buprenorphine has also produced insignificant effects on respiration.[211] No additive effects on respiratory depression have been observed when buprenorphine is administered along with another pure μ opioid receptor agonist; buprenorphine has also been shown to produce a dose-related blockade of opioid agonist effects.[213,214]

The abrupt termination of buprenorphine has produced subjective reports of a mild to moderate withdrawal syndrome that occurs within the first 3 days, peaks between days 3 and 5, and gradually diminishes over days 8 to 10.[205,215] On the basis of this evidence it has been suggested that buprenorphine produces a relatively low level of physical dependence.[170,213,216,217]

Naltrexone

Naltrexone was synthesized in 1963 in response to the need for a potent, orally active, longer-acting opioid antagonist as naloxone did not satisfy the latter two criteria. Naltrexone is increasingly being used in the treatment of opioid and alcohol dependence. Due to its longer duration of action, possibly due to the presence of an active metabolite 6ß-naltrexol, it is suited to maintenance therapy, with a single oral dose (normally 50 mg) taken daily.

Absorption, metabolism, and pharmacokinetics

Naltrexone is rapidly and almost completely absorbed following oral administration,[218,219] however it undergoes extensive first-pass metabolism.[220] Oral bioavailability has varied considerably, ranging from 5%[221] to 20%,[222] to 60%,[218] as a consequence of inherent differences between investigations.[223] Plasma concentrations peak at approximately one hour after oral administration. Verebey et al[222] investigated the disposition of oral naltrexone in both acute and chronic administration in a cohort of opioid-free former heroin users. Following administration of an acute dose of naltrexone (100 mg), the peak plasma concentrations of naltrexone and the major metabolite in humans, 6β-naltrexol, were 43.6±29.9 ng/ml at 1 hour and 87.2±25.0 ng/ml at 2 hours, respectively. On chronic dosing, peak concentrations at 1 hour were 46.4±29.9 ng/ml (naltrexone) and 158.4±89.9 ng/ml (6β-naltrexol).

The half-life for naltrexone ranges from 2 to 6 hours,[221,222] it has a total clearance from 1.5 l/min[221] to 3.3 l/min,[218] the unbound fraction in plasma is 20%, and the volume of distribution is about 15 l/kg.[223] In humans, following oral administration, naltrexone is extensively reduced to 6β-naltrexol, the weaker antagonist,[224–226] but is present in higher concentrations with a longer half-life than naltrexone (between 7.5 and 16.8 hours[227,228]). Between 30 and 60 minutes after naltrexone administration, plasma concentrations of 6β-naltrexol have been reported to be 10 to 30 times higher than naltrexone.[221] Hence, the antagonist activity is likely to be mediated by both naltrexone and 6β-naltrexol. The comparatively higher plasma concentration of the metabolite and its prolonged presence in the systemic circulation are thought to contribute to the longer duration of action associated with naltrexone.[209,222,224] However, recent findings have shown that there is considerable interindividual variation in the kinetics of 6β-naltrexol formation that could influence concentrations of this metabolite.[228] Both naltrexone and 6β-naltrexol undergo extensive glucuronide conjugation. Naltrexone is eliminated primarily by hepatic metabolism[219] and approximately 60% of a naltrexone dose is excreted in urine, mostly as 6β-naltrexol.

Naltrexone does not accumulate with chronic dosing in healthy volunteers, and there is no difference in the time to peak plasma concentration between single and repeated administration.[221,222] A small degree of 6β-naltrexol accumulation may be expected due to its longer half-life. In former opioid-dependent subjects, half-lives of both naltrexone and 6β-naltrexol decreased after 1 month of chronic treatment.[222] Ferrari et al[219] investigated changes in naltrexone pharmacokinetics during chronic dosing in a larger sample of opioid-free former heroin users. This study revealed that naltrexone disposition did not significantly change over chronic (3 month) dosing. There was a marginal decrease in naltrexone half-life during the first month of dosing, however this remained stable over the subsequent study period. There were no significant differences in 6β-naltrexol half-life over the course of the study. There are no drug interaction studies involving the pharmacokinetics of naltrexone but it is recommended not to coadminister disulfiram as both are hepatotoxic.

Pharmacodynamics

Naltrexone has a higher affinity for μ than κ or δ opioid receptors. A comparison of the in vitro potency of naltrexone and 6β-naltrexol reported that the metabolite was more potent than naltrexone (K_i=94±25 pM vs K_i=420±150 pM).[228] Naltrexone is structurally similar to naloxone and nalorphine, but in rodent and primate in vivo studies has been shown to have an antagonistic potency 12 times that of nalorphine, and 2.5 times that of naloxone or cyclazocine.[229] In vivo studies have reported that 6β-naltrexol is one twelfth to one eighty-fifth as potent as the parent drug in achieving the same degree of antagonism.[224–226]

Naltrexone has been shown to reduce drug-seeking behavior by blocking the euphoria and reinforcement associated with self-administration of opioids.[230,231] Naltrexone blocks both subjective and objective responses to opioid agonist administration. In human studies, the antagonist properties of naltrexone have been investigated with single oral doses and subcutaneous injection in opioid-dependent and ex-dependent individuals.[227,232,233] Resnick et al[227] found that 20 mg to 200 mg oral naltrexone produced a dose-related antagonism of the euphoric effects of intravenous heroin (25 mg) for up to 72 hours. A dose of 100 mg of oral naltrexone was associated with prolonged blockade of opioid effect in response to 25 mg intravenous heroin challenge. At 24 hours post dose, naltrexone was associated with 96% blockade of opioid effect. Blockade had only marginally reduced at 48 hours post dosing (86.5%), and considerable blockade was still evident at 72 hours post dosing (46.6%). At 72 hours, objective opioid effects such as miosis became apparent before subjective effects such as euphoria. The authors reported that the lowest plasma naltrexone concentration associated with significant blockade of opioid effects was 2.0 ng/ml, and this was considered the minimum concentration for therapeutic use, achieving a blockade of 86.5% of opioid effects associated with 25 mg intravenous heroin challenge.

While naltrexone has been reported to be a 'pure' opioid antagonist with no agonist activity,[234] in some human studies mild agonist effects, such as pupillary miosis, have been found,[222,233] although the findings have been inconsistent. It has been proposed, however, that any agonist effects observed with naltrexone may not be clinically significant and, in fact, the relative absence of agonist effects accounts for the high drop-out rates associated with outpatients maintained on naltrexone.[235] There have been some reports that at ultra low concentrations (pM to nM), opioid antagonists, including naltrexone, may enhance the analgesic effects of opioid agonists.[236,237] However, reports have been inconsistent, and further research is required to explore this relationship and determine the underlying mechanism for any analgesic synergism that may be observed.

At the clinical dose of 50 mg, no toxic effects have been evident in rats, dogs, rabbits, or monkeys. In humans, this dose can cause nausea, possibly with vomiting, and dizziness. Other commonly reported adverse effects include lethargy, headache, insomnia, anxiety, sleepiness, and dizziness, although these are usually transient and subside within 1 to 2 weeks of treatment.[238] Hepatotoxicity is rare,[239,240] and more likely to occur with doses exceeding 50 mg daily.

Single-dose naltrexone (50–100 mg) has been associated with a significant increase in circulating luteinizing hormone in healthy volunteers,[241,242] abstinent heroin users,[243] and in heroin-dependent individuals chronically dosed with naltrexone (50 mg).[244] Multiple-dose naltrexone (100–150 mg) has also been associated with a significant increase in plasma cortisol[245] and β-endorphin[246] concentrations in abstinent heroin users. A significant increase in cortisol, testosterone, and prolactin has also been observed following single-dose naltrexone (50–100 mg) in healthy volunteers.[242]

Conclusion

A diverse range of opioid drugs has been developed for treatment of dependence. These range from full agonists such as methadone to the partial agonist buprenorphine and the antagonist naltrexone. In addition to differences in efficacy, each of the drugs has particular pharmacologic characteristics that need to be considered if they are to be used effectively in clinical practice. There is also an increasing diversity of formulations of those drugs resulting in pharmacokinetic properties that have advantages in the clinical setting.

References

1. King A, Miller N. Medications of abuse: opioids. In: Ott P, ed. Handbook of Substance Abuse: Neurobehavioural Pharmacology. New York: Plenum Press, 1998.
2. Benedetti C, Premuda L. The history of opium and its derivatives. In: Giron G, ed. Opioid Analgesia. New York: Raven Press, 1990: 1–35.
3. Guilland J, Robinson R. The morphine group. Part I. A discussion of the constitutional problems. J Chem Soc 1923; 123: 980–98.
4. Hughes J, Smith TW, Kosterlitz HW et al. Identification of two related pentapeptides from the brain with potent opiate agonist activity. Nature 1975; 258: 577–9.
5. Cabot PJ, Cater L, Gaiddon C, et al. Immune cell-derived β-endorphin: production, release and control of inflammatory pain in rats. J Clin Invest 1997; 100(1): 142–8.
6. Miller BC, Thiele DL, Rodd D, Hersh LB, Cottman GL. Active ß-endorphin metabolites generated by T-cell ectopeptidases. Adv Exp Med Biol 1995; 373: 49–56.
7. Czlonkowski A, Stein C, Herz A. Peripheral mechanisms of opioid antinociception in inflammation: involvement of cytokines. Eur J Pharmacol 1993; 242(3): 229–35.
8. Zadina JE, Martin-Schild S, Gerall AA, et al. Endomorphins: novel endogenous mu-opiate receptor agonists in regions of high mu-opiate receptor density. Ann NY Acad Sci 1999; 897: 136–44.
9. Pert C, Snyder S. Opiate receptor: demonstration in nervous tissues. Science 1973; 179: 1011–14.
10. Simon E, Hiller J, Edelman I. Stereospecific binding of the potent analgesic 3H-eporphine to rat brain homogenate. Proc Natl Acad Sci 1973; 70: 1947–9.
11. Terenius L. Stereospecific interaction between narcotic analgesics and a synaptic plasma membrane fraction of rat cerebral cortex. Acta Pharm and Tox 1973; 32: 317–20.

12. Martin W, Eades C, Thompson J, Huppler R, Gilbert P. The effects of morphine and nalorphine-like drugs in the nondependent and morphine dependent chronic spinal dog. J Pharmacol Exp Ther 1976; 197: 517–32.
13. Kosterlitz HW, Lord J, Paterson S, Waterfield AA. Effects of changes in the structure of enkephalins and of narcotic analgesic drugs on their interactions with mu and delta receptors. Br J Pharmacol 1980; 68: 333–42.
14. Lord J, Waterfield AA, Hughes J, Kosterlitz HW. Endogenous opioid peptides: multiple agonists and receptors. Nature 1977; 267: 495–9.
15. Evans CJ, Keith DE, Jr., Morrison H, Magendzo K, Edwards RH. Cloning of a delta opioid receptor by functional expression. Science 1992; 258(5090): 1952–5.
16. Satoh M, Minami M. Molecular pharmacology of the opioid receptors. Pharmacol Ther 1995; 68(3): 343–64.
17. Dhawan B, Cesselin F, Raghubir R, et al. International Union of Pharmacology. XII. Classification of opioid receptors. Pharmacol Rev 1996; 48(4): 567–93.
18. Brown G, Yang K, Ouerfelli O, Standifer K, Byrd D, Pasternak G. 3H-Morphine-6β-glucuronide binding in brain membranes and MOR-1-trasnfected cell line. J Exp Pharma Ther 1997; 282(3): 1291–7.
19. Brown G, Yany K, King M, et al. 3-Methoxynaltrexone, a selective heroin/morphine-6β-glucuronide antagonist FEBS Lett 1997; 412: 35–8.
20. Rossi G, Leventhal L, Pan Y-X, et al. Antisense mapping of MOR-1 in rats: distinguishing between morphine and morphine-6β-glucuronide antinociception. J Pharmacol Exp Ther 1997; 281: 109–14.
21. Rossi GC, Pan YX, Brown GP, Pasternak GW. Antisense mapping of the MOR-1 opioid receptor: evidence for alternative splicing and a novel morphine-6 beta-glucuronide receptor. FEBS Lett 1995; 369(2–3): 192–6.
22. Pan YX. Identification and characterization of a novel promoter of the mouse mu opioid receptor gene (Oprm) that generates eight splice variants. Gene 2002; 295(1): 97–108.
23. Bolan EA, Pan YX, Pasternak GW. Functional analysis of MOR-1 splice variants of the mouse mu opioid receptor gene Oprm. Synapse 2004; 51(1): 11–18.
24. King M, Su W, Chang A, Zuckerman A, Pasternak GW. Transport of opioids from the brain to the periphery by P-glycoprotein: peripheral actions of central drugs. Nat Neurosci 2001; 4(3): 268–74.
25. Childers SR. Opiate-inhibited adenylate cyclase in rat brain membranes depleted of Gs-stimulated adenylate cyclase. J Neurochem 1988; 50(2): 543–53.
26. Childers SR, Fleming L, Konkoy C, et al. Opioid and cannabinoid receptor inhibition of adenylyl cyclase in brain. Ann NY Acad Sci 1992; 654: 33–51.
27. Minami M, Satoh M. Molecular biology of the opioid receptors: structures, functions and distributions. Neurosci Res 1995; 23(2): 121–45.

28. Williams JT, Christie MJ, Manzoni O. Cellular and synaptic adaptations mediating opioid dependence. Physiol Rev 2001; 81(1): 299–343.
29. Collett B. Opioid tolerance: the clinical perspective. Br J Anaesth 1998; 81: 58–68.
30. Plummer JL, Cmielewski PL, Reynolds GD, Gourlay GK, Cherry DA. Influence of polarity on dose–response relationships of intrathecal opioids in rats. Pain 1990; 40(3): 339–47.
31. O'Brien C. Drug addiction and drug abuse. In: Limbird L, ed. Goodman & Gilman: The Pharmacological Basis of Therapeutics. 9th edn. New York: MacGraw-Hill 1996: 557–77.
32. Elliott K, Minami N, Kolesnikov YA, Pasternak GW, Inturrisi CE. The NMDA receptor antagonists, LY274614 and MK-801, and the nitric oxide synthase inhibitor, NG-nitro-l-arginine, attenuate analgesic tolerance to the mu-opioid morphine but not to kappa opioids. Pain 1994; 56(1): 69–75.
33. Nestler EJ. Molecular neurobiology of addiction. Am J Addict 2001; 10: 201–17.
34. Pasternak GW. Nitric oxide and opioid tolerance. NIDA Res Monogr 1995; 147: 182–94.
35. Kolesnikov YA, Pick CG, Pasternak GW. NG-nitro-l-arginine prevents morphine tolerance. Eur J Pharmacol 1992; 221(2–3): 399–400.
36. Kolesnikov YA, Pick CG, Ciszewska G, Pasternak GW. Blockade of tolerance to morphine but not to kappa opioids by a nitric oxide synthase inhibitor. Proc Natl Acad Sci USA 1993; 90(11): 5162–6.
37. Aley KO, Levine JD. Dissociation of tolerance and dependence for opioid peripheral antinociception in rats. J Neurosci 1997; 17(10): 3907–12.
38. Dambisya Y, Lee T. Role of nitric oxide in the induction and expression of morphine tolerance and dependence in mice. Br J Pharmacol 1996; 117(5): 914–8.
39. Beck O, Boreus LO, Lafolie P, Jacobsson G. Chiral analysis of methadone in plasma by high-performance liquid chromatography. J Chromatogr 1991; 570(1): 198–202.
40. Gourevitch MN, Hartel D, Tenore P, et al. Three oral formulations of methadone. A clinical and pharmacodynamic comparison. J Subst Abuse Treat 1999; 17(3): 237–41.
41. Dale O, Hoffer C, Sheffels P, Kharasch ED. Disposition of nasal, intravenous, and oral methadone in healthy volunteers. Clin Pharmacol Ther 2002; 72(5): 536–45.
42. Meresaar U, Nilsson MI, Holmstrand J, Änggård E. Single dose pharmacokinetics and bioavailability of methadone in man studied with a stable isotope method. Eur J Clin Pharmacol 1981; 20(6): 473–8.
43. Nilsson MI, Änggård E, Holmstrand J, Gunne L-M. Pharmacokinetics of methadone during maintenance treatment: adaptive changes during the induction phase. Eur J Pharmacol 1982; 22(4): 343–9.
44. Inturrisi CE, Verebely K. Disposition of methadone in man after a single oral dose. Clin Pharmacol Ther 1972; 13(6): 923–30.

45. Nilsson MI, Meresaar U, Anggard E. Clinical pharmacokinetics of methadone. Acta Anaesthesiol Scand Suppl 1982; 74: 66–9.
46. de Vos JW, Geerlings PJ, van den Brink W, Ufkes JG, van Wilgenburg H. Pharmacokinetics of methadone and its primary metabolite in 20 opiate addicts. Eur J Clin Pharmacol 1995; 48(5): 361–6.
47. Foster DJ, Somogyi AA, Dyer KR, White JM, Bochner F. Steady-state pharmacokinetics of (R)- and (S)-methadone in methadone maintenance patients. Br J Clin Pharmacol 2000; 50(5): 427–40.
48. Beckett AH, Taylor JF, Casy AF, Hassan MM. The biotransformation of methadone in man: synthesis and identification of a major metabolite. J Pharm Pharmacol 1968; 20(10): 754–62.
49. Iribarne C, Berthou F, Baird S, et al. Involvement of cytochrome P450 3A4 enzyme in the N-demethylation of methadone in human liver microsomes. Chem Res Toxicol 1996; 9(2): 365–73.
50. Moody DE, Alburges ME, Parker RJ, Collins JM, Strong JM. The involvement of cytochrome P450 3A4 in the N-demethylation of L-alpha-acetylmethadol (LAAM), norLAAM, and methadone. Drug Metab Dispos 1997; 25(12): 1347–53.
51. Foster DJ, Somogyi AA, Bochner F. Methadone N-demethylation in human liver microsomes: lack of stereoselectivity and involvement of CYP3A4. Br J Clin Pharmacol 1999; 47(4): 403–12.
52. Wang JS, DeVane CL. Involvement of CYP3A4, CYP2C8, and CYP2D6 in the metabolism of (R)- and (S)-methadone in vitro. Drug Metab Dispos 2003; 31(6): 742–7.
53. Gerber JG, Rhodes RJ, Gal J. Stereoselective metabolism of methadone N-demethylation by cytochrome P4502B6 and 2C19. Chirality 2004; 16(1): 36–44.
54. Dyer KR, White JM. Patterns of symptom complaints in methadone maintenance patients. Addiction 1997; 92(11): 1445–55.
55. Shinderman M, Maxwell S, Brawand-Amey M, Golay KP, Baumann P, Eap CB. Cytochrome P4503A4 metabolic activity, methadone blood concentrations, and methadone doses. Drug Alcohol Depend 2003; 69(2): 205–11.
56. Eap CB, Buclin T, Baumann P. Interindividual variability of the clinical pharmacokinetics of methadone: implications for the treatment of opioid dependence. Clin Pharmacokinet 2002; 41(14): 1153–93.
57. Davis MP, Walsh D. Methadone for relief of cancer pain: a review of pharmacokinetics, pharmacodynamics, drug interactions and protocols of administration. Support Care Cancer 2001; 9(2): 73–83.
58. Eich-Hochli D, Oppliger R, Golay KP, Baumann P, Eap CB. Methadone maintenance treatment and St. John's Wort – a case report. Pharmacopsychiatry 2003; 36(1): 35–7.
59. Weschules DJ, Bain KT. A systematic review of opioid conversion ratios used with methadone for the treatment of pain. Pain Medicine. 2008 Jun 18 [epub ahead of print].
60. Kreek MJ. Methadone disposition during the perinatal period in humans. Pharmacol Biochem Behav 1979; 11 Suppl: 7–13.

61. Pond SM, Kreek MJ, Tong TG, Raghunath J, Benowitz NL. Altered methadone pharmacokinetics in methadone-maintained pregnant women. J Pharmacol Exp Ther 1985; 233(1): 1–6.
62. Iribarne C, Dreano Y, Bardou LG, Menez JF, Berthou F. Interaction of methadone with substrates of human hepatic cytochrome P450 3A4. Toxicology 1997; 117(1): 13–23.
63. Boulton DW, Arnaud P, DeVane CL. A single dose of methadone inhibits cytochrome P-4503A activity in healthy volunteers as assessed by the urinary cortisol ratio. Br J Clin Pharmacol 2001; 51(4): 350–4.
64. Verebely K, Volavka J, Resnick R. Methadone in man: pharmacokinetic and excretion studies in acute and chronic treatment phases. Fed Proc 1975; 34: 814.
65. Rostami-Hodjegan A, Wolff K, Hay AW, Raistrick D, Calvert R, Tucker GT. Population pharmacokinetics of methadone in opiate users: characterization of time-dependent changes. Br J Clin Pharmacol 1999; 48(1): 43–52.
66. Wu D, Otton SV, Sproule BA, et al. Inhibition of human cytochrome P450 2D6 (CYP2D6) by methadone. Br J Clin Pharmacol 1993; 35(1): 30–4.
67. Shiran MR, Chowdry J, Rostami-Hodjegan A, et al. A discordance between cytochrome P450 2D6 genotype and phenotype in patients undergoing methadone maintenance treatment. Br J Clin Pharmacol 2003; 56(2): 220–4.
68. Kristensen K, Christensen CB, Christrup LL. The mu1, mu2, delta, kappa opioid receptor binding profiles of methadone stereoisomers and morphine. Life Sci 1995; 56(2): PL45–50.
69. Magnan J, Paterson SJ, Tavani A, Kosterlitz HW. The binding spectrum of narcotic analgesic drugs with different agonist and antagonist properties. Naunyn Schmiedebergs Arch Pharmacol 1982; 319(3): 197–205.
70. Codd EE, Shank RP, Schupsky JJ, Raffa RB. Serotonin and norepinephrine uptake inhibiting activity of centrally acting analgesics: structural determinants and role in antinociception. J Pharmacol Exp Ther 1995; 274(3): 1263–70.
71. Gorman AL, Elliott KJ, Inturrisi CE. The d- and l-isomers of methadone bind to the non-competitive site on the N-methyl-d-aspartate (NMDA) receptor in rat forebrain and spinal cord. Neurosci Lett 1997; 223(1): 5–8.
72. Donzanti BA, Warwick RO. Effect of methadone and morphine on serotonin uptake in rat periaqueductal gray slices. Eur J Pharmacol 1979; 59(1–2): 107–10.
73. Larsen JJ, Hyttel J. 5-HT-uptake inhibition potentiates antinociception induced by morphine, pethidine, methadone and ketobemidone in rats. Acta Pharmacol Toxicol (Copenh) 1985; 57(3): 214–18.
74. Nilsson MI, Grönbladh L, Widerlov E, Änggård E. Pharmacokinetics of methadone in methadone maintenance treatment: characterization of therapeutic failures. Eur J Clin Pharmacol 1983; 25(4): 497–501.
75. Eap CP, Cuendt C, Baumann P. Binding of d-methadone, L-methadone, and dl-methadone to proteins in plasma of healthy volunteers: role of the variants of alpha 1-acid blycoprotein. Clin Pharmacol Ther 1990; 47: 338–46.

76. Wilkins JN, Ashofteh A, Setoda D, Wheatley WS, Huigen H, Ling W. Ultrafiltration using the Amicon MPS-1 for assessing methadone plasma protein binding. Ther Drug Monit 1997; 19(1): 83–7.
77. Gourlay GK, Wilson PR, Glynn CJ. Pharmacodynamics and pharmacokinetics of methadone during the perioperative period. Anesthesiology 1982; 57(6): 458–67.
78. Kristensen K, Blemmer T, Angelo HR, et al. Stereoselective pharmacokinetics of methadone in chronic pain patients. Ther Drug Monit 1996; 18(3): 221–7.
79. Olsen GD, Wendel HA, Livermore JD, Leger RM, Lynn RK, Gerber N. Clinical effects and pharmacokinetics of racemic methadone and its optical isomers. Clin Pharmacol Ther 1977; 21(2): 147–57.
80. Anggard E, Nilsson MI, Holmstrand J, Gunne LM. Pharmacokinetics of methadone during maintenance therapy: pulse labeling with deuterated methadone in the steady state. Eur J Clin Pharmacol 1979; 16(1): 53–7.
81. Inturrisi CE, Colburn WA, Kaiko RF, Houde RW, Foley KM. Pharmacokinetics and pharmacodynamics of methadone in patients with chronic pain. Clin Pharmacol Ther 1987; 41(4): 392–401.
82. Wolff K, Hay AW, Raistrick D, Calvert R. Steady-state pharmacokinetics of methadone in opioid addicts. Eur J Clin Pharmacol 1993; 44(2): 189–94.
83. Foster DJ, Somogyi AA, White JM, Bochner F. Population pharmacokinetics of (R)-, (S)- and rac-methadone in methadone maintenance patients. Br J Clin Pharmacol 2004; 57(6): 742–55.
84. Scott CC, Robbins EB, Chen KK. Pharmacologic comparison of the optical isomers of methadone. J Pharmacol Exp Ther 1948; 199: 103–16.
85. Isbell H, Eisenman AJ. Physical dependence liability of drugs of the methadone series and of 6-methyldihydromorphine. Fed Proc 1948; 7: 162.
86. Davis AM, Inturrisi CE. d-Methadone blocks morphine tolerance and N-methyl-d-aspartate-induced hyperalgesia. J Pharmacol Exp Ther 1999; 289(2): 1048–53.
87. Kreek MJ. Medical safety and side effects of methadone in tolerant individuals. JAMA 1973; 223(6): 665–8.
88. Longwell B, Kestler RJ, Cox TJ. Side effects in methadone patients: a survey of self-reported complaints. Int J Addict 1979; 14(4): 485–94.
89. Goldstein A, Judson BA. Proceedings: Efficacy and side effects of three widely different methadone doses. Proc Natl Conf Methadone Treat 1973; 1: 21–44.
90. Gil M, Sala M, Anguera I, et al. QT prolongation and Torsades de Pointes in patients infected with human immunodeficiency virus and treated with methadone. Am J Cardiol 2003; 92(8): 995–7.
91. Krantz MJ, Mehler PS. Synthetic opioids and QT prolongation. Arch Intern Med 2003; 163(13): 1615; author reply.
92. Dyer KR, Foster DJR, White JM, Somogyi AA, Menelaou A, Bochner F. Steady-state pharmacokinetics and pharmacodynamics in methadone maintenance patients: comparison of those who do and do not experience withdrawal

and concentration–effect relationships. Clin Pharmacol Ther 1999; 65(6): 685–94.

93. Dyer KR, White JM, Foster DJ, Bochner F, Menelaou A, Somogyi AA. The relationship between mood state and plasma methadone concentration in maintenance patients. J Clin Psychopharmacol 2001; 21(1): 78–84.
94. Woods JH, Medzihradsky F, Smith CB, Winger GD, France CP. Evaluation of new compounds for opioid activity (1991). NIDA Res Monogr 1992; 119: 559–603.
95. Bertalmio AJ, Medzihradsky F, Winger G, Woods JH. Differential influence of N-dealkylation on the stimulus properties of some opioid agonists. J Pharmacol Exp Ther 1992; 261(1): 278–84.
96. Horng JS, Smits SE, Wong DT. The binding of the optical isomers of methadone, alpha-methadol, alpha-acetylmethadol and their N-demethylated derivatives to the opiate receptors of rat brain. Res Commun Chem Pathol Pharmacol 1976; 14(4): 621–9.
97. Newcombe DAL, Irvine RJ, Salem A. In vitro characterisation of the relative potency of levo-alpha-acetylmethadol (LAAM) and its nor-metabolites. Proceedings of the Joint Meeting of the Australasian Society of Clinical and Experimental Pharmacologists and Toxicologists and the British Pharmacological Society 2000; 7: 111.
98. Nickander R, Booher R, Miles H. Alpha-1-acetylmethadol and its N-demethylated metabolites have potent opiate action in the guinea pig isolated ileum. Life Sci 1974; 14(10): 2011–17.
99. Foldes FF, Shiwaku Y, Matsuo S, Morita K. The influence of methadone derivatives on the isolated myenteric plexus-longitudinal muscle preparation of the guinea-pig ileum. Third Congress of the Hungarian Pharmacological Society 1979: 165–1780.
100. Smits SE. The analgesic activity of alpha-1-acetylmethadol and two of its metabolites in mice. Res Commun Chem Pathol Pharmacol 1974; 8(3): 575–8.
101. Umans JG, Inturrisi C. Analgesic activity of methadone, l-alpha-acetylmethadol and its normetabolites after intracerebroventricular administration to mice. Res Comm Sub Abuse 1981; 2: 291–302.
102. Vaupel DB, Jasinski DR. l-alpha-Acetylmethadol, l-alpha-acetyl-*N*-normethadol and l-alpha-acetyl-*N,N*-dinormethadol: comparisons with morphine and methadone in suppression of the opioid withdrawal syndrome in the dog. J Pharmacol Exp Ther 1997; 283(2): 833–42.
103. Finkle BS, Jennison TA, Chinn DM, Ling W, Holmes ED. Plasma and urine disposition of 1-alpha-acetylmethadol and its principal metabolites in man. J Anal Toxicol 1982; 6(2): 100–5.
104. Henderson GL, Wilson BK, Lau DH. Plasma l-alpha-acetylmethadol (LAAM) after acute and chronic administration. Clin Pharmacol Ther 1977; 21(1): 16–25.
105. Billings RE, McMahon RE, Blake DA. l-Acetylmethadol (LAM) treatment of opiate dependence: plasma and urine levels of two pharmacologically active metabolites. Life Sci 1974; 14(8): 1437–46.

106. Kaiko RF, Inturrisi CE. Disposition of acetylmethadol in relation to pharmacologic action. Clin Pharmacol Ther 1975; 18(1): 96–103.
107. Oda Y, Kharasch ED. Metabolism of methadone and levo-alpha-acetylmethadol (LAAM) by human intestinal cytochrome P450 3A4 (CYP3A4): potential contribution of intestinal metabolism to presystemic clearance and bioactivation. J Pharmacol Exp Ther 2001; 298(3): 1021–32.
108. Neff JA, Moody DE. Differential N-demethylation of l-alpha-acetylmethadol (LAAM) and norLAAM by cytochrome P450s 2B6, 2C18, and 3A4. Biochem Biophys Res Commun 2001; 284(3): 751–6.
109. Moody DE, Walsh SL, Rollins DE, Neff JA, Huang W. Ketoconazole, a cytochrome P450 3A4 inhibitor, markedly increases concentrations of levo-acetyl-alpha-methadol in opioid-naive individuals. Clin Pharmacol Ther 2004; 76(2): 154–66.
110. McCance-Katz EF, Rainey PM, Smith P, et al. Drug interactions between opioids and antiretroviral medications: interaction between methadone, LAAM, and delavirdine. Am J Addict 2006; 15(1): 23–34.
111. Welsh CJ, Cargiulo T. Nevirapine induced opioid withdrawal in a patient previously stable on Levo-Alpha-Acetyl-Methadol (LAAM). J Mainten Addict 2003; 2(3): 51–6.
112. Kaiko RF, Chatterjie N, Inturrisi CE. Simultaneous determination of acetylmethadol and its active biotransformation products in human biofluids. J Chromatogr 1975; 109(2): 247–58.
113. Newcombe DA, Bochner F, White JM, Somogyi AA. Evaluation of levo-alpha-acetylmethdol (LAAM) as an alternative treatment for methadone maintenance patients who regularly experience withdrawal: a pharmacokinetic and pharmacodynamic analysis. Drug Alcohol Depend 2004; 76(1): 63–72.
114. Ling W, Rawson RA, Compton MA. Substitution pharmacotherapies for opioid addiction: from methadone to LAAM and buprenorphine. J Psychoactive Drugs 1994; 26(2): 11–28.
115. Misra AL, Mule SJ, Bloch R, Bates TR. Physiological disposition and biotransformation of l-alpha-[2–3H]acetylmethadol (LAAM) in acutely and chronically treated monkeys. J Pharmacol Exp Ther 1978; 206(2): 475–91.
116. Fraser HF, Isbell H. Actions and addiction liabilities of alpha-acetyl-methadols in man. J Pharmacol Exp Ther 1952; 105(4): 458–65.
117. Walsh SL, Johnson RE, Cone EJ, Bigelow GE. Intravenous and oral l-alpha-acetylmethadol: pharmacodynamics and pharmacokinetics in humans. J Pharmacol Exp Ther 1998; 285(1): 71–82.
118. Keats AS, Beecher HK. Analgesic activity and toxic effects of acetylmethadol isomers in man. J Pharmacol Exp Ther 1952; 105(2): 210–15.
119. Jaffe JH, Schuster CR, Smith BB, Blachley PH. Comparison of acetylmethadol and methadone in the treatment of long-term heroin users. A pilot study. JAMA 1970; 211(11): 1834–6.
120. Ling W, Charuvastra C, Kaim SC, Klett CJ. Methadyl acetate and methadone as maintenance treatments for heroin addicts. A Veterans Administration cooperative study. Arch Gen Psychiat 1976; 33(6): 709–20.

121. Levine R, Zaks A, Fink M, Freedman AM. Levomethadyl acetate. Prolonged duration of opioid effects, including cross tolerance to heroin, in man. JAMA 1973; 226(3): 316–18.
122. Houtsmuller EJ, Walsh SL, Schuh KJ, Johnson RE, Stitzer ML, Bigelow GE. Dose–response analysis of opioid cross-tolerance and withdrawal suppression during LAAM maintenance. J Pharmacol Exp Ther 1998; 285(2): 387–96.
123. Fudala PJ, Vocci F, Montgomery A, Trachtenberg AI. Levomethadyl acetate (LAAM) for the treatment of opioid dependence; a multisite, open-label study of LAAM safety and an evaluation of the product labeling and treatment regulations. J Mainten Addict 1997; 1: 9–39.
124. Judson BA, Goldstein A. Symptom complaints of patients maintained on methadone, LAAM (methadyl acetate), and naltrexone at different times in their addiction careers. Drug Alcohol Depend 1982; 10(2–3): 269–82.
125. White J, Danz C, Kneebone J, La Vincente S, Newcombe D, Ali R. Relationship between LAAM-methadone preference and treatment outcomes. Drug Alcohol Depend 2002; 66: 295–301.
126. Marcovici M, O'Brien CP, McLellan AT, Kacian J. A clinical, controlled study of l-alpha-acetylmethadol in the treatment of narcotic addiction. Am J Psychiatry 1981; 138(2): 234–6.
127. Anonymous. FDA warns about Orlaam T01-15. Print Media. April 2001: 301-827-6242.
128. Anonymous. EMEA public statement on the recommendations to suspend the marketing authorisation for ORLAAM (levoacetylmethadol) in the European Union. The European Agency for the Evaluation of Medicinal Products. April 2001.
129. Deamer RL, Wilson DR, Clark DS, Prichard JG. Torsades de pointes associated with high dose levomethadyl acetate (ORLAAM). J Addict Dis 2001; 20(4): 7–14.
130. Inturrisi CE. Clinical pharmacology of opioids for pain. Clin J Pain 2002; 18(4 Suppl): S3–13.
131. Musto DF, Ramos MR. Notes on American medical history: a follow-up study of the New Haven morphine maintenance clinic of 1920. N Engl J Med 1981; 304(18): 1071–7.
132. Waldorf D, Orlick M, Reinarman C. Morphine Maintenance, the Shreveport Clinic 1919–1923. Washington: The Drug Abuse Council, 1974.
133. Moldavanyi A, Ladewig D, Affentranger P, Natsch C, Stohler R. Morphine maintenance treatment of opioid-dependent out-patients. Eur Addict Res 1996; 2: 208–12.
134. Uchtenhagen A, Dobler-Mikola A, Gutzwiller F. Medical prescription of narcotics. Background and immediate results of a Swiss national project. Eur Addict Res 1996; 2: 201–7.
135. Derks J. The Amsterdam morphine-dispensing experiment. Med Law 1990; 9(2): 841–53.
136. Derks J. The efficacy of the Amsterdam morphine-dispensing programme. In: Mann RD, ed. Drug Misuse and Dependence. Park Ridge, NJ: Parthenon 1990: 85–108.

137. Andersen G, Christrup L, Sjogren P. Relationships among morphine metabolism, pain and side effects during long-term treatment: an update. J Pain Symptom Manage 2003; 25(1): 74–91.
138. Osborne R, Joel S, Trew D, Slevin M. Morphine and metabolite behavior after different routes of morphine administration: demonstration of the importance of the active metabolite morphine-6-glucuronide. Clin Pharmacol Ther 1990; 47(1): 12–19.
139. Sawe J. High-dose morphine and methadone in cancer patients. Clinical pharmacokinetic considerations of oral treatment. Clin Pharmacokinet 1986; 11(2): 87–106.
140. Milne RW, Nation RL, Somogyi AA. The disposition of morphine and its 3- and 6-glucuronide metabolites in humans and animals, and the importance of the metabolites to the pharmacological effects of morphine. Drug Metab Rev 1996; 28(3): 345–472.
141. Adams JU, Paronis CA, Holtzman SG. Assessment of relative intrinsic activity of mu-opioid analgesics in vivo by using beta-funaltrexamine. J Pharmacol Exp Ther 1990; 255(3): 1027–32.
142. Ivarsson M, Neil A. Differences in efficacies between morphine and methadone demonstrated in the guinea pig ileum: a possible explanation for previous observations on incomplete opioid cross-tolerance. Pharmacol Toxicol 1989; 65(5): 368–71.
143. Samuelsson H, Hedner T, Venn R, Michalkiewicz A. CSF and plasma concentrations of morphine and morphine glucuronides in cancer patients receiving epidural morphine. Pain 1993; 52(2): 179–85.
144. Wolff T, Samuelsson H, Hedner T. Morphine and morphine metabolite concentrations in cerebrospinal fluid and plasma in cancer pain patients after slow-release oral morphine administration. Pain 1995; 62(2): 147–54.
145. Osborne R, Thompson P, Joel S, Trew D, Patel N, Slevin M. The analgesic activity of morphine-6-glucuronide. Br J Clin Pharmacol 1992; 34(2): 130–8.
146. Skarke C, Darimont J, Schmidt H, Geisslinger G, Lotsch J. Analgesic effects of morphine and morphine-6-glucuronide in a transcutaneous electrical pain model in healthy volunteers. Clin Pharmacol Ther 2003; 73(1): 107–21.
147. Murthy BR, Pollack GM, Brouwer KL. Contribution of morphine-6-glucuronide to antinociception following intravenous administration of morphine to healthy volunteers. J Clin Pharmacol 2002; 42(5): 569–76.
148. Frances B, Gout R, Monsarrat B, Cros J, Zajac JM. Further evidence that morphine-6 beta-glucuronide is a more potent opioid agonist than morphine. J Pharmacol Exp Ther 1992; 262(1): 25–31.
149. Paul D, Standifer KM, Inturrisi CE, Pasternak GW. Pharmacological characterization of morphine-6 beta-glucuronide, a very potent morphine metabolite. J Pharmacol Exp Ther 1989; 251(2): 477–83.
150. Yaksh TL, Harty GJ, Onofrio BM. High dose of spinal morphine produces a nonopiate receptor-mediated hyperesthesia: clinical and theoretic implications. Anesthesiology 1986; 64(5): 590–7.

151. Yaksh TL, Harty GJ. Pharmacology of the allodynia in rats evoked by high dose intrathecal morphine. J Pharmacol Exp Ther 1988; 244(2): 501–7.
152. Gong QL, Hedner T, Hedner J, Bjorkman R, Nordberg G. Antinociceptive and ventilatory effects of the morphine metabolites: morphine-6-glucuronide and morphine-3-glucuronide. Eur J Pharmacol 1991; 193(1): 47–56.
153. Gourlay GK, Cherry DA, Onley MM, et al. Pharmacokinetics and pharmacodynamics of twenty-four-hourly Kapanol compared to twelve-hourly MS Contin in the treatment of severe cancer pain. Pain 1997; 69(3): 295–302.
154. Gourlay GK. Sustained relief of chronic pain. Pharmacokinetics of sustained release morphine. Clin Pharmacokinet 1998; 35(3): 173–90.
155. Bochner F, Somogyi AA, Christrup LL, Larsen LI, Danz C, Elbaek K. Comparative pharmacokinetics of two modified-release oral morphine formulations (Reliadol and Kapanol) and an immediate-release morphine tablet (Morfin 'DAK') in healthy volunteers. Clinical Drug Investigation 1999; 17(1): 59–66.
156. Broomhead A, West R, Eglinton L, et al. Comparative single-dose pharmacokinetics of sustained-release and modified-release morphine sulphate capsules under fed and fasting conditions. Clin Drug Invest 1997; 13(3): 162–70.
157. Broomhead A, West R, Kadirgamanathan G, Knox K, Krueger D, Malick J. Comparative bioavailability of sustained-release morphine sulfate capsules versus pellets. Clinical Drug Invest 1997; 14(2): 137–45.
158. Maccarone C, West RJ, Broomhead AF, Hodsman GP. Single-dose pharmacokinetics of Kapanol, a new oral sustained-release morphine formulation. Drug Invest 1994; 7(5): 262–74.
159. Mitchell TB, White JM, Somogyi AA, Bochner F. Comparative pharmacodynamics and pharmacokinetics of methadone and slow-release oral morphine for maintenance treatment of opioid dependence. Drug Alcohol Depend 2003; 72: 85–94.
160. Eder H, Kraigher D, Peternell A, et al. Delayed release morphine and methadone for maintenance therapy in opioid dependence. Drug Alcohol Depend 2002; 66(Suppl. 1): 50.
161. Kraigher D, Ortner R, Eder H, Schindler S, Fischer G. Slow release of morphine hydrochloride for maintenance therapy of opioid dependence. Wien Klin Wochenschr 2002; 114(21–22): 904–10.
162. Giacomuzzi SM, Riemer Y, Ertl M, et al. Substitution treatment and quality of life: methadone vs. retard morphine sulfate – a comparative study. Suchtmed 2001; 3: 1–7.
163. Fischer G, Presslich O, Diamant K, Schneider C, Pezawas L, Kasper S. Oral morphine-sulphate in the treatment of opiate dependent patients. Alcoholism 1996; 32(1): 35–43.
164. Fischer G, Jagsch R, Eder H, et al. Comparison of methadone and slow-release morphine maintenance in pregnant addicts. Addict 1999; 94(2): 231–9.

165. Brewer C. Recent developments in maintenance prescribing and monitoring in the United Kingdom. Bull NY Acad Med 1995; 72(2): 359–70.
166. Sherman JP. Managing heroin addiction with a long-acting morphine product (Kapanol). Med J Aust 1996; 165(4): 239.
167. Lewis JW. Ring C-bridged derivatives of thebaine and oripavine. Adv Biochem Psychopharmacol 1973; 8: 123–36.
168. Cowan A, Lewis JW, Macfarlane IR. Agonist and antagonist properties of buprenorphine, a new antinociceptive agent. Br J Pharmacol 1977; 60(4): 537–45.
169. Cowan A. Update on the general pharmacology of buprenorphine. In: Lewis JW, ed. Buprenorphine Combating Drug Abuse with a Unique Opioid. New York: Wiley-Liss, Inc, 1995: 31–47.
170. Jasinski DR, Pevnick JS, Griffith JD. Human pharmacology and abuse potential of the analgesic buprenorphine: a potential agent for treating narcotic addiction. Arch Gen Psychiat 1978; 35(4): 501–16.
171. Mendelson J, Fernandez E, Welm MS, Upton RA, Chin BA, Jones RT. Bioavailability of oral and sublingual buprenorphine and naloxone tablets. Clin Pharmacol Ther 2001; 69(2): 29.
172. Brewster D, Humphrey MJ, McLeavy MA. The systemic bioavailability of buprenorphine by various routes of administration. J Pharm Pharmacol 1981; 33(8): 500–6.
173. Everhart ET, Cheung P, Shwonek P, et al. Subnanogram-concentration measurement of buprenorphine in human plasma by electron-capture capillary gas chromatography: application to pharmacokinetics of sublingual buprenorphine. Clin Chem 1997; 43(12): 2292–302.
174. Kuhlman JJ, Jr., Lalani S, Magluilo J, Jr., Levine B, Darwin WD. Human pharmacokinetics of intravenous, sublingual, and buccal buprenorphine. J Anal Toxicol 1996; 20(6): 369–78.
175. Nath RP. Buprenorphine pharmacokinetics: relative bioavailability of sublingual tablet and liquid formulations. J Clin Pharmacol 1999; 39(6): 619–23.
176. Compton P, Ling W, Moody D, Chiang N. Pharmacokinetics, bioavailability and opioid effects of liquid versus tablet buprenorphine. Drug Alcohol Depend 2006; 82(1): 25–31.
177. Strain EC, Moody DE, Stoller KB, Walsh SL, Bigelow GE. Relative bioavailability of different buprenorphine formulations under chronic dosing conditions. Drug Alcohol Depend 2004; 74(1): 37–43.
178. Walsh SL, Preston KL, Stitzer ML, Cone EJ, Bigelow GE. Clinical pharmacology of buprenorphine: ceiling effects at high doses. Clin Pharmacol Ther 1994; 55(5): 569–80.
179. Everhart ET, Cheung P, Shwonek P, et al. Subnanogram-concentration measurement of buprenorphine in human plasma by electron-capture capillary gas chromatography: application to pharmacokinetics of sublingual buprenorphine. Clin Chem 1997; 43(12): 2292–302.
180. Mendelson J, Upton RA, Everhart ET, Jacob P, 3rd, Jones RT. Bioavailability of sublingual buprenorphine. J Clin Pharmacol 1997; 37(1): 31–7.

181. Nath RP, Upton RA, Everhart ET, et al. Buprenorphine pharmacokinetics: relative bioavailability of sublingual tablet and liquid formulations. J Clin Pharmacol 1999; 39(6): 619–23.
182. Schuh KJ, Johanson CE. Pharmacokinetic comparison of the buprenorphine sublingual liquid and tablet. Drug Alcohol Depend 1999; 56(1): 55–60.
183. McAleer SD, Mills RJ, Polack T, et al. Pharmacokinetics of high-dose buprenorphine following single administration of sublingual tablet formulations in opioid naive healthy male volunteers under a naltrexone block. Drug Alcohol Depend 2003; 72(1): 75–83.
184. Ciraulo DA, Hitzemann RJ, Somoza E, et al. Pharmacokinetics and pharmacodynamics of multiple sublingual buprenorphine tablets in dose-escalation trials. J Clin Pharmacol 2006; 46(2): 179–92.
185. Cone EJ, Gorodetzky CW, Yousefnejad D, Buchwald WF, Johnson RE. The metabolism and excretion of buprenorphine in humans. Drug Metab Dispos 1984; 12(5): 577–81.
186. Huang P, Kehner GB, Cowan A, Liu-Chen LY. Comparison of pharmacological activities of buprenorphine and norbuprenorphine: norbuprenorphine is a potent opioid agonist. J Pharmacol Exp Ther 2001; 297(2): 688–95.
187. Chang Y, Moody DE, McCance-Katz EF. Novel metabolites of buprenorphine detected in human liver microsomes and human urine. Drug Metab Dispos 2006; 34(3): 440–8.
188. Picard N, Cresteil T, Djebli N, Marquet P. In vitro metabolism study of buprenorphine: evidence for new metabolic pathways. Drug Metab Dispos 2005; 33(5): 689.
189. King CD, Green MD, Rios GR, et al. The glucuronidation of exogenous and endogenous compounds by stably expressed rat and human UDP-glucuronosyltransferase 1.1. Arch Biochem Biophys 1996; 332(1): 92–100.
190. Green MD, King CD, Mojarrabi B, Mackenzie PI, Tephly TR. Glucuronidation of amines and other xenobiotics catalyzed by expressed human UDP-glucuronosyltransferase 1A3. Drug Meta Dispos 1998; 26(6): 507–12.
191. Zhang W, Ramamoorthy Y, Tyndale RF, Sellers EM. Interaction of buprenorphine and its metabolite norbuprenorphine with cytochromes p450 in vitro. Drug Metab Dispos 2003; 31(6): 768–72.
192. Lintzeris N, Mitchell TB, Bond A, Nestor L, Strang J. Interactions on mixing diazepam with methadone or buprenorphine in maintenance patients. J Clin Psychopharmacol 2006; 26(3): 274–83.
193. Lintzeris N, Mitchell TB, Bond AJ, Nestor L, Strang J. Pharmacodynamics of diazepam co-administered with methadone or buprenorphine under high dose conditions in opioid dependent patients. Drug Alcohol Depend 2007; 91(2–3): 187–94.
194. Thummel KE, Wilkinson GR. In vitro and in vivo drug interactions involving human CYP3A. Annu Rev Pharmacol Toxicol 1998; 38: 389–430.
195. Reynaud M, Petit G, Potard D, Courty P. Six deaths linked to concomitant use of buprenorphine and benzodiazepines. Addiction 1998; 93(9): 1385–92.

196. Iribarne C, Berthou F, Carlhant D, et al. Inhibition of methadone and buprenorphine N-dealkylations by three HIV-1 protease inhibitors. Drug Metab Dispos 1998; 26(3): 257–60.
197. McCance-Katz EF, Moody DE, Morse GD, et al. Interactions between buprenorphine and antiretrovirals. I. The nonnucleoside reverse-transcriptase inhibitors efavirenz and delavirdine. Clin Infect Dis 2006; 43(S4): 224–34.
198. McCance-Katz EF, Moody DE, Smith PF, et al. Interactions between buprenorphine and antiretrovirals. II. The protease inhibitors nelfinavir, lopinavir/ritonavir, and ritonavir. Clin Infect Dis 2006; 43(S4): 235–46.
199. Johnson RE, Strain EC, Amass L. Buprenorphine: how to use it right. Drug Alcohol Depend 2003; 70(2 Suppl): S59–77.
200. Mégarbane B, Marie N, Pirnay S, et al. Buprenorphine is protective against the depressive effects of norbuprenorphine on ventilation. Toxicol Appl Pharmacol 2006; 212(3): 256–67.
201. Hambrook JM, Rance MJ. The interaction of buprenorphine with the opiate receptor: lipophilicity as a determining factor in drug-receptor kinetics. In: Kosterlitz HW, ed. Opiates and Endogenous Opioid Peptides. Amsterdam: Elsevier/North-Holland Biomedical Press, 1976: 295–301.
202. Schuh KJ, Walsh SL, Bigelow GE, Preston KL, Stitzer ML. Buprenorphine, morphine and naloxone effects during ascending morphine maintenance in humans. J Pharmacol Exp Ther 1996; 278(2): 836–46.
203. Walsh SL, June HL, Schuh KJ, Preston KL, Bigelow GE, Stitzer ML. Effects of buprenorphine and methadone in methadone-maintained subjects. Psychopharmacology (Berl). 1995; 119(3): 268–76.
204. Strain EC, Preston KL, Liebson IA, Bigelow GE. Acute effects of buprenorphine, hydromorphone and naloxone in methadone-maintained volunteers. J Pharmacol Exp Ther 1992; 261(3): 985–93.
205. Kuhlman JJ, Jr., Levine B, Johnson RE, Fudala PJ, Cone EJ. Relationship of plasma buprenorphine and norbuprenorphine to withdrawal symptoms during dose induction, maintenance and withdrawal from sublingual buprenorphine. Addiction 1998; 93(4): 549–59.
206. Iribarne C, Picart D, Dreano Y, Bail JP, Berthou F. Involvement of cytochrome P450 3A4 in N-dealkylation of buprenorphine in human liver microsomes. Life Sci 1997; 60(22): 1953–64.
207. Walter DS, Inturrisi CE. Absorption, distribution, metabolism, and excretion of buprenorphine in animals and humans. In: Lewis JW, ed. Buprenorphine Combating Drug Abuse with a Unique Opioid. New York: Wiley-Liss, Inc, 1995: 113–35.
208. Bullingham RE, McQuay HJ, Moore A, Bennett MR. Buprenorphine kinetics. Clin Pharmacol Ther 1980; 28(5): 667–72.
209. Bullingham RE, McQuay HJ, Moore RA. Clinical pharmacokinetics of narcotic agonist-antagonist drugs. Clin Pharmacokinet 1983; 8(4): 332–43.
210. Walsh SL, Eissenberg T. The clinical pharmacology of buprenorphine: extrapolating from the laboratory to the clinic. Drug Alcohol Depend 2003; 70(2 Suppl): S13–27.

211. Lopatko OV, White JM, Huber A, Ling W. Opioid effects and opioid withdrawal during a 24 h dosing interval in patients maintained on buprenorphine. Drug Alcohol Depend 2003; 69(3): 317–22.
212. Ward J, Mattick RP, Hall W, eds. Methadone Maintenance Treatment and Other Opioid Replacement Therapies. Australia: Hardwood Academic Publishers, 1998.
213. Mello NK, Mendelson JH. Buprenorphine suppresses heroin use by heroin addicts. Science 1980; 207(4431): 657–9.
214. Bickel WK, Stitzer ML, Bigelow GE, Liebson IA, Jasinski DR, Johnson RE. Buprenorphine: dose-related blockade of opioid challenge effects in opioid dependent humans. J Pharmacol Exp Ther 1988; 247(1): 47–53.
215. Fudala PJ, Jaffe JH, Dax EM, Johnson RE. Use of buprenorphine in the treatment of opioid addiction. II. Physiologic and behavioral effects of daily and alternate-day administration and abrupt withdrawal. Clin Pharmacol Ther 1990; 47(4): 525–34.
216. Mello NK, Mendelson JH, Kuehnle JC. Buprenorphine effects on human heroin self-administration: an operant analysis. J Pharmacol Exp Ther 1982; 223(1): 30–9.
217. Bickel WK, Stitzer ML, Bigelow GE, Liebson IA, Jasinski DR, Johnson RE. A clinical trial of buprenorphine: comparison with methadone in the detoxification of heroin addicts. Clin Pharmacol Ther 1988; 43(1): 72–8.
218. Wall ME, Brine DR, Perez-Reyes M. Metabolism and disposition of naltrexone in man after oral and intravenous administration. Drug Metab Dispos 1981; 9(4): 369–75.
219. Ferrari A, Bertolotti M, Dell'Utri A, Avico U, Sternieri E. Serum time course of naltrexone and 6 beta-naltrexol levels during long-term treatment in drug addicts. Drug Alcohol Depend 1998; 52(3): 211–20.
220. Kogan MJ, Verebey K, Mule SJ. Estimation of the systemic availability and other pharmacokinetic parameters of naltrexone in man after acute and chronic oral administration. Res Commun Chem Pathol Pharmacol 1977; 18(1): 29–34.
221. Meyer MC, Straughn AB, Lo MW, Schary WL, Whitney CC. Bioequivalence, dose-proportionality, and pharmacokinetics of naltrexone after oral administration. J Clin Psychiatry 1984; 45(9 Pt 2): 15–19.
222. Verebey K, Volavka J, Mule SJ, Resnick RB. Naltrexone: disposition, metabolism, and effects after acute and chronic dosing. Clin Pharmacol Ther 1976; 20(3): 315–28.
223. Gonzalez JP, Brogden RN. Naltrexone. A review of its pharmacodynamic and pharmacokinetic properties and therapeutic efficacy in the management of opioid dependence. Drugs 1988; 35(3): 192–213.
224. Cone EJ, Gorodetzky CW, Yeh SY. The urinary excretion profile of naltrexone and metabolites in man. Drug Metab Dispos 1974; 2(6): 506–12.
225. Chatterjie N, Fujimoto JM, Inturrisi CE, et al. Isolation and stereochemical identification of a metabolite of naltrexone from human urine. Drug Metab Dispos 1974; 2(5): 401–5.

226. Fujimoto JM, Roerig S, Wang RI, Chatterjie N, Inturrisi CE. Narcotic antagonist activity of several metabolites of naloxone and naltrexone tested in morphine dependent mice. Proc Soc Exp Biol Med 1975; 148(2): 443–8.
227. Resnick RB, Volavka J, Freedman AM, Thomas M. Studies of EN-1639A (naltrexone): a new narcotic antagonist. Am J Psychiat 1974; 131(6): 646–50.
228. Porter SJ, Somogyi AA, White JM. Kinetics and inhibition of the formation of 6beta-naltrexol from naltrexone in human liver cytosol. Br J Clin Pharmacol 2000; 50(5): 465–71.
229. Valentino RJ, Katz JL, Medzihradsky F, Woods JH. Receptor binding, antagonist, and withdrawal precipitating properties of opiate antagonists. Life Sci 1983; 32(25): 2887–96.
230. Gold MS, Dackis CA, Pottash AL, et al. Naltrexone, opiate addiction, and endorphins. Med Res Rev 1982; 2(3): 211–46.
231. Roth RH, Elsworth JD, Redmond DE, Jr. Clonidine suppression of noradrenergic hyperactivity during morphine withdrawal by clonidine: biochemical studies in rodents and primates. J Clin Psychiatry 1982; 43(6 Pt 2): 42–6.
232. Charney DS, Redmond DE, Jr., Galloway MP, et al. Naltrexone precipitated opiate withdrawal in methadone addicted human subjects: evidence for noradrenergic hyperactivity. Life Sci 1984; 35(12): 1263–72.
233. Martin WR, Jasinski DR, Mansky PA. Naltrexone, an antagonist for the treatment of heroin dependence. Effects in man. Arch Gen Psychiat 1973; 28(6): 784–91.
234. Ginzburg HM, MacDonald MG. The role of naltrexone in the management of drug abuse. Med Toxicol 1987; 2(2): 83–92.
235. Mello NK, Mendelson JH, Bree MP. Naltrexone effects on morphine and food self-administration in morphine-dependent rhesus monkeys. J Pharmacol Exp Ther 1981; 218(2): 550–7.
236. Powell KJ, Abul-Husn NS, Jhamandas A, Olmstead MC, Beninger RJ, Jhamandas K. Paradoxical effects of the opioid antagonist naltrexone on morphine analgesia, tolerance, and reward in rats. J Pharmacol Exp Ther 2002; 300(2): 588–96.
237. La Vincente SF, White JM, Somogyi AA, Bochner F, Chapleo CB. Enhanced buprenorphine analgesia with the addition of ultra-low-dose naloxone in healthy subjects. Clin Pharmacol Ther 2008; 83: 144–52.
238. Australian medicines handbook. Adelaide 2004.
239. Sax DS, Kornetsky C, Kim A. Lack of hepatotoxicity with naltrexone treatment. J Clin Pharmacol 1994; 34(9): 898–901.
240. Brahen LS, Capone TJ, Capone DM. Naltrexone: lack of effect on hepatic enzymes. J Clin Pharmacol 1988; 28(1): 64–70.
241. Mendelson JH, Ellingboe J, Kuehnle J, Mello NK. Heroin and naltrexone effects on pituitary-gonadal hormones in man: tolerance and supersensitivity. NIDA Res Monogr 1979; 27: 302–8.
242. Volavka J, Mallya A, Bauman J, et al. Hormonal and other effects of naltrexone in normal men. Adv Exp Med Biol 1979; 116: 291–305.
243. Mirin SM, Meyer RE, McNamee HB. Psychopathology and mood during heroin use: acute vs chronic effects. Arch Gen Psychiat 1976; 33(12): 1503–8.

244. Mendelson JH, Ellingboe J, Kuehnle JC, Mello NK. Heroin and naltrexone effects on pituitary-gonadal hormones in man: interaction of steroid feedback effects, tolerance and supersensitivity. J Pharmacol Exp Ther 1980; 214(3): 503–6.
245. Kosten TR, Kreek MJ, Ragunath J, Kleber HD. Cortisol levels during chronic naltrexone maintenance treatment in ex-opiate addicts. Biol Psychiat 1986; 21(2): 217–20.
246. Kosten TR, Kreek MJ, Ragunath J, Kleber HD. A preliminary study of beta endorphin during chronic naltrexone maintenance treatment in ex-opiate addicts. Life Sci 1986; 39(1): 55–9.

chapter 3

Services for heroin withdrawal: A review

Nicholas Lintzeris, Linda Gowing, and James Bell

Introduction

In Irving Welsh's novel *Trainspotting*, a tale of heroin users in Edinburgh, the protagonist decides at one point that he is going to detoxify from heroin. He tells his friends that he is going away for the weekend, equips himself with numerous cans of soup and a blanket, and locks himself in a room in his parents' house, where he shivers and sweats for a few days. He does so because he is feeling increasingly out of control with his increased level of heroin use and, having just experienced an overdose, detoxification allows him to interrupt this period of heavy heroin use, regain control – and, indeed, regain the capacity to enjoy heroin use again.

It may be protested that this was a work of fiction, and therefore unreliable compared to scientific reports. However, the 'scientific' literature on detoxification has an Alice-in-Wonderland quality – everything works, and yet nothing works – irrespective of the technique used, most people relapse. Withdrawal can be managed with antagonists or agonists, and with a range of other preparations or practices – and, indeed, with no treatment at all. The process of detoxification can take anywhere from 24 hours to several months. Untreated, heroin withdrawal is not life-threatening, but there have been reports of death associated with some detoxification techniques. Set against these 'scientific' findings, Welsh's account seems increasingly grounded in reality. The technique he describes is safe, economical, and is probably as effective as any other means of withdrawing from heroin. Importantly, such an approach challenges service providers with the critical question – why are we providing detoxification services at all?

Heroin withdrawal

Heroin withdrawal is a specific syndrome following the cessation or reduction in heavy and prolonged heroin use. Characteristic features of the heroin withdrawal syndrome are shown in Table 3.1.

Physical symptoms generally commence 8 to 12 hours after last heroin use, peak in severity at about 36 to 72 hours, and generally subside by day 7. There have been reports that dysphoria, anxiety, sleep disturbances and increased cravings may be protracted for 6 months or longer.[1,2] However, persistent cravings and sleep and mood disturbances lasting for weeks or months are common following the cessation of various drug classes including alcohol, opiates, stimulants, and benzodiazepines, and, as such, may not be part of a drug-specific withdrawal syndrome, but rather may represent difficulties in adjusting to life without drugs.[3]

Heroin withdrawal is rarely (if ever) life-threatening on its own, although it can complicate concomitant medical or psychiatric conditions. For this reason, management of withdrawal in people with acute illnesses – such as drug users hospitalized with endocarditis or psychosis – is an important part of management in general health care settings. In those settings, the objective in treating withdrawal is to minimize withdrawal severity.

Table 3.1 Features of the heroin withdrawal syndrome

- Increased sweating, lacrimation (watery eyes), rhinorrhea (runny nose), urinary frequency, diarrhea, abdominal cramps, nausea, vomiting
- Muscle spasm leading to headaches, back aches, leg cramps, arthralgia
- Piloerection ('goosebumps'), dilated pupils, elevated blood pressure, tachycardia
- Anxiety, irritability, dysphoria (low mood), disturbed sleep
- Increased cravings for opiates

This minimizes the risks of patients discharging themselves or injecting drugs while hospitalized, and helps to clarify the cause of signs and symptoms.

The role and objectives of elective detoxification

The term 'detoxification' was originally used to describe elective withdrawal from drugs on the grounds that it involved the removal of toxins from the body. A preferable phrase is 'withdrawal management', although use of the word detoxification has become increasingly entrenched. Indeed, detoxification has become part of popular culture, and lifestyle magazines regularly promote the concept with stories such as 'The seven-day detox diet'. The concept underlying such stories appears to be a period of renunciation (such as not eating junk food) with a view to improving health and well-being – but no assumption of lasting abstinence. This may well be becoming the dominant paradigm of detoxification, and fits quite well with the actual role and benefits of detoxification from heroin.

Many heroin users undergo withdrawal without seeking assistance from services.[4] However, the striking feature of elective detoxification is that it is consumer-driven – there is a brisk demand for detoxification from heroin. One reason for the steady consumer demand is the community perception that detoxification is important. Parents and partners are often anxious to get drug-using people into 'detox'. Many people see entering detoxification as a critical 'first step', because the person is acknowledging that they have a problem. Bundled up in the notion of detoxification are some less clear assumptions – that detoxification, by releasing the grip that heroin has on an individual, will be a cure; or, more moderately, that entering detoxification is a way of connecting heroin users with the treatment system, and beginning a path to recovery.

Data on what actually happens to patients seeking an episode of detoxification are available from ATOS – the recent Australian Treatment Outcome Study.[5] One hundred and seventy-one subjects commencing detoxification from heroin were interviewed at baseline, 3 months post treatment, and 12 months post treatment. In addition, cohorts of heroin users entering methadone treatment, residential rehabilitation, and heroin users not in treatment were interviewed, allowing for comparisons of outcomes. Eighty-three percent of the detoxification cohort was reinterviewed at 12 months. During the 12 months between first and last interview, 92% of subjects had used heroin, and 15% had overdosed at least once. Eighty-nine percent entered a further episode of treatment, having a mean of 3.1 episodes of treatment, and spending a median time of 74 days in treatment during the 12 months. At the 12-month interview, 50% were currently in treatment, a figure remarkably close to the 45% of residential rehabilitation cohort, and 45% of no-treatment cohort, who were in treatment at 12 months.

These figures are consistent with the repeated observation that detoxification is seldom, if ever, a cure of addiction; and rather than a first step into long-term treatment, detoxification tends to function as a revolving door. The reality of detoxification is summed up by Judd et al:[6] 'although detoxification is often the route into treatment, many who begin detoxification do not complete it, and many completers do not go on to more definitive treatment. Some enter detoxification only to lower their level of dependence and make their habit cheaper; others fully believe that detoxification is all that is necessary and that they will be able to remain drug-free.' In the light of these findings, it is possible to identify different, though not necessarily mutually exclusive, understandings of the role of detoxification services: including detoxification as a 'cure' for heroin use; detoxification as the 'first step' in a longer-term process of rehabilitation towards abstinence; detoxification as a means of facilitating a safe and comfortable reversal of neuroadaptation (physical dependence); or detoxification as a means by which users can reduce their level of heroin use and dependence in order to reduce some of the more deleterious effects of dependent drug use.

Given the heterogeneity of heroin users and their circumstances at treatment entry, each of these 'aspirations' may be valid for different individuals, or for the same individual at different times. An unfortunate limitation of research examining the efficacy of detoxification services is that it has often been unclear as to the primary goal of the detoxification program being examined, or studies have often used measures that prioritize particular outcomes and ignore others. The following framework is proposed for the objectives of detoxification services:

1. *To interrupt a pattern of heavy and regular drug use.* Complete cessation of heroin use is generally considered the optimal outcome regarding drug use during a detoxification attempt, and is usually a prerequisite

of inpatient admission. However, continued heroin use is possible in outpatient settings, and reduction in heroin use during detoxification may still represent a positive and worthwhile outcome for some clients.

2. *To alleviate the symptoms and distress of withdrawal.* Palliation of the discomfort of withdrawal is an important reason for clients presenting for treatment. Reduced withdrawal severity may also alleviate demands upon community supports and service providers.
3. *To prevent the development of severe withdrawal sequelae and complications.* The three dimensions of safety particularly pertinent to heroin detoxification are:
   (i) deterioration or complications in concomitant medical or psychiatric conditions (e.g., precipitation of acute psychosis in a patient with schizophrenia);
   (ii) severe adverse events of the detoxification treatment (e.g. methadone toxicity, anesthesia-related complications in antagonist-assisted detoxification); and
   (iii) increased risk of overdose following detoxification.[7,8]
4. *To provide linkages to appropriate post-withdrawal services that address the client's drug use, physical, psychological, and social needs.* Heroin dependence is generally a chronic relapsing condition, and long-term participation in treatment is usually required in order to achieve long-term benefits. An important role therefore of detoxification services is to facilitate linkages with post-withdrawal services.

These objectives can also serve as a template for evaluating the effectiveness of detoxification services. In addition, there are important 'process' measures fundamental in health service evaluation, including accessibility of services, retention in (or completion of) detoxification treatment, service costs, and measures of client satisfaction.

The incorporation of multiple treatment objectives and outcome measures allows for the possibility that some detoxification approaches may have advantages in achieving certain treatment goals, but may be less successful in meeting others. Clinically, the emphasis placed upon different objectives relates to the context in which detoxification services are provided. For example, issues regarding safety and prevention of complications are paramount in non-elective detoxification services provided to heroin users undergoing hospitalization for a concomitant medical condition. Alternatively, elective detoxification services provided at the commencement of a long-term rehabilitation program (e.g., a therapeutic community or naltrexone treatment) should focus upon post-withdrawal treatment induction as its primary outcome. Identification of the strengths and weaknesses of different detoxification approaches may also assist the process of client–treatment matching.

Patient factors impacting upon detoxification outcomes

Whereas anecdotal reports and conventional 'wisdom' suggest that withdrawal severity is related to duration and levels of heroin use, research findings directly examining this issue are equivocal. Whilst associations between withdrawal severity and quantity of opiate use have been reported,[9,10] most researchers have found no significant association between baseline heroin consumption and subsequent withdrawal severity.[11–13] Smolka and Schmidt also identified a relationship between route of administration and withdrawal severity, with greater withdrawal reported by those injecting, rather than smoking, equivalent amounts of heroin.[10]

Psychologic factors have been shown to impact considerably upon withdrawal severity and treatment retention. Phillips and colleagues examined a range of client and treatment factors in heroin and methadone users undergoing a 21-day methadone-assisted withdrawal.[11] Methadone dose at the commencement of the withdrawal and duration of opioid use were not predictive of withdrawal severity, whereas level of neuroticism and expectancy regarding withdrawal severity were significantly associated with withdrawal severity. Similar findings have been reported for individuals undergoing withdrawal from methadone maintenance treatment. Kosten and colleagues found higher scores for depression at baseline (as measured by the Beck Depression Inventory) to be a significant predictor of failure at attempts to withdraw from methadone maintenance treatment.[14] Kanof et al reported that subjects with increasing levels of dysphoria during the withdrawal episode (but not necessarily high scores at baseline) complained of greater withdrawal discomfort and had less success in completing withdrawal; however, directions of causality cannot be determined from such findings as dysphoria may have been a consequence of withdrawal discomfort.[15]

Predictors of outcome for detoxification were examined from pooled studies of inpatient and outpatient randomized controlled trials (RCTs) (comparing buprenorphine to symptomatic medication), examining client and treatment factors in 344 subjects.[16] Whilst treatment factors (inpatient versus outpatient setting and medication type) were related to treatment outcomes (retention, heroin use), no significant relationship was found between treatment outcome and age, gender, race, education, employment, marital status, legal problems, baseline depression, or length or severity of drug use. The only client factors related to treatment outcome were tobacco use (poorer outcomes), and severe baseline anxiety (better outcomes).

Perhaps one of the most important factors impacting upon detoxification outcomes is the extent to which clients presenting for treatment are committed to long-term abstinence and have the psychologic and social resources available to achieve abstinence. These can be difficult parameters to measure in both clinical and research settings, and, as such, their importance may be underestimated in the literature.

Interventions for heroin withdrawal

The delivery of heroin detoxification services includes assessment and planning, treatment settings, supportive care, pharmacotherapy, and facilitating post-withdrawal linkages. The role of pharmacotherapies is described in the following section.

Assessment

The two main objectives of assessment are to ascertain valid information in order to identify the most suitable treatment plan for the client, and to engage the client in the treatment process – including the establishment of rapport and facilitation of treatment plans. The process of assessment and client selection for withdrawal programs (and research studies) can have a considerable impact upon outcomes.[17]

Settings for withdrawal

Heroin detoxification can be located in intensive inpatient units such as general or psychiatric hospital wards, specialist addiction detoxification units, in community residential units (providing supported accommodation with limited medical staffing or monitoring), or in ambulatory settings including outpatient and home-based services. Non-elective withdrawal also occurs in a range of settings, such as prisons or police cells.

There are advantages and disadvantages to different treatment settings. A systematic review of detoxification programs using reducing methadone doses reported that 78% of opiate (heroin and/or methadone)-dependent subjects attempting inpatient methadone withdrawal completed the regimen (referring to the proportion of subjects reaching 0 mg of methadone), compared to 31% of outpatient attempts ($p<0.001$).[18] Two RCTs have compared inpatient (in specialist addiction units) to outpatient detoxification. Gossop and colleagues compared outcomes for subjects allocated to a 21-day inpatient reduction or to an 8-week outpatient reduction regimen.[19] The inpatient group had a significantly higher completion rate (81% compared to 17%). However, the outpatient group had a significantly higher rate of post-withdrawal treatment retention than the inpatient group, suggesting that inpatient services may result in better short-term outcomes; however, outpatient detoxification may be associated with a more seamless transition between detoxification and post-withdrawal services. Wilson and colleagues compared outcomes for 40 heroin users randomly assigned to either an inpatient or outpatient 10-day methadone reduction regimen.[20] The authors reported that few subjects completed either regimen, and 98% of subjects had relapsed to heroin use within 2 months of treatment. Given the poor completion rates for both groups, the authors concluded that outpatient services were a more cost-effective treatment approach.

Whilst inpatient detoxification may be associated with better immediate outcomes, improved long-term outcomes, such as long-term abstinence or treatment retention, have not been clearly demonstrated.[21] Given the limited availability of, and greater expense generally associated with intensive inpatient services, the clinical indications for heroin detoxification to be conducted in intensive inpatient settings are generally limited to patients with conditions requiring intensive medical support, such as the presence of concomitant medical or psychiatric conditions, or concurrent withdrawal from heavy alcohol or benzodiazepine use.[22–25] Community residential units are suited to those individuals with inadequate social supports and for those with repeated failure at outpatient withdrawal attempts.

Ambulatory detoxification is generally suitable for most heroin users who have adequate social supports and without severe dependence on other drugs, or medical or psychiatric co-morbidity.

Supportive care

Supportive care refers to the provision of psychosocial support during the withdrawal episode and is an important component of detoxification services, particularly as psychologic factors appear to have a considerable impact upon withdrawal severity and outcomes. Supportive care involves regular monitoring, provision of information, and counseling.

Monitoring includes frequent review of the client to identify their general progress and motivation, severity of withdrawal symptoms (which can be facilitated by the use of withdrawal scales), drug use (particularly in an outpatient context), response to the medication(s), and complications. This is important for the individualization of treatment such as the titration of medication doses or tailoring of ancillary services, and for ongoing treatment planning. Validated scales such as the Subjective and Objective Opiate Withdrawal Scales[26] may assist in this process. Evidence from other medical disciplines suggests that encouraging clients to self-monitor their progress during treatment (such as symptom severity, side-effects) improves treatment adherence.[27–29]

The provision of information to clients regarding the nature and duration of withdrawal, treatment procedures, and coping strategies can enhance outcomes. In a randomized trial, the structured provision of information to clients undergoing an inpatient 21-day methadone taper resulted in enhanced treatment retention and less severe withdrawal severity than in subjects receiving information on request.[30]

Counseling during the detoxification episode is generally aimed at supporting the client through the detoxification period and facilitating post-withdrawal linkages. Strategies should be employed that provide symptomatic relief, such as allaying cravings, mood (anxiety, dysphoria) and sleep disturbances, and to maintain motivation, although there has been limited formal evaluation of such approaches.

The role of more structured psychosocial interventions in detoxification has recently been the subject of a systematic review.[31] Eight randomized trials were identified that have examined structured psychosocial interventions during methadone or buprenorphine detoxification regimens compared to medication regimens 'alone'. The studies examined behavioral interventions (contingency management[32–36] or community reinforcement strategies;[37] family therapy,[38] or psychotherapeutic interventions).[39] Meta-analyses indicate significant benefits when any psychosocial treatment is added in achieving:

- completion of treatment (RR=1.68, 95% confidence interval [CI] 1.11–2.55),
- abstinence rates following detoxification (RR=2.43, 95% CI 1.61–3.66), and
- a non-significant trend towards less heroin use in treatment (R=0.77, 95% CI 0.59–1.01).

These studies examined the role of behavioral interventions during gradual methadone or buprenorphine reduction regimens, which may not be readily generalized to alternative (e.g. inpatient) settings or detoxification approaches. More research is required examining the role of psychosocial interventions in detoxification.

The evidence regarding 'alternative' therapies such as acupuncture remains unclear, largely due to poor research methodologies.[40,41] However, such approaches are popular among some clients who testify to their value in reducing the severity of withdrawal symptoms and cravings.

Pharmacotherapies for heroin withdrawal

Numerous pharmacologic approaches have been used to manage opiate withdrawal during the past century.[42] Many approaches had been introduced with considerable initial enthusiasm, only for most approaches to be abandoned as concerns regarding their effectiveness or safety emerged, or newer approaches developed. The changes in 'conventional' clinical practice and 'wisdom' over time emphasize the need for thorough evaluation of pharmacotherapies and an evidence-based approach to clinical practice.

Medication regimens for heroin withdrawal in the contemporary research literature can be broadly classified into four approaches:

- reducing doses of an opioid agonist, usually methadone;
- partial opioid agonists, usually buprenorphine;

- symptomatic medications, most notably the α_2 adrenergic agonists (clonidine and lofexidine), which aim to reduce the severity of withdrawal symptoms, without fundamentally changing the course of the withdrawal syndrome;
- opioid antagonists, predominantly naloxone or naltrexone.

Key issues regarding the use of these medications for the management of heroin detoxification, and relevant comparative RCTs are presented here. Each of these medication approaches has been the subject of recent systematic Cochrane reviews for managing opiate withdrawal; including the use of α_2 adrenergic agonists,[43] buprenorphine,[44] methadone,[45] and antagonist-assisted withdrawal.[46,47] These Cochrane reviews have incorporated studies of patients withdrawing from heroin and/or methadone. As the focus of this chapter is the management of heroin withdrawal, greater attention is given to the trials that have only (or largely) examined patients undergoing detoxification from heroin. The use of other symptomatic medications (such as benzodiazepines, antidepressants) will also be briefly described as they are frequently used in clinical practice, although there is limited research evidence regarding their use.

Methadone and other opioid agonists

Methadone is an agonist at μ opiate receptors and can fully substitute for heroin in dependent individuals, thereby preventing heroin withdrawal. Although there is considerable variation in the manner in which methadone has been used in the treatment of heroin withdrawal, the general clinical principles involve:

1. Initial titration of the methadone dose to prevent features of heroin withdrawal (usually in the range of 30 to 60 mg daily).
2. Reduction in the methadone dose over a period of time. From 10 to 21 days of methadone tapering is frequently described in the research literature, extending to longer programs in some cases (e.g. 6-week to 6-month reduction regimens).
3. Adjuvant symptomatic medications are often employed towards the end of the methadone reduction regimen, corresponding to the period when withdrawal severity is greatest.

The use of methadone delays the emergence of peak opiate withdrawal symptoms and prolongs the duration of withdrawal symptoms compared to unmedicated heroin withdrawal. Methadone generally prevents significant withdrawal symptoms until the dose is reduced below a certain threshold (often in the range of 10 to 20 mg), at which point opiate withdrawal symptoms emerge. Withdrawal symptoms peak at about the time of the last methadone dose or in the first few days after the cessation of methadone. Peak withdrawal severity is generally less than for unassisted heroin withdrawal, although withdrawal discomfort tends to persist for approximately 7 to 14 days following a 10- to 21-day methadone reduction regimen.[48–51] The prolonged withdrawal discomfort is among the main limitations of using methadone for heroin withdrawal, particularly in detoxification programs of short duration (e.g. inpatient settings).

A consistent finding in the studies of methadone-assisted heroin detoxification is the high rate of relapse to heroin use following cessation of methadone doses. The few studies that have reported post-withdrawal outcomes suggest very high rates of relapse to heroin use – for example, in a review of outpatient methadone-assisted heroin withdrawal studies (n=20) conducted in the USA in the 1970s, between 0% and 38% of subjects in these studies were abstinent at follow-up several months later.[52] These authors concluded that detoxification alone does not lead to prolonged abstinence in most heroin users. The authors of the recent Cochrane review[45] made similar conclusions.

From the perspective of safety, methadone is generally well tolerated by heroin-dependent individuals, although there are concerns regarding methadone toxicity and diversion.

The use of methadone to assist heroin withdrawal is well suited to facilitating continued methadone treatment as a maintenance program, particularly for those clients who do not cease their heroin use during the withdrawal episode, or relapse to heroin use on discontinuing methadone treatment. However, the prolonged withdrawal following the cessation of methadone can be a barrier to entry into abstinence-oriented post-withdrawal treatment modalities. For example, the commencement of naltrexone is generally recommended 10 to 14 days after the last methadone dose,[53] while many residential rehabilitation programs will not accept clients until several days after the cessation of methadone.

Treatment factors impacting upon outcomes

The manner in which methadone-assisted detoxification programs are delivered impacts upon outcomes. However, the capacity to identify an 'optimal' approach for the use of methadone in heroin detoxification is limited by the wide variation between studies. Nevertheless, it is possible to identify important treatment variables.

The treatment setting

Historically, long-term inpatient withdrawal programs involving gradual methadone reductions over weeks were not uncommon. Studies examining such programs indicated that inpatient withdrawal programs using methadone generally resulted in a greater rate of program 'completion' than outpatient-based programs, although longer-term benefits have not been identified. Indeed, a trend in recent years has been towards shorter inpatient detoxification programs, often no longer than 7 to 10 days. This restricts the utility of methadone as a detoxification medication, given that withdrawal symptoms persist for several days beyond the last methadone dose. Despite anecdotal reports of programs using brief inpatient methadone regimens (3 to 5 days), only one controlled trial[54] has compared a brief methadone regimen (3 day methadone versus 3 day buprenorphine vs clonidine). However, this study is difficult to interpret, as it was conducted in medically ill HIV-positive patients, with approximately half of all patients receiving morphine doses as 'rescue' medication for pain relief.

The initial stabilization period on methadone prior to dose reduction

Initial stabilization on methadone can disrupt a pattern of heavy daily heroin use, enhance the client's sense of self-efficacy, and improve their capacity to cope with subsequent withdrawal symptoms.[55] Although not systematically examined in the research literature, the extent of continued heroin use during the period of initial stabilization on methadone may impact upon subsequent withdrawal outcomes. In a study examining a 90-day outpatient methadone reduction regimen for heroin users, subjects who continued to use heroin during the initial 2-week stabilization period had worse outcomes than those subjects who had ceased heroin use during stabilization.[56] There may be advantages in enabling sufficient time (and methadone doses) during the initial stabilization period to ensure cessation of heroin use, prior to dose reduction, although further research on this issue is required.

The rate and frequency of dose reduction

There are both advantages and limitations with methadone detoxification programs of different duration. Shorter reduction regimens appear to be associated with greater peak withdrawal discomfort, shorter duration of withdrawal symptoms,[48] and greater 'completion' rates with subjects reaching 0 mg of methadone in line with the protocol.[18] However, the higher completion rates for shorter regimens may merely reflect that longer programs have more time in which subjects can relapse to heroin use and/or drop out of treatment. Some authors have argued against rapid reduction regimens (e.g. 10 to 21 days), stating that many individuals are prematurely withdrawn and consequently resume heroin use, and that longer programs may be associated with the benefits afforded by longer periods of adequate methadone doses.[52] Unfortunately, most studies of outpatient reduction regimens have reported very low rates of abstinence from heroin following the cessation of methadone, regardless of the duration of the reduction regimen. A randomized trial comparing linear and inverse exponential methadone dose reductions[49] showed greater overall withdrawal discomfort in the exponential group (largely early in the reduction regimen), although there were no significant differences on other outcomes.

The flexibility (patient involvement) in dose reductions

The literature examining the impact of flexibility (or patient involvement) in dosing reduction regimens is equivocal. Two studies have reported higher 'completion' rates (subjects reaching 0 mg of methadone) for fixed (physician-regulated) than patient-regulated reduction regimens,[4,57] although the findings regarding outcomes such as rates of heroin use are mixed. A larger study of 108 heroin-dependent adults using a 22-week methadone reduction regimen[58] showed no difference on any outcome measure between subjects randomly assigned to physician- or client-regulated dose reduction.

The level of psychosocial and supportive care

The research literature regarding the role of psychosocial interventions in heroin detoxification was identified earlier. The provision of information to patients enhances outcomes.[30] Most research has examined the role of contingency management during gradual dose reduction regimens, which appears to enhance short-term outcomes (such as less heroin use and greater treatment retention), however few studies have demonstrated long-term improvements after methadone is discontinued. Another randomized trial examined the impact of structured counseling regarding post-withdrawal treatment options in the context of an outpatient methadone-assisted withdrawal for heroin users.[39] The structured counseling group had a significantly greater uptake of alternative treatment options (48%) compared to those only receiving information on request (12%). These findings suggest the importance of providing information and post-detoxification treatment planning as structured components of detoxification treatment. More complex behavioral interventions such as contingency management or community reinforcement may be more difficult to incorporate into 'routine' detoxification services.

The use of adjuvant symptomatic medications

Systematic evaluation of adjuvant medications in addition to methadone reductions has been limited. The use of a high-dose clonidine regimen throughout a 10-day inpatient methadone reduction resulted in higher drop-out rates than the placebo and methadone group, due to the hypotensive side effects of clonidine.[59] Little systematic research has examined the use of benzodiazepines in this context. Diazepam was found to enhance treatment retention and reduce heroin use during an outpatient methadone regimen when compared to the tricyclic antidepressant doxepin.[60] Srisurapanont and colleagues found amitriptyline and lorazepam to be equally effective in managing sleep disturbances during withdrawal from methadone maintenance treatment.[61] This evidence suggests minimal advantage in using adrenergic agonists during a methadone reduction regimen, although there may be some advantages in using benzodiazepines in methadone reduction regimens under carefully monitored conditions.

The availability of transfer to maintenance substitution treatment (and the extent to which this is encouraged by treatment staff)

Many clients undergoing methadone-assisted heroin withdrawal will take up the option of transferring to methadone maintenance treatment if it is available.[39] Importantly, the enhanced long-term outcome associated with methadone maintenance treatment warrants its promotion to all clients undergoing heroin detoxification, particularly in circumstances where other effective treatment modalities are not being considered. However, the decision for a client to discontinue a detoxification regimen and transfer to methadone maintenance complicates the interpretation of withdrawal outcomes, and detoxification research studies have not usually included (or reported) such options in their protocols.

Other opioid agonists in the management of heroin withdrawal

A number of other opioid agonists have also been used and evaluated for heroin withdrawal, most notably propoxyphene and levo-alpha-acetylmethadol (LAAM).

Propoxyphene has been described in a number of trials of heroin withdrawal.[62–64] Propoxyphene and methadone were directly compared in an outpatient RCT of 72 heroin users using 21-day reduction regimens.[64] Subjects randomized to methadone reported significantly less severe withdrawal features and had higher treatment retention rates, although similar rates of heroin use were reported during the withdrawal episode. The initial enthusiasm shown with propoxyphene has been tempered with more recent reports of adverse events and abuse of the medication.[65–67]

LAAM, a long-acting synthetic opioid, was compared to methadone for heroin withdrawal in an RCT of 61 male heroin users using a 9-week outpatient treatment protocol, with comparable outcomes between the two groups.[68]

A recent study examined the role of dihydrocodeine, which has historically been widely used in parts of the UK for treating heroin dependence, despite concerns regarding misuse and diversion. Wright et al[69] compared outcomes in 60 illicit opioid-dependent patients randomized to either dihydrocodeine or buprenorphine in an outpatient setting, with up to 15-day medication regimens. The buprenorphine group had better outcomes regarding detox completion, heroin use, and long-term abstinence (at 3 and 6 months' follow-up), suggesting buprenorphine to be superior to dihydrocodeine.

The role of tincture of opium for treating opiate withdrawal in opium users has been examined in phase II research, suggesting that it may be a useful strategy in countries where opium use is more culturally accepted, although further research is required.[70]

Buprenorphine

Buprenorphine is a partial opioid agonist, with high affinity and low intrinsic activity at the μ opiate receptor. The rationale for the use of buprenorphine for heroin detoxification is not dissimilar to methadone: the use of an opiate substitute in reducing doses to modify the severity of withdrawal discomfort. Clinical and research experience with the use of buprenorphine for detoxification is still emerging. Nevertheless, there have been a number of comparative trials comparing buprenorphine with other detoxification medications.

Buprenorphine compared to symptomatic medications

Ten RCTs, involving over 800 subjects, have compared buprenorphine to the α-adrenergic agonist clonidine for the management of heroin (with or without methadone) detoxification.[54,71–75] Meta-analysis by the Cochrane review[44] of key findings indicates that, compared to clonidine, buprenorphine has greater efficacy on a range of key outcomes:

- Buprenorphine was significantly more effective in reducing peak withdrawal severity (standardized mean difference of 0.61; 95% CI=0.36–0.86, $p<0.001$),[72,74,75] and reducing global withdrawal severity (standardized mean difference of 0.59; 95% CI=0.39–0.79, $p<0.001$).[76,77]
- Buprenorphine had significantly higher detoxification completion rates in both inpatient (relative risk [RR]=2.06; confidence interval [CI]=1.03–4.14)[71,76,78–80] and outpatient settings (RR=1.46; CI=1.07–1.99).[73,75–77,81] Combined, buprenorphine has a significantly greater rate of completion than clonidine-assisted detoxification (RR=1.67; CI=1.24–2.25).
- Buprenorphine had a significantly higher uptake of post-detoxification treatment,[75] a finding not reported in other studies.

As yet, fewer studies have compared buprenorphine with lofexidine. A large study of outpatient heroin withdrawal[82] compared a 4-day lofexidine regimen to a 7-day buprenorphine regimen in 210 patients randomized to the two groups, and in 271 patients who self-selected their medication (not reported here). Sixty-five percent of the buprenorphine group completed the withdrawal regimen, and 40% of those followed up were abstinent at 1 month after detox, compared to 46% in the lofexidine group and 32% abstinent at 1 month. Withdrawal severity was significantly lower in the buprenorphine group. Similar findings were reported in a controlled non-randomized trial[83] that reported outcomes in 69 heroin users presenting for outpatient detoxification. Outcomes were better for the buprenorphine group (n=38), with less severe withdrawal and higher rates of completion.

One small inpatient RCT has compared buprenorphine to oxazepam, with carbamazepine used in both groups.[84] The buprenorphine group reported significantly less severe withdrawal than the benzodiazepine group, with comparable completion rates.

Buprenorphine compared to methadone

Four RCTs and two non-randomized trials have compared buprenorphine to methadone for opiate detoxification.[54,85–87] Bickel and colleagues compared a gradual outpatient reduction regimen using either buprenorphine or methadone.[85] Unfortunately, the study is difficult to interpret due to the small sample size, the fact that all patients dropped out or relapsed to regular heroin use before completing the reduction regimen, there was no follow-up post medication, and morphine was available for severe breakthrough withdrawal symptoms. In an open label inpatient RCT, Petitjean and colleagues reported more severe withdrawal in the buprenorphine group at the beginning, but significantly less severe withdrawal at the completion of the dosing regimen, compared to the methadone group.[86] The methadone group had greater overall peak and more prolonged withdrawal severity. Completion rates were comparable between the groups. Seifert and colleagues compared reducing doses of buprenorphine to methadone in a 14-day inpatient blinded RCT with 26 subjects.[87] Medication was given for the first 10 days. There was a non-significant trend for greater completion amongst buprenorphine (64%) compared to methadone (42%) patients. The buprenorphine group reported less severe withdrawal in the second week of the withdrawal regimen. Umbricht and colleagues compared the efficacy of 3-day regimens of buprenorphine, clonidine, and methadone in reducing withdrawal severity and pain in 55 heroin-dependent HIV-positive patients hospitalized for medical reasons on an inpatient AIDS service.[54] Pain relief and withdrawal severity were comparable for the three groups, although the availability of morphine for breakthrough pain complicates the interpretation of the findings.

Ebner et al[88] examined completion rates in 93 adolescents withdrawing from opioids (methadone and/or heroin) using either buprenorphine or methadone (self-selected) in adolescents in an inpatient setting. Buprenorphine has a higher completion rate (38%) compared to methadone (24%), although this did not reach statistical significance. Reed and colleagues[89] likewise compared self-selected buprenoprhine or methadone reductions in an inpatient setting for withdrawal in 123 methadone and/or heroin users (with 28% also codependent to benzodiazepines). The authors reported significantly lower withdrawal severity in the buprenorphine-treated group, and significantly greater withdrawal completion in the buprenorphine-treated patients codependent to benzodiazepines. There was no difference in completion between methadone and buprenorphine for non-benzodiazepine codependent patients.

A non-randomized controlled trial comparing tramadol and buprenorphine[90] suggested that tramadol may be an effective option for patients with low levels of withdrawal severity, however the tramadol group required greater use of breakthrough medication.

In summary, available data suggest that buprenorphine may result in less severe and less prolonged rebound withdrawal at the completion of short dosing regimens compared with methadone. This may be particularly attractive for inpatient or other settings where the capacity for extended follow-up after the completion of medication is limited (e.g. correctional facilities). Further research is required to better understand the relative benefits of buprenorphine and methadone for detoxification.

Delivering buprenorphine detoxification treatment

Duration of treatment

The optimal duration of reduction regimens has not yet been established for methadone or buprenorphine. Five RCTs have examined this issue with buprenorphine:

- Amass and colleagues compared a rapid-reduction (n=5, over 2 to 3 weeks) compared to a slow-reduction regimen (n=3, over 36 days).[91] The rapid-taper group reported greater heroin use and more severe withdrawal.

- Wang and Young compared a rapid reduction (n=16, over 14 days), compared to a slow reduction (n=7, over 8 weeks).[92] The rapid-taper group had more severe withdrawal symptoms, and 38% completed the regimen heroin free, compared to milder symptoms and less heroin use (71% opiate free) in the gradual taper.
- Conversely, another study reported greater completion rates (36%) in a rapid-reduction group (n=39, 9 days) than in a slow-reduction (n=19, 28 days) group (21%).[93] There were no differences in rates of heroin use during the detoxification or at 3-month follow-up.
- Assadi and colleagues compared a rapid buprenorphine inpatient detoxification regimen (24 mg administered intramuscularly over 24 hours) compared to a 5-day dose reduction regimen, with generally comparable outcomes.[94]
- Hopper et al[95] randomized 20 patients to undergo a 1-day buprenophine regimen (32 mg sublingual), compared to 32 mg buprenorphine administered over 3 days in an inpatient setting. There were no differences in completion rates (90%) or withdrawal severity between the groups.

By comparing reports of withdrawal severity across trials, Lintzeris and colleagues have argued that longer duration and higher doses of buprenorphine may be associated with the emergence of greater withdrawal severity (or rebound withdrawal) upon the cessation of buprenorphine treatment.[96] This has not been adequately addressed in randomized inpatient trials.

Buprenorphine doses

The optimal doses in detoxification programs are likewise unclear – with only two studies having compared subjects on different buprenorphine doses.[97,98] Liu and colleagues[97] allocated heroin users by their severity of dependence to 'low' (average dose of 2 mg), 'medium' (2.9 mg), and 'high' dose (3.6 mg) buprenorphine, and demonstrated no significant difference between groups, which may reflect the minimal difference in doses between the groups, or may reflect that patients with higher levels of dependence require higher doses. Oreskovich and colleagues[98] randomly assigned 30 heroin users to either high-dose buprenorphine (daily doses of 8 mg, 8 mg, 8 mg, 4 mg, 2 mg), low-dose buprenorphine (2 mg, 4 mg, 8 mg, 4 mg, 2 mg) or a clonidine regimen. Both buprenorphine groups reported lower withdrawal severity compared to clonidine ($p=0.001$), and whilst withdrawal severity was less in the high-dose than low-dose buprenorphine group, the difference was not significant, which may reflect the small study size. Further research is required to identify optimal buprenorphine doses. Nevertheless, there is considerable research demonstrating that daily buprenorphine doses of 4 mg or more per day are more effective in suppressing withdrawal and heroin use than lower doses, and that outcomes are optimized when using doses in the range of 8 to 16 mg per day (see reference 96 for review). Most contemporary approaches have recommended using maximum doses in the range of 8 to 16 mg per day for detoxification.[99,100]

Buprenorphine preparations

The development of alternative buprenorphine preparations has also been examined in the research literature for the management of heroin withdrawal. Lanier and colleagues[101] reported findings from an open-label study of a single buprenorphine patch (applied for 7 days) in managing opiate withdrawal in 12 inpatient heroin users. The authors reported that the approach was well tolerated, with a marked reduction of withdrawal severity. In another open-label phase II study of 5 heroin users,[102] a depot intramuscular buprenorphine injection produced adequate relief of opiate withdrawal, and continued to produce some opioid blockade for 6 weeks following administration. Both these approaches appear promising as mechanisms to deliver buprenorphine-assisted withdrawal with less inconvenience than daily attendance at a clinic or pharmacy for dosing.

Post-detoxification treatment options following buprenorphine

A number of studies have examined post-detoxification treatment uptake following buprenorphine. When given the opportunity, it appears that many patients attempting a detoxification episode with buprenorphine choose to remain in longer-term buprenorphine maintenance treatment.[75,103,104]

Another post-detoxification option is treatment with naltrexone, an opioid antagonist licensed for relapse prevention. Due to buprenorphine's high affinity for μ opiate receptors, naltrexone can be initiated without considerable delays or severe precipitated withdrawal. O'Connor et al reported comparable rates of induction onto naltrexone treatment when comparing naltrexone-assisted rapid detoxification and buprenorphine detoxification regimens in an outpatient RCT.[74] Similar findings were reported by Collins et al[80] in a study of 106 heroin users randomized to either anesthesia-assisted rapid detoxification, buprenorphine, or clonidine regimens, with subsequent 12-week naltrexone treatment. The rapid detox and buprenorphine-assisted naltrexone induction were comparable to naltrexone induction and retention, and superior to the clonidine group. Studies have reported the initiation of naltrexone whilst patients are still taking buprenorphine, or within 3 days of stopping buprenorphine.[74,80,105–109]

The relative merits of early naltrexone induction (commencing naltrexone within 24 hours of the last buprenorphine dose) include greater withdrawal severity following first naltrexone dose, but greater rates of induction onto naltrexone; whereas delaying the introduction of naltrexone until 3 to 5 days after the last buprenorphine dose results in less severe peak withdrawal, but is potentially associated with greater relapse prior to commencing naltrexone.[108,109]

Alpha adrenergic agonists

A number of α_2 adrenergic agonists have been investigated for the management of heroin withdrawal, including clonidine, lofexidine, guanfacine, and guanabenz acetate; although only two, clonidine and lofexidine, are widely used clinically, and the discussion will be limited to these medications.

The main mechanism of action postulated for the alpha adrenergic agonists is that they reduce the noradrenergic hyperactivity in the locus coeruleus seen during opiate withdrawal,[110] although other neurotransmitter systems may be implicated, including serotonin and cholinergic systems.[111] Alpha adrenergic agonists appear to be more effective in reducing certain withdrawal features, such as restlessness and the 'autonomic' features of withdrawal including diarrhea, nausea, abdominal cramps, sweating, rhinorrhea, and lacrimation. However, alpha adrenergic agonists appear less beneficial in alleviating sleep disturbances, dysphoria, body and muscle aches, or cravings.[112,113]

The time frame of withdrawal symptoms when using alpha adrenergic agonists is comparable to unmedicated heroin withdrawal, peaking in severity within the first 2 to 4 days of heroin cessation, with most objective features resolved within 5 to 7 days, although subjective symptoms generally persist for longer. This facilitates shorter treatment programs and enhances the capacity for induction onto naltrexone as a post-withdrawal treatment option.

Clonidine dosing regimens generally involve titration of the dose according to the client's experience of withdrawal symptoms and side-effects. The main adverse events reported are features of hypotension experienced as dizziness, fainting, light-headedness, fatigue or lethargy, and dry mouth. It is the former cluster of side-effects that frequently restricts upper dosing levels, and indeed has often limited the use of clonidine in outpatient settings where clients can be less readily monitored. Whilst most authors suggest doses of clonidine should be individually titrated, maximum dosing levels of 1 to 1.2 mg (or 15 µg/kg/day) orally per day (in three or four divided doses) have been frequently used in research[114,115] and recommended in clinical guidelines.[23,111]

Lofexidine has the advantage in producing less hypotensive side-effects than clonidine, thereby improving its safety and applicability in the outpatient context. Three RCTs comparing lofexidine to clonidine in inpatient settings have shown similar efficacy regarding withdrawal severity and completion rates.[116–118]

Efficacy of alpha adrenergic agonists

The research evidence from RCTs comparing the efficacy of clonidine or lofexidine and methadone in managing heroin withdrawal is limited. Separate Cochrane reviews have identified the controlled trials comparing methadone and alpha adrenergic agonists.[31,43] Comparisons of clonidine and methadone for the management of heroin detoxification include controlled trials.[54,119–123] Randomized trials[50,124] and one non-randomized controlled trial[125] have compared lofexidine and methadone.

Several other randomized trials[126,127] examined subjects withdrawing from either heroin or methadone maintenance programs, without differentiating the findings according to the primary drug of dependence; consequently, these studies are difficult to interpret in considering the management of heroin withdrawal, and will not be considered in detail in this report.

The first published controlled trial comparing clonidine with methadone for the management of heroin withdrawal was by Cami and colleagues, with 30 heroin users enrolled in a 12-day inpatient program.[119] The study demonstrated comparable completion rates between clonidine and an 8- to 10-day reduction regimen of methadone. The clonidine group experienced greater peak symptoms early in the withdrawal regimen, with resolution of withdrawal symptoms by discharge. In contrast, the methadone subjects reported less peak withdrawal severity, but were still complaining of withdrawal symptoms on discharge.

Similar findings have been reported in most other randomized trials comparing methadone and adrenergic agonist medications. No significant differences were reported regarding completion rates in two trials with small subject numbers ($n=22$,[120] and $n=16$[123]) nor in a larger randomized trial of 200 subjects,[122] albeit a proportion of these subjects were undergoing treatment involuntarily and therefore completion rates are difficult to interpret. These studies consistently demonstrated that methadone subjects reported delayed peak withdrawal severity compared to those subjects randomized to clonidine.

The randomized trial of San and colleagues is the only one to report a difference in retention rates between the two medications.[121] The 12-day inpatient trial compared 3 groups: methadone, clonidine, and guanfacine (another adrenergic agonist), and continued to recruit subjects until 30 successful withdrawals had occurred for each condition, with methadone having the highest completion rate: 75% of subjects commencing methadone successfully completed the regimen, compared to 48% of subjects commencing guanfacine and 44% of subjects commencing clonidine. Again, the methadone group complained of less severe withdrawal early in the withdrawal (days 2 to 5), however, had more symptoms towards the end of the admission.

Trials comparing lofexidine and methadone reductions have demonstrated similar general findings. Bearn and colleagues examined 10-day inpatient regimens of lofexidine versus methadone reductions in 86 heroin and/or methadone users over a 21-day inpatient detoxification.[50] There were comparable completion rates for the two groups (69% lofexidine group, 77% methadone group), with greater withdrawal severity early in the lofexidine group and more prolonged withdrawal in the methadone group. Howells and colleagues demonstrated comparable withdrawal outcomes in an RCT comparing methadone and lofexidine conducted in a prison context, which limits the capacity to interpret completion rates.[124] One controlled trial in which patients self-allocated to a 5-day high-dose lofexidine, 10-day 'standard' lofexidine or 10-day methadone regimen demonstrated a quicker resolution of symptoms in the rapid, high-dose lofexidine group.[50]

Unfortunately, there have been no randomized trials comparing methadone reductions to alpha adrenergic agonists for the management of heroin withdrawal in outpatient settings. Studies examining outpatient withdrawal from methadone maintenance treatment suggest that completion rates with clonidine may be comparable[115,128] or inferior[127] to methadone reductions.

Clonidine has been shown to result in better outcomes than placebo for the management of inpatient heroin withdrawal,[129,130] with less withdrawal severity than tranquilizers (chlordiazepoxide and chlorpromazine),[131] and with comparable outcomes to a combination of mianserin and carbamazepine for management of withdrawal.[132]

Despite the methodologic problems of comparing outcomes between studies, there is sufficient evidence to suggest that clonidine and lofexidine are effective pharmacotherapies for heroin withdrawal. Although not successful in reducing all the features of withdrawal, such as cravings, alpha adrenergic agonists nevertheless have an advantage over methadone in not prolonging the duration of the withdrawal syndrome. The use of clonidine outside of inpatient settings is somewhat restricted by its side-effect profile, particularly by inexperienced service providers. Whilst side-effects are less of a concern with lofexidine, it has limited availability outside of Europe.

Accelerated detoxification using opioid antagonists

The opioid antagonists naloxone and naltrexone have been used to accelerate the onset and reduce the duration of acute heroin withdrawal. It is postulated that shortening the withdrawal process reduces the risk (or opportunity) of relapse to heroin use, and enables earlier initiation onto post-withdrawal treatment involving naltrexone for relapse prevention.

The compression of acute withdrawal symptoms is associated with a considerable increase in the severity of withdrawal, such that other medications are required to make the process tolerable for clients. Whilst the techniques used have varied considerably,[133–135] two broad approaches have been described:

- Rapid detoxification (ROD) procedures in which the patient is only mildly sedated – antagonists are combined with symptomatic medications such as clonidine, benzodiazepines, and anti-emetics. Rapid detoxification programs have been provided in a variety of treatment settings, ranging from intensive hospital settings to supervised outpatient day programs.
- Ultra rapid detoxification (URD) procedures in which the client is inducted onto antagonists whilst under general anesthesia or heavy sedation in a highly supervised hospital setting.

Following the acute withdrawal process, a comprehensive post-withdrawal program involving continuation in naltrexone treatment and structured counseling for several months is generally recommended by service providers.

Rapid detoxification

Several RCTs have been published comparing rapid detoxification to conventional approaches for heroin withdrawal. Gerra and colleagues[130] compared four randomly assigned outpatient conditions in 152 heroin users: (a) clonidine only, (b) naltrexone plus clonidine, (c) naloxone plus clonidine, and (d) placebo. Outcomes reported included withdrawal severity, proportion of subjects taking naltrexone on day 8 (withdrawal completion rates), and post-withdrawal outcomes at 6-month follow-up. The study reported very high levels of retention in withdrawal treatment for all groups (74% for placebo and over 90% for the other three groups). Unfortunately the study report had a number of methodologic flaws, including lack of clarity regarding the method of randomization, the proportion of subjects reporting continued heroin use (the proportions of all urine samples testing positive were reported), and the handling of missing data such as treatment drop-outs. The mean proportions (± standard deviations) of morphine-positive urine results during the first 5 days were 30 ± 21% for the clonidine group, 5 ± 6% for the naltrexone–clonidine group, 11 ± 7% for the naloxone–clonidine group, and 48 ± 8% for the placebo group. At 6-month follow-up, the mean proportion of positive morphine urine results was 60 ± 7% in the clonidine group, 74 ± 12% in the placebo group, 20 ± 5% for the naloxone–clonidine group, and 18 ± 4% for the naltrexone–clonidine group.

Despite problems in the way this study was reported, the findings suggest that there are no immediate benefits in using opioid antagonists during withdrawal compared to using clonidine on its own, given the very similar proportions of individuals in the clonidine and antagonist–clonidine groups who were inducted onto naltrexone by the end of the first week. The study findings did indicate a significant difference with regard to post-withdrawal outcomes, suggesting that the early use of antagonists during withdrawal may enhance retention in longer-term naltrexone treatment. However, the study reported remarkably high rates of withdrawal completion and post-withdrawal abstinence rates for all groups – including 74% completion rates for outpatient heroin withdrawal using placebo! As identified earlier, the findings of this study may be difficult to generalize to broader populations of heroin users undergoing withdrawal treatment – subjects in this study were concurrently recruited into a 6-month naltrexone study, suggesting that they were highly motivated to achieve and maintain abstinence, with good psychosocial supports during and after the withdrawal episode.

Another randomized trial of rapid detoxification was conducted in an outpatient primary care setting in the USA.[74] This study examined short-term withdrawal outcomes in 162 heroin-dependent users randomly allocated to three groups: (a) clonidine only during the first 7 days, receiving naltrexone on day 8; (b) naltrexone commencing on day 2 at 12.5 mg, increasing to 50 mg daily by day 3, together with clonidine; and (c) buprenorphine from days 1 to 3 with clonidine and naltrexone commenced on day 4 at 25 mg, increasing to 50 mg by day 5. Findings regarding the use of buprenorphine were considered earlier in this chapter; the data regarding clonidine compared to clonidine–naltrexone indicated that the two regimens were comparable with regard to rates of induction onto naltrexone (both in terms of proportion taking a full 50 mg dose and the proportion in treatment at day 8), and had similar severity of reported heroin withdrawal. Unfortunately, the report did not indicate the proportions of subjects using heroin during the withdrawal episode, the need for 'rescue' medications during withdrawal, the incidence of adverse events, nor the proportion of subjects in the clonidine group who remained in naltrexone treatment beyond one dose. Nevertheless, the study demonstrated that antagonist-assisted withdrawal is possible in an outpatient setting, with comparable short-term outcomes to a conventional clonidine regimen.

Arnold-Rees and Hulse[136] reported an RCT comparing clonidine to rapid opioid detoxification (using clonidine–naloxone under sedation) in 80 heroin users. The ROD had greater completion of withdrawal and uptake of oral naltrexone, however, at 4-week follow-up, oral naltrexone compliance and abstinence were similar between the two groups.

Buntwal and colleagues compared a naltrexone–lofexidine combination to lofexidine alone over a 7-day regimen in an inpatient setting with 22 mixed heroin/methadone-dependent users.[137] The naltrexone–lofexidine combination was associated with a more rapid resolution of the opiate withdrawal syndrome than the lofexidine-only group, however there were no significant differences in the proportion of patients completing detoxification. In a similar study by the same research group,[138] a naloxone–lofexidine combination was compared to placebo–lofexidine in an inpatient double-blinded RCT with 89 heroin- and/or methadone-dependent users. As with the previous study, there were no significant differences with regards to completion rates or length of stay, although the naloxone–lofexidine group had lower withdrawal severity towards the end of the detoxification period.

There has been considerable variation in the reported outcomes of cohort studies employing rapid detoxification. 'Successful' withdrawal outcomes have usually been defined as the proportion of subjects receiving a full dose of naltrexone (e.g. 50 mg) after several days (usually day 3 to day 8). Completion rates have been reported as high as 100% to as low as 7% remaining in inpatient treatment at 2 weeks,[139] with a mean completion rate of 83%.[134]

Unfortunately, few studies have included any significant follow-up information. The findings of the study by Gerra and colleagues[130] were previously discussed. Bell and colleagues conducted rapid detoxification in an inpatient setting on 15 heroin-dependent users and 15 methadone clients, with outcomes reported at day 7 and at 3 months.[140] The methadone group performed better at 3 months than the heroin group, a finding consistent with previous research with clonidine- and methadone-assisted withdrawal programs. The majority (n=13; 87%) of the heroin users were taking naltrexone at day 7, and 10 (67%) were taking naltrexone after 4 weeks. At 3-month follow up, 4 (27%) were taking naltrexone (of whom one was not using heroin), 5 (37%) were in methadone treatment, 4 (27%) had relapsed into dependent heroin use, one person was abstinent but not in treatment, and one person was dead. Seoane and colleagues reported that 93% of 300 heroin users self reported to be opiate-free and provided an opiate-negative urine test 1 month after a rapid withdrawal procedure.[141]

The pattern of withdrawal symptoms using rapid detoxification is related to the procedure utilized. The typical profile reported is that of severe withdrawal following the initial dose of antagonist medication, with symptoms abating thereafter, although many studies have described continued subjective withdrawal symptoms persisting for several days after the first dose of opioid antagonist.[142,143] To this extent, the claims that rapid detoxification procedures markedly reduce the duration of withdrawal symptoms may be exaggerated. Rather, antagonist-assisted withdrawal regimens appear to be a useful means of inducting heroin users into antagonist treatment early in the treatment process, thereby reducing drop-out rates and diminishing the capacity for continued heroin use in those clients for whom long-term treatment with naltrexone is indicated.

The increased severity of withdrawal associated with certain rapid detoxification procedures is potentially associated with severe adverse events, including dehydration and renal failure,[144] and delirium in 20% of ROD cases.[145]

Ultra rapid detoxification

This procedure entails the introduction of opioid antagonists under heavy sedation and/or general anesthesia. The evidence base regarding this approach is emerging, with several published RCTs, case series (albeit with markedly different outcomes), and systematic reviews.[134,146]

McGregor and colleagues compared outcomes for heroin-dependent users randomized to receive either a 1-day precipitated withdrawal procedure using naloxone under anesthetic (n=51), or a standard 7-day inpatient detoxification using symptomatic medications including clonidine ($n=50$).[147] All subjects were offered naltrexone plus supportive counseling for 9 months after detoxification. Significantly more of the precipitated withdrawal group completed withdrawal, commenced naltrexone, and stayed in treatment for the first 3 months, however there were no significant differences between the groups at 6- or 12-month follow-up, by which time subjects in treatment were engaged in methadone maintenance treatment, highlighting the limited long-term retention associated with naltrexone treatment.

An RCT in 270 patients[148] compared antagonist-induced withdrawal with or without general anesthesia, in which identical treatment regimens were employed apart from the level of sedation. There were no differences in abstinence rates at 1 month (approximately 60% in both groups), however more severe adverse events and a 1.5-fold increase in cost were associated with the treatment regimen incorporating general anesthesia.

Similar findings were reported in an Australian comparison[149] of heroin users undergoing anesthesia and sedated detoxification regimens. Similar proportions (72% and 60%, respectively) were on naltrexone and opiate-free 10 days later, suggesting no additional benefit from anesthesia.

Collins and colleagues[80] compared withdrawal and post-withdrawal outcomes in 106 dependent heroin users randomized to either buprenorphine-, clonidine- or anesthesia-assisted withdrawal conducted in an inpatient setting, followed by 12 weeks of naltrexone treatment. Detoxification completion and mean withdrawal severities were comparable across the three treatments, however the buprenorphine- and anesthesia-assisted detox approaches had significantly higher rates of naltrexone induction (94% anesthesia, 97% buprenorphine) than the clonidine group (21%). Treatment retention over 12 weeks was not significantly different among groups (20% retained in the anesthesia-assisted group, 24% in the buprenorphine-assisted group, and 9% in the clonidine-assisted group). Of concern, however, was the finding that the anesthesia procedure was associated with three potentially life-threatening adverse events (including pulmonary edema and psychiatric hospitalization). The study highlights the concerns regarding URD given the safety concerns and costs involved, and the comparable treatment outcomes for buprenorphine-assisted withdrawal.

A retrospective (non-randomized) controlled study[150] compared outcomes for all patients who underwent UROD over a 6-month period ($n=139$) compared to all patients who underwent the conventional 30-day inpatient detoxification (n=87) during the same period. There were no significant differences in demographic or substance use issues between the patients presenting to the two services, with the exception of significantly fewer recent arrests in the UROD group. All of the patients undergoing UROD completed detoxification, compared to 81% of the conventional group. Attempts were made to follow-up subjects by telephone approximately 18 months later, with 60% of UROD and 92% of conventional treatment patients being contacted. A greater proportion of patients in the conventional treatment group were abstinent at follow-up (42%) than in the UROD group (22%). Similar proportions of patients in each treatment group had requested further treatment. Duration of education received was the only significant patient characteristic that served as a predictor of abstinence for either group.

Rabinowitz and colleagues compared long-term outcomes in 30 patients who underwent URD and were then prescribed naltrexone for relapse prevention, compared to 33 patients detoxified who used a 1-month inpatient clonidine regimen and were then provided with counseling after care.[151] At approximately 13-month follow-up there were similar self-reported rates of relapse to regular heroin use for the one-third of subjects available for follow-up.

The emerging evidence regarding 'ultra rapid' or antagonist-accelerated withdrawal under anesthesia/heavy sedation suggests that it does not provide additional benefits with regards to naltrexone induction rates or longer-term outcomes compared to rapid detoxification under minimal sedation, or indeed buprenorphine-assisted withdrawal. Furthermore, URD is associated with greater cost and intensity of service provision, and increased risk of serious adverse events with reports of anesthesia-related deaths[152] and complications requiring prolonged hospitalization.[80,141,148,153,154] Given the availability of less dramatic alternatives, it is unlikely that URD procedures will have a significant role for heroin detoxification.

The role of antagonist-accelerated withdrawal for heroin users is yet to be established in the research literature. This approach does have the advantage of inducting heroin users into a form of post-withdrawal treatment – naltrexone maintenance treatment for relapse prevention – although concerns regarding safety and associated costs of URD suggest there is a limited role for this particular approach. Unfortunately, naltrexone treatment is not particularly attractive to many heroin users who may be contemplating withdrawal, nor is it particularly effective in retaining heroin users in treatment compared to substitution maintenance treatment, and no better than placebo in double-blinded randomized trials (see the Cochrane review of antagonists for opioid relapse prevention[155]). The development of sustained-release naltrexone products (e.g. depot injections, implants) may alter the future role of naltrexone, however they are not currently indicated for treating opiate dependence. As such, antagonist-accelerated approaches to withdrawal treatment are likely to only be indicated for individuals who are suited to longer-term naltrexone treatment, such as opiate users highly motivated for abstinence and with good social support systems.

Summary of management of heroin withdrawal

In summary, each of the main pharmacologic approaches for heroin withdrawal reviewed thus far is well suited to particular treatment populations and clinical settings; however, they each have their limitations when the broader objectives and outcomes of withdrawal services are considered.

Methadone-assisted withdrawal has been shown to be a safe, effective, and acceptable approach. The initial period of stability afforded by methadone prior to the onset of significant withdrawal symptoms enables heroin users to distance themselves from daily heroin use. Methadone-assisted withdrawal has an advantage in that clients are engaged in a treatment modality that can be easily continued into a longer-term methadone maintenance program, thereby facilitating linkage with post-withdrawal treatment. Unfortunately, methadone delays and prolongs the withdrawal syndrome, which limits its use in brief inpatient settings, and complicates induction onto naltrexone as a post-withdrawal approach for those clients considering longer-term abstinence from all opiates. Methadone also carries considerable negative stigma among certain groups of heroin users, health professionals, and the broader community, and is associated with considerable regulatory control that limits the capacity for its widespread use in certain countries. For example, fewer than 5% of general practitioners are authorized to prescribe methadone in Australia, whereas methadone is restricted to specialist clinics in the USA.

Most research literature regarding symptomatic medication approaches has focused upon the use of the alpha adrenergic antagonist clonidine, and more recently lofexidine. These medications have the advantage over methadone in not prolonging the withdrawal syndrome, thereby making them well suited to brief inpatient withdrawal programs. Their use does not delay induction onto naltrexone as a post-withdrawal medication, although the use of symptomatic medications for withdrawal is perhaps less likely to facilitate post-withdrawal referrals into substitution maintenance treatment to the same extent as methadone-assisted withdrawal treatment. The high incidence of side-effects, particularly hypotension and lethargy, and their inability to relieve cravings and mood disturbances reduces their safety and effectiveness in outpatient settings. Lofexidine has a lower incidence of hypotension-related side-effects; however, it is not registered in most countries, is considerably more expensive than clonidine, and has not been shown to significantly improve treatment outcomes compared to clonidine.

There is increasing evidence regarding the safety and efficacy of buprenorphine for heroin detoxification. Buprenorphine appears to result in greater detoxification completion rates, less withdrawal severity, and less heroin use than symptomatic medications. Further research is required to compare methadone and buprenorphine reduction regimens, although current evidence suggests that buprenorphine results in less withdrawal discomfort, particularly at the completion of a medication reduction regimen, compared to methadone. Perhaps the real advantage of buprenorphine as a detoxification medication is its greater flexibility regarding post-withdrawal treatment options – buprenorphine can be continued into a maintenance program, or patients can commence rehabilitation programs or naltrexone treatment without significant delays after stopping buprenorphine. This flexibility may be particularly important given the difficulties in developing long-term treatment plans for patients when they first present to treatment, often in crisis – stabilization on buprenorphine for several days allows the opportunity for treatment planning, without restricting ongoing treatment options.

The research evidence regarding the safety and efficacy of opioid antagonist-assisted withdrawal approaches has not been clearly established, although these approaches have gained in popularity in certain areas, and there are clinicians with considerable experience in delivering these detoxification techniques. Ultimately, antagonist-assisted withdrawal is likely to only be of benefit to those heroin users contemplating long-term naltrexone treatment for relapse prevention, and estimates would suggest that this represents a minority of heroin users presenting to conventional treatment services.

Managing withdrawal in practice

Tailoring detoxification approaches for individuals

The application of evidence-based medicine is not about identifying from systematic reviews or meta-analyses which is the 'best' medication approach for treating all patients with a particular condition, nor is it about the development of 'cook book' recipes of medication regimens.[156] Rather, the application of evidence-based practice in clinical decision-making regarding the management of heroin detoxification for individuals must take into consideration a number of factors routinely confronted in clinical scenarios by service users and service providers. These include:

- The evidence regarding the safety and efficacy of different detoxification methods.
- The patient's physical, psychological and social conditions and needs.
- The resources available for detoxification, including treatment settings, the level of staff expertise, the extent of supervision, monitoring and support available during detoxification, and the time frame in which withdrawal is to be conducted.
- The preferences and consent of *informed* patients.
- The post-withdrawal treatment options being considered for each patient.

Table 3.2 examines the relative advantages of the four different medication approaches for heroin detoxification against each of the four objectives of detoxification, and also against factors such as 'setting' and 'cost'. A number of clinical scenarios can serve to highlight the importance of each of these:

- A heroin user who must continue to function in his/her daily routine may have difficulties attempting antagonist-accelerated or symptomatic withdrawal due to the severity of withdrawal or the sedating effects of the medications. (S)he should perhaps consider a gradual reduction

Table 3.2 A comparison of medication approaches against objectives of detoxification services

Treatment objectives	*Methadone-assisted withdrawal*	*Adrenergic agonists (clonidine, lofexidine)*	*Buprenorphine-assisted withdrawal*	*Antagonist-accelerated withdrawal*
To alleviate the severity of withdrawal discomfort.	Delays onset of peak withdrawal symptoms until ~ time of last dose. Symptoms persist for ~ 7 to 14 days following last methadone dose (depending upon the duration of methadone treatment).	Relief of symptoms without delaying or prolonging withdrawal syndrome. Particularly effective in reducing 'autonomic' features, but less impact upon cravings, muscle cramps, sleep, or mood problems. Ancillary medications (e.g. benzodiazepines) often required for refractory withdrawal symptoms.	Good relief of withdrawal symptoms. Using short courses (<2 weeks), symptoms peak in severity usually prior to second dose, with mild rebound withdrawal. More prolonged courses (weeks) have more severe and prolonged rebound withdrawal, often lasting for several days.	Peak symptoms increase in severity and occur after initial antagonist dose. Peak withdrawal features of short duration (<48 h), and require sedation (typically benzodiazepines) and other medications (typically adrenergic agonists). Residual low level symptoms often persist for several days.

To prevent the development of severe withdrawal sequelae and complications, including adverse events, overdoses or abuse of medication.	Greater control over timing of peak withdrawal symptoms allows time to stabilize concomitant medical or psychiatric conditions. Risk of overdose in combination with other sedative drugs, or if initial methadone doses are too high (e.g. poor assessment and monitoring). Methadone toxicity is potentially fatal.	Side-effects (e.g. hypotension and sedation) are poorly tolerated in some individuals, and can limit use of effective doses. Risk of overdose if too high doses taken, and/or in combination with other sedatives. Clonidine abuse has been reported and overdose can be fatal. Risk for abuse and/or diversion of ancillary medications.	Greater control over timing of peak withdrawal symptoms allows time to stabilize concomitant medical or psychiatric conditions. Risk of overdose in combination with other sedative drugs. Extent of abuse of buprenorphine is related to system of dispensing. Supervised dispensing limits abuse (e.g. injection) and diversion, however increases costs and inconvenience of service delivery.	The marked increase in withdrawal severity may complicate concomitant medical or psychiatric conditions. High incidence of (anticipated) side-effects requiring management (e.g. severe agitation, intractable vomiting, diarrhea, dehydration, delirium). Uncommon, but severe risks associated with heavy sedation or anesthesia (e.g. death, respiratory infections).

(*Continued*)

Table 3.2 (*Continued*)

Treatment objectives	*Methadone-assisted withdrawal*	*Adrenergic agonists (clonidine, lofexidine)*	*Buprenorphine-assisted withdrawal*	*Antagonist-accelerated withdrawal*
	Extent of abuse of methadone is related to system of dispensing. Supervised dispensing limits abuse (e.g. injection) and diversion of methadone, however increases costs and inconvenience of service delivery.	Short duration of action requires multiple doses per day, and take-home medication in outpatient settings, increasing the risk of abuse/non-compliance and/or diversion.		Risk of heroin overdose following the cessation of naltrexone (probably due to reduced tolerance to opioids), and from ancillary sedatives (e.g. benzodiazepines, clonidine).
To interrupt a pattern of regular and heavy heroin use.	Methadone substitutes for heroin. It reduces heroin use by relieving withdrawal symptoms and cravings. Dosages used in detoxification do not generally block the effects of additional heroin use. Moderate and prolonged rebound withdrawal often	Adrenergic agonists can indirectly reduce heroin use by alleviating withdrawal symptoms, but with minimal impact upon cravings and no 'blockade' of the effects of additional heroin use. Adrenergic agonists do not prolong withdrawal, thereby reducing the period of time	Buprenorphine substitutes for heroin. It reduces heroin use by relieving withdrawal symptoms and cravings and blockading the effects of additional heroin use. Mild rebound withdrawal and short prolongation of withdrawal (when used in short courses) reduces	Naltrexone is very effective in reducing heroin use by blocking the effects of additional heroin use and reducing cravings. Few patients on naltrexone continue to use heroin regularly. Early establishment of receptor blockade reduces

	associated with high rates of relapse upon the discontinuation of methadone.	required for the reversal of tolerance.	opportunity for relapse to heroin use.	the opportunity for relapse to heroin use.
To facilitate linkages to post-withdrawal services	Ideally suited to facilitating links to longer-term methadone maintenance treatment. Patients who do not cease their heroin use during the withdrawal should generally not discontinue methadone. The use of methadone complicates the commencement of opiate-free post-withdrawal treatment. Naltrexone should usually be delayed for at least 7 to 10 days. Similarly, drug-free residential rehabilitation programs generally do not admit patients until the	Well suited to subjects considering drug-free post-withdrawal treatment modalities, such as residential rehab or naltrexone treatment. The sedating properties of clonidine and other common ancillary symptomatic medications (e.g. benzodiazepines), and the reduction of opioid tolerance associated with symptomatic detoxification require that additional caution be exercised in commencing substitution maintenance treatment, in	Ideally suited to a range of post-withdrawal treatment options. Buprenorphine can be continued as a maintenance program for those individuals unable or unwilling to consider complete abstinence from all opioids. Naltrexone can be commenced without significant delays, either during a short course of buprenorphine, or soon after its discontinuation. The limited prolongation of withdrawal should not delay	Ideally suited to those heroin users who wish to continue in long-term naltrexone treatment. A limitation of this approach is that a considerable proportion of patients will discontinue naltrexone within days or weeks, and relapse to heroin use. Induction into substitution maintenance treatment is potentially complicated following naltrexone treatment due to the reversal of opioid tolerance, and the sedating properties of common ancillary

(*Continued*)

Table 3.2 (*Continued*)

Treatment objectives	*Methadone-assisted withdrawal*	*Adrenergic agonists (clonidine, lofexidine)*	*Buprenorphine-assisted withdrawal*	*Antagonist-accelerated withdrawal*
	resolution of withdrawal symptoms (e.g. 5 to 10 days after last dose). Many patients will relapse to heroin use in the intervening period.	order to prevent sedation and overdose.	entry into drug-free residential rehabilitation programs or other counseling programs.	medications (clonidine, benzodiazepines). Additional caution must be exercised in commencing maintenance substitution treatment.
Setting	Can easily be accommodated in an outpatient setting. Restricted use in inpatient settings due to the prolongation of withdrawal, and the increasingly shorter admission times available in inpatient detoxification units.	Ideally suited to short-term residential detoxification programs, where greater monitoring of side-effects and dose titration is possible. Risks of side-effects, abuse, and/or diversion of medication require some degree of supervision in outpatient settings, and staff with some expertise in their use.	Suited to either short or longer gradual reduction regimens in outpatient settings. Supervised dispensing limits abuse or diversion potential. Short courses of buprenorphine (<1 week) are well suited to residential detoxification programs.	Ideally suited to residential settings due to the severity of withdrawal symptoms, levels of monitoring required, and the need for large amounts of ancillary medications. Rapid opiate withdrawal with minimal sedation can be performed in outpatient settings, although this requires considerable staffing resources and supervision by family or friends in a stable environment. Extended day care desirable.

Cost and accessibility	Methadone is an opioid drug, often with restrictions regarding which service providers can prescribe and dispense the medication. This limits the availability and access to treatment.	Few restrictions in the use of these medications, and they are widely available. Widespread prescribing of ancillary symptomatic medications for detoxification (in particular benzodiapezines) may contribute to abuse, diversion, and the expensive phenomenon of 'doctor shopping'.	Buprenorphine is an opioid medication, often with restrictions regarding which service providers can prescribe and dispense the medication. This limits the availability and access to treatment.	Ultra rapid procedures require intensive hospital settings and anesthesia, thereby increasing cost, and restricting accessibility. Supportive home environments and suitable support people are not available for many heroin users, limiting the accessibility of this treatment. Service providers need considerable resources and expertise, and generally should only be attempted by specialists, thereby limiting its accessibility.

regimen using methadone or buprenorphine, thereby postponing the more severe withdrawal features until support strategies such as leave from work or respite child-care can be organized.

- The heroin user who is not interested in long-term naltrexone treatment should not be subjected to the expense and risks associated with opioid antagonist-accelerated withdrawal. Alternatively, a patient who is keen to commence long-term naltrexone treatment should avoid methadone-assisted withdrawal, as this will delay naltrexone induction.
- A heroin user who is ambivalent regarding detoxification or maintenance substitution treatment should consider detoxification using either methadone or buprenorphine, which can be continued if long-term abstinence is not an immediate option.

Integrating withdrawal services within the service system

There are many reports on managing heroin withdrawal, and having reviewed the salient evidence, it is helpful to draw back and place withdrawal management in perspective.

People generally present for detoxification at times of crisis, when their drug use has escalated and is experienced as being out of control. Undoubtedly, some people at that time are seeking to become abstinent from heroin, and embrace a new lifestyle. Others probably say they want abstinence because that is how they will be offered medication to manage withdrawal symptoms. Others will present for methadone-assisted detoxification because there is no maintenance available, or because there has been a sudden interruption of their heroin supply. At best, most people present with ambivalence, and their motivation to lifestyle change is often poorly sustained.

In Australia, and in some other countries, detoxification services, especially residential ones, have often operated separately and/or independently from other treatment services, particularly those delivering methadone maintenance treatment. Thus, there was not only a cultural divide between services oriented to abstinence, and those oriented to maintenance, but also a physical divide in every sense of the word, with services operated from different premises and often by different organizations. This lack of integration of services unwittingly mirrored the internal conflict and ambivalence of service users.

In recent years, two developments have challenged this traditional divide between services. The first has been the advent of buprenorphine for use in detoxification. Because a single daily dose of buprenorphine is safe and offers good symptomatic control of withdrawal, people can be managed successfully as outpatients, diminishing the need for more costly residential care. More importantly, buprenorphine has been used in a way that blurs the traditional distinction between detoxification and maintenance. Consumers have been inducted onto buprenorphine, and encouraged to remain in treatment for as long as they perceived that the benefits of receiving treatment outweighed the disadvantages of attending daily for supervised administration. The majority of subjects presenting for elective detoxification from heroin and treated in this way with buprenorphine have elected to remain in treatment beyond one month.[49,64]

The second development has been a greater awareness of the need for specialist multimodal services offering comprehensive treatment – assessment, detoxification, maintenance, counseling, welfare assistance, medical and psychiatric care, and access to long-term residential services. Such integrated services provide a setting in which treatment planning becomes a key part of assessment, avoiding the problem expressed in the phrase 'When the only tool you have is a hammer, all problems start to look like nails'.

Conclusion

Withdrawal arises from the cessation or reduction in opioid use in dependent individuals. Withdrawal services aim to interrupt a pattern of heavy use, relieve the discomfort of withdrawal, minimize complications during withdrawal, and facilitate linkages to ongoing services. As with most chronic conditions, a short-term intervention such as a detoxification, on its own, is rarely associated with long-term behavior change. Nevertheless, detoxification may serve as a gateway into longer-term treatment; and even those who do not continue in treatment may yet benefit from a reduction in their level of use and related harms.

The key principles of delivering safe and effective detoxification services include an appropriate setting, regular monitoring, and supportive care. Medications can assist detoxification outcomes, and in particular reducing doses of opioids such as methadone or buprenorphine, or symptomatic medications (such as clonidine) have a sufficient evidence base to recommend their use. The selection of treatment approaches for individual patients includes a consideration of the physical, psychologic, and social needs of the individual, the goals, motivations, and preferences of the patient, available resources, and an understanding of the relative benefits and problems associated with each of the different medication approaches.

References

1. Himmelsbach CK. The morphine abstinence syndrome: its nature and treatment. Ann Intern Med 1941; 15: 829–39.
2. Martin W, Jasinski D. Physiological parameters of morphine dependence in man – tolerance, early abstinence, protracted abstinence. J Psychiat Res 1969; 7: 9–17.
3. Hartnoll RL. Opiates: prevalence and demographic factors. Addiction 1994; 89(11): 1377–83.
4. Dawe S, Griffiths P, Gossop M, Strang J. Should opiate addicts be involved in controlling their own detoxification? A comparison of fixed versus negotiable schedules. Brit J Addict 1991; 86(8): 977–82.
5. Teesson M, Ross J, Darke S, et al. Twelve month outcomes of the treatment of heroin dependence: findings from the Australian Treatment Outcome Study (ATOS) New South Wales. Sydney: University of New South Wales, National Drug and Alcohol Research Centre; 2003.
6. Judd LL, Marston MG, Attkisson C, et al. Effective medical treatment of opiate addiction. J Am Med Assn 1998; 280(22): 1936–43.
7. Gearing F, Schweitzer M. An epidemiologic evaluation of long-term methadone maintenance treatment for heroin addiction. Am J Epidemiol 1974; 100(2): 101–12.
8. Strang J, McCambridge J, Best D, et al. Loss of tolerance and overdose mortality after inpatient opiate detoxification: follow up study. BMJ 2003; 326: 959–60.
9. Andrews L, Himmelsbach C. Relation of the intensity of the morphine abstinence syndrome to dosage. J Exp Pharmacol Ther 1944; 81: 288–93.
10. Smolka M, Schmidt LG. The influence of heroin dose and route of administration on the severity of the opiate withdrawal syndrome. Addictions 1999; 94(8): 1191–8.
11. Phillips GT, Gossop M, Bradley B. The influence of psychological factors on the opiate withdrawal syndrome. Brit J Psychiat 1986; 149: 235–8.
12. Gossop M, Bradley B, Phillips G. An investigation of withdrawal symptoms shown by opiate addicts during and subsequent to a 21-day in-patient methadone detoxification procedure. Addict Behav 1987; 12(1): 1–6.

13. Gossop M, Battersby M, Strang J. Self-detoxification by opiate addicts. A preliminary investigation. Br J Psychiat 1991; 159: 208–12.
14. Kosten TR, Morgan C, Kleber HD. Phase II clinical trials of buprenorphine: detoxification and induction onto naltrexone. In: Blaine JD, ed. Buprenorphine: An Alternative Treatment for Opioid Dependence. NIDA Research Monograph Series. Rockville, M.D.: US Department of Health and Human Services; 1992; 101–19.
15. Kanof P, Aronson M, Ness R. Organic mood syndrome associated with detoxification from methadone maintenance. Am J Psychiat 1993; 150(3): 423–8.
16. Ziedonis DM, Amass L, Steinberg M, et al. Predictors of outcome for short-term medically supervised opioid withdrawal during a randomized, multicenter trial of buprenorphine-naloxone and clonidine in the NIDA clinical trials network Drug Alcohol Dependence. Drug Alcohol Depen 2008; in press.
17. Blaine JD, Ling W, Kosten TR, O'Brien CP, Chiarello RJ. Establishing the efficacy and safety of medications for the treament of drug dependence and abuse: methodological issues. In: Prien RF, Robinson DS, eds. Clinical Evaluation of Psychotropic Drugs: Principles and Guidelines. New York: Raven Press Ltd; 1994.
18. Gowing L, Ali R, White J. The Management of Opioid Withdrawal: An Overview of the Research Literature. Drug and Alcohol Services Council Reseach Series Monograph No 9. Adelaide, Australia; 2000.
19. Gossop M, Johns A, Green L. Opiate withdrawal: inpatient versus outpatient programmes and preferred versus random assignment to treatment. Brit Med J 1986; 293: 103–4.
20. Wilson B, Elms R, Thomson C. Outpatient vs hospital detoxification: an experimental comparison. Int J Addict 1975; 10(1): 13–21.
21. Day E, Ison J, Strang J. Inpatient versus other settings for detoxifcation for opioid dependence. Cochrane Database Syst Rev 2005; Issue 2 (Art. No. CD004580).
22. Frank L, Pead J. New concepts in drug withdrawal. A resource handbook. Melbourne: The University of Melbourne; 1995.
23. NSW Health Department. NSW Detoxification Clinical Practice Guidelines. Sydney: NSW Health Department; 1999.
24. Chang G, Kosten T. Detoxification. In: Lowinson J, Ruiz P, Millman R, Langrod J, eds. Substance Abuse: A Comprehensive Textbook. Third ed. Baltimore, Maryland: Williams and Wilkins; 1997; 377–81.
25. American Society of Addiction Medicine. Patient Placement Criteria for Treatment of Psychoative Substance Abuse Disorders. Washington DC: American Society of Addiction Medicine; 1991.
26. Handelsman L, Cochrane KJ, Aronson MJ, Ness RA, Rubinstein KJ, Kanof PD. Two new rating scales for opiate withdrawal. Am J Drug Alcohol Ab 1987; 13(3): 293–308.
27. Fishman S, Wilsey B, Yang J, Reisfield G, Bandman T, Borsook D. Adherence monitoring and drug surveillance in chronic opioid therapy. J Pain Symptom Manag 2000; 20(4): 293–307.

28. Waeber B, Burnier M, Brunner H. How to improve adherence with prescribed treatment in hypertensive patients? J Cardiovasc Pharm 2000; 35 (Suppl 3): S23–6.
29. Denolle T, Waeber B, Kjeldsen S, Parati G, Wilson M, Asmar R. Self-measurement of blood pressure in clinical trials and therapeutic applications. Blood Press Monit 2000; 5(2): 145–9.
30. Green L, Gossop M. Effects of information on the opiate withdrawal syndrome. Brit J Addict 1988; 83(3): 305–9.
31. Amato L, Minozzi S, Davoli M, Vecchi S, Ferri M, Mayet S. Psychosocial and pharmacological treatments versus pharmacological treatments for opioid detoxification. Cochrane Database Syst Rev 2004; 4(CD005031).
32. Hall S, Bass A, Hargreaves WA, Loeb P. Contingency management and information feedback on outpatient heroin detoxification. Behav Ther 1979; 10: 443–51.
33. McCaul M, Stitzer M, Bigelow G, Liebson I. Contingency management interventions: effects on treatment outcome during methadone detoxification. J Appl Behav Anal 1984; 17(1): 35–43.
34. Robles E, Stitzer M, Strain E, Bigelow G, Silverman K. Voucher-based reinforcement of opiate abstinence during methadone detoxification. Drug Alcohol Depen 2002; 65(2): 179–89.
35. Higgins ST, Stitzer ML, Bigelow GE, Liebson I. Contingent methadone dose increases as a method for reducing illicit opiate use in detoxification patients. NIDA Research Monograph 1984; 55: 178–83.
36. Higgins ST, Stitzer ML, Bigelow GE, Liebson I. Contingent methadone delivery: effects on illicit opiate use. Drug Alcohol Depen 1986; 17: 3111–22.
37. Bickel WK, Amass L, Higgins ST, Badger GJ, Esch RA. Effects of adding behavioral treatment to opioid detoxification with buprenorphine. J Consult Clin Psychol 1997; 65(5): 803–10.
38. Yandoli D, Eisler I, Robbins C, Mulleady G, Dare C. A comparative study of family therapy in the treatment of opiate users in a London clinic. The Association of Family Therapy and Systematic Practice 2002; 24(4): 402–22.
39. Rawson R, Mann A, Tennant F, Clabough D. Efficacy of psychotherapeutic counselling during 21-day ambulatory heroin detoxification. Drug Alcohol Depen 1983; 12(2): 197–200.
40. Alling F, Johnson B, Elmoghazy E. Cranial electrostimulation (CES) use in the detoxification of opiate-dependent patients. J Subst Abuse Treat 1990; 7(3): 173–80.
41. Brewington V, Smith M, Lipton D. Acupuncture as a detoxification treatment: an analysis of controlled research. J Subst Abuse Treat 1994; 11(4): 289–307.
42. Kleber H, Riordan C. The treatment of narcotic withdrawal: a historical review. J Clin Psychiatry 1982; 43 (6): 30–4.
43. Gowing L, Farrell M, Ali R, White J. Alpha2 adrenergic agonists for the management of opioid withdrawal. Cochrane Database Syst Rev 2004; Issue 4 (Art No. CD002024).

44. Gowing L, Ali R, White J. Buprenorphine for the management of opioid withdrawal. Cochrane Database Syst Rev 2004; 4: CD002025.
45. Amato L, Davoli M, Minozzi S, Ali R, Ferri MMF. Methadone at tapered doses for the management of opioid withdrawal. Cochrane Database Syst Rev 2008; Issue 1 (Art No. CD 003409).
46. Gowing L, Ali R, White J. Opioid antagonists under heavy sedation or anaesthesia for opioid withdrawal. Cochrane Database Syst Rev 2002; 2: CD002022.
47. Gowing L, Ali R, White J. Opioid antagonists with minimal sedation for opioid withdrawal. Cochrane Database Syst Rev 2002; 2: CD002021.
48. Gossop M, Griffiths P, Bradley BP, Strang J. Opiate withdrawal symptoms in response to 10 day and 21 day methadone withdrawal programmes. Brit J Psychiat 1989; 154: 360–3.
49. Strang J, Gossop M. Comparsion of linear versus inverse exponential methadone reduction curves in the detoxification of opiate addicts. Addict Behav 1990; 15(6): 541–7.
50. Bearn J, Gossop M, Strang J. Randomised double-blind comparison of lofexidine and methadone treatment for in-patient opiate detoxification. Drug Alcohol Depen 1996; 43: 87–91.
51. Kasvikis Y, Bradley B, Gossop M, Griffiths P, Marks I. Clonidine versus long and short term methadone aided withdrawal from opiates: an uncontrolled comparison. Int J Addict 1990; 25(10): 1169–78.
52. Maddux J, Desmond D, Esquivel M. Outpatient methadone withdrawal for heroin dependence. Am J Drug Alcohol Abuse 1980; 7(3–4): 323–33.
53. Bell J, Kimber J, Lintzeris N, et al. Clinical Guidelines and Procedures for the Use of Naltrexone in the Treatment of Opioid Dependence. Canberra: National Drug Strategy, Commonwealth Department of Health and Aged Care; 2003.
54. Umbricht A, Hoover D, Tucker M, Leslie J, Chaisson R, Preston K. Opioid detoxification with buprenorphine, clonidine, or methadone in hospitalized heroin-dependent patients with HIV infection. Drug Alcohol Depen 2003; 69(3): 263–72.
55. Holgate F, O'Reilly S, Carnegie J, Murray T, McLoughlin S. Guidelines for the delivery of alcohol and drug specific counselling interventions. Melbourne: Victorian Department of Human Services; 1996 July Contract No.: Document Number.
56. Stitzer M, McCaul M, Bigelow G, Liebson I. Treatment outcome in methadone detoxification: Relationship to initial levels of opiate use. Drug Alcohol Depen 1983; 12(3): 259–67.
57. Fulwiler R, Hargreaves W, Bortman R. Detoxification from heroin using self vs physician regulation of methadone dose. Int J Addict 1979; 14(2): 289–98.
58. Senay EC, Dorus W, Showalter C. Methadone detoxification: self versus physician regulation. Am J Drug Alcohol Ab 1984; 10(3): 361–74.
59. Ghodse H, Myles J, Smith SE. Clonidine is not a useful adjunct to methadone gradual detoxification in opioid addiction. Brit J Psychiat 1994; 165(3): 370–4.

60. McCaul M, Stitzer M, Bigelow G, Liebson I. Outpatient methadone detoxification: effects of diazepam and doxepin as adjunct medications. NIDA Research Monograph 1984; 55: 191–6.
61. Srisurapanont M, Jarusuraisin N. Amitriptylline vs. lorazepam in the treatment of opiate withdrawal insomnia: a randomised double-blind study. Acta Psychiat Scand 1998; 97(3): 233–5.
62. Inaba D, Gay G, Whitehed C, Newmeyer J, Bergin D. The use of propoxyphene napsylate in the treatment of heroin and methadone addiction. Western J Med 1974; 121(2): 106–11.
63. Tennant F, Russell B, Tate J, Bleich R. Comparative valuation of propoxyphene napsylate (Darvon-N) and placebo in heroin detoxification. Int J Addict 1977; 12(4): 565–74.
64. Tennant F, Russell B, Casas S, Bleich R. Heroin detoxification – a comparison of propoxyphene and methadone. JAMA 1975; 232(10): 1019–22.
65. Dore G. The dangers of dextropropoxyphene. Aust NZ J Psychiatry 1996; 30(6): 864–6.
66. Matusiewicz S, Wallace W, Crompton G. Hypersensitivity pneumonitis associated with co-proxamol (paracetamol + dextropropoxyphene) therapy. Postgrad Med J 1999; 75(886): 475–6.
67. Jonasson B, Jonasson U, Saldeen T. The manner of death among fatalities where dextropropoxyphene caused or contributed to death. Forensic Sci Int 1998; 96(2–3): 181–7.
68. Sorensen JL, Hargreaves WA, Weinberg JA. Withdrawal from heroin in three or six weeks: comparison of LAAM versus methadone. Arch Gen Psychiat 1982; 39: 167–71.
69. Wright NMJ, Sheard L, Tompkins CNE, Adams CE, Allgar VL, Oldham NS. Buprenorphine versus dihydrocodeine for opiate detoxification in primary care: a randomised controlled trial. BMC Fam Pract 2007; 8(3).
70. Jittiwutikarn J, Ali R, White J, Bochner F, Somogyi AA, Foster DJR. Comparison of tincture of opium and methadone to control opioid withdrawal in a Thai treatment centre. Brit J Pharmacol 2004; 58(5): 536–41.
71. Cheskin LJ, Fudala PJ, Johnson RE. A controlled comparison of buprenorphine and clonidine for acute detoxification from opioids. Drug Alcohol Depen 1994; 36(2): 115–21.
72. Nigam AK, Ray R, Tripathi BM. Buprenorphine in opiate withdrawal: a comparison with clonidine. J Subst Abuse Treat 1993; 10(4): 391–4.
73. Janiri L, Mannelli P, Persico A, Serretti A, Tempesta E. Opiate detoxification of methadone maintenance patients using lefetamine, clonidine and buprenorphine. Drug Alcohol Depen 1994; 36: 139–45.
74. O'Connor P, Carroll KM, Shi JM, Schottenfeld RS, Kosten TR, Rounsaville BJ. Three methods of opioid detoxification in a primary care setting. A randomized trial. Ann Intern Med 1997; 127(7): 526–30.
75. Lintzeris N, Bell J, Bammer G, Jolley D, Rushworth L. A randomised controlled trial of buprenorphine in the ambulatory management of heroin withdrawal. Addiction 2002; 97: 1395–404.
76. Ling W, Amass L, Shoptaw S, et al. A multi-center randomized trial of buprenorphine-naloxone versus clonidine for opioid detoxification: findings

from the National Institute on Drug Abuse Clinical Trials Network. Addiction 2005; 100(8): 1090–100.

77. O'Connor PG, Carroll KM, Shi JM, Schottenfeld RS, Kosten TR, Rounsaville BJ. Three methods of opioid detoxification in a primary care setting: a randomized trial. Ann Intern Med 1997; 127(7): 526–30.
78. Nigam AK, Ray R, Tripathi M. Buprenorphine in opiate withdrawal: a comparison with clonidine. J Subst Abuse Treat 1993; 10: 391–4.
79. Collins E, Whittington R, Heitler N, Kleber H, editors. Randomized comparison of buprenorphine-, clonidine- and anesthesia-assisted heroin detoxification and naltrexone induction. From Addiction to Abstinence: new pharmacological techniques for making and maintaining the change. 7th International Stapleford Conference on Addiction Management; 2002 November 13–15 2002; Nijmegen, the Netherlands.
80. Collins ED, Kleber HD, Whittington RA, Heitler NE. Anesthesia-assisted vs buprenorphine- or clonidine-assisted heroin detoxification and naltrexone induction: a randomized trial. JAMA 2005; 294(8): 903–13.
81. Fingerhood MI, Thompson MR, Jasinski DR. A comparison of clonidine and buprenorphine in the outpatient treatment of opiate withdrawal. Subst Ab 2001; 22(3): 193–9.
82. Raistrick D, West D, Finnegan O, Thistlethwaite G, Brearley R, Banbury J. A comparison of buprenorphine and lofexidine for community opiate detoxification: results from a randomize controlled trial. Addiction 2005; 100: 1860–7.
83. White R, Alcorn R, Feinmann C. Two methods of community detoxification from opiates: an open-label comparison of lofexidine and buprenorphine. Drug Alcohol Depen 2001; 65(1): 77–83.
84. Schneider U, Paetzold W, Eronat V, et al. Buprenorphine and carbamazepine as a treatment for detoxification of opiate addicts with multiple drug misuse: a pilot study. Addict Biol 2000; 5(1): 65–9.
85. Bickel WK, Stitzer ML, Bigelow GE, Liebson IA, Jasinski DR, Johnson RE. A clinical trial of buprenorphine: comparison with methadone in the detoxification of heroin addicts. Clin Pharmacol Ther 1988; 43(1): 72–8.
86. Petitjean S, Stohler R, Deglon JJ, et al. Double-blind randomized trial of buprenorphine and methadone in opiate dependence. Drug Alcohol Depen 2001; 62: 97–104.
87. Seifert J, Metzner C, Paetzold W, et al. Detoxification of opiate addicts with multiple drug abuse: a comparison of buprenorphine vs. methadone. Pharmacopsychiatry 2002; 35(5): 159–64.
88. Ebner R, Schreiber W, Zierer C. Buprenorphin oder Methadon im Entzug junger Opiatabhangiger. Psychiatrische Praxis 2004; 31(Suppl 1): S108–10.
89. Reed LJ, Glasper A, de Wet CJ, Bearn J, Gossop M. Comparison of buprenorphine and methadone in the treatment of opioid withdrawal: possible advantages of buprenorphine in the treatment of opiate-benzodiazepine codependent patients? J Clin Psychopharmacol 2007; 27: 188–92.
90. Tamaskar R, Parran TJ, Heggi A, Brateanu A, Rabb M, Yu J. Tramadol versus buprenorphine for the treatment of opiate withdrawal: a retrospective cohort control study. J Addict Dis 2003; 22(4): 5–12.

91. Amass L, Bickel WK, Higgins ST, Hughes JR. A preliminary investigation of outcome following gradual or rapid buprenorphine detoxification. In: Magura S, Rosenblum A, eds. Experimental Therapeutics in Addiction Medicine. The Haworth Press; 1994; 33–45.
92. Wang RIH, Young LD, eds. Double-blind controlled detoxification from buprenorphine. CPDD 1995; 1995. NIDA.
93. Pycha C, Resnick RB, Galanter M, eds. Buprenorphine: Rapid and slow dose-reductions for heroin detoxification. Problems of drug dependence, 1993: Proceedings of the 55th Annual Scientific Meeting, the College on Problems of Drug Dependence NIDA Research Monograph Series; 1993; Rockville, USA. srb-in1: National Institute on Drug Abuse.
94. Assadi S, Hafezi M, Mokri A, Razzaghi E, Ghaeli P. Opioid detoxification using high doses of buprenorphine in 24 hours: a randomized, double blind, controlled clinical trial. J Subst Abuse Treat 2004; 27(1): 75–82.
95. Hopper JA, Wu J, Martus W, Pierre JD. A randomized trial of one-day vs. three-day buprenorphine inpatient detoxification protocols for heroin dependence. J Opioid Manag 2005; 1(1): 31–5.
96. Lintzeris N, Bammer G, Rushworth L, Jolley D, Whelan G. Buprenorphine dosing regimen for inpatient heroin withdrawal: a symptom triggered dose titration study. Drug Alcohol Depen 2003; 70(3): 287–94.
97. Liu ZM, Cai ZJ, Wang XP, Ge Y, Li CM. Rapid detoxification of heroin dependence by buprenorphine. Acta Pharm Sinic 1997; 18(2): 112–14.
98. Oreskovich MR, Saxon AJ, Ellis ML, Malte CA, Reoux JP, Knox PC. A double-blind, double-dummy, randomized, prospective pilot study of the partial mu opiate agonist, buprenorphine, for acute detoxification from heroin. Drug Alcohol Depen 2005; 77(1): 71–9.
99. Lintzeris N, Clark N, Muhleisen P, et al. National Clinical Guidelines on the Use of Buprenorphine in the Management of Heroin Dependence. Canberra: National Drug Strategy, Commonwealth of Australia; 2001.
100. Ford C, Morton S, Lintzeris N, Bury J, Gerada C. Guidance for the use of buprenorphine for the treatment of opioid dependence in primary care. London: Royal College General Practitioners, UK; 2003.
101. Lanier RK, Umbricht A, Harrison JA, Nuwayser ES, Bigelow GE. Opioid detoxification via single 7-day application of a buprenorphine transdermal patch: an open-label evaluation. Psychopharmacology 2008; 198(2): 149–58.
102. Sobel BF, Sigmon SC, Walsh SL, et al. Open-label trial of an injection depot formulation of buprenorphine in opioid detoxification. Drug Alcohol Depen 2004; 73(1): 11–22.
103. Vignau J. Preliminary assessment of a 10-day rapid detoxification programme using high dosage buprenorphine. Eur Addict Res 1998; 4(Suppl 1): 29–31.
104. Gibson A, Doran C, Bell J, Ryan A, Lintzeris N. A comparison of buprenorphine treatment in clinic and primary care settings: a randomised trial. Med J Australia 2003; 179(1): 38–42.
105. Kosten TR, Morgan C, Kleber HD. Treatment of heroin addicts using buprenorphine. Am J Drug Alcohol Ab 1991; 17(2): 119–28.

106. Kosten TR, Kleber HD. Buprenorphine detoxification from opioid dependence: a pilot study. Life Sci 1988; 42(6): 635–41.
107. Mann D, Montoya ID, Contoreggi C, Ellison PA, Lange WR, Preston K, eds. Inpatient medically supervised opioid withdrawal with buprenorphine alone or in combination with naltrexone. CPDD 1994; 1994; Washington.
108. Umbricht A, Montoya ID, Hoover DR, Demuth KL, Chiang CT, Preston KL. Naltrexone shortened opioid detoxification with buprenorphine. Drug Alcohol Depen [clinical trial] 1999; 56(3): 181–90.
109. Lintzeris N, Bammer G, Bell J, Rushworth L, Main N, eds. Commencing naltrexone treatment following brief buprenorphine regimens for heroin withdrawal in inpatient and ambulatory settings. 63rd Annual Scientific Meeting of the College on Problems of Drug Dependence; 2001; Scottsdale, USA.
110. Maldonado R. Participation of noradrenergic pathways in the expression of opiate withdrawal: biochemical and pharmacological evidence. Neuroscience Biobehav Rev 1997; 21: 91–104.
111. Greenstein RA, Fudala PJ, O'Brien CP. Alternative pharmacotherapies for opiate addiction. In: Substance abuse: A comprehensive textbook. 1997; 415–25.
112. Jasinski D, Johnson R, Kocher T. Clonidine in morphine withdrawal. Differential effects on signs and symptoms. Arch Gen Psychiat 1985; 42: 1063–5.
113. Gossop M. Clonidine and the treatment of the opiate withdrawal syndrome. Drug Alcohol Depen 1988; 21(3): 253–9.
114. Washton A, Resnick R. Clonidine vs. methadone for opiate detoxification: double-blind outpatient trials. NIDA Res Monogram 1981; 34: 89–94.
115. Kleber H, Riordan C, Rounsaville B, et al. Clonidine in outpatient detoxification from methadone maintenance. Arch Gen Psychiat 1985; 42: 391–4.
116. Lin SK, Strang J, Su LW, Tsai CJ, Hu WH. Double-blind randomised controlled trial of lofexidine versus clonidine in the treatment of heroin withdrawal. Drug Alcohol Depen 1997; 48: 127–33.
117. Kahn A, Muford J, Rogers G, Beckford H. Double-blind study of lofexidine and clonidine. Drug Alcohol Depen 1997; 44(1): 57–61.
118. Carnwath T, Hardman J. Randomised double-blind comparison of lofexidine and clonidine in the out-patient treatment of opiate withdrawal. Drug Alcohol Depen 1998; 50: 251–4.
119. Cami J, De Torress S, San L, Sole A, Guerra D, Ugena B. Efficacy of clonidine and methadone in the rapid detoxification of patients dependent on heroin. Clin Pharmacol Ther 1985; 38: 336–41.
120. Vilalta J, Treserra J, Garcia-Esteve L, Garcia-Giralt M, Cirera E. Methadone, clonidine and levomepromazine in the treatment of opiate abstinence syndrome: double-blind clinical trial in heroin-addicted patients admitted to a general hospital for organic pathology. Med Clin-Barcelona 1987; 88(17): 674–6.
121. San L, Cami J, Peri J, Mata R, Porta M. Efficacy of clonidine, guanfacine and methadone in the rapid detoxification of heroin addicts: a controlled clinical trial. Brit J Addict 1990; 85(1): 141–7.

122. Jiang Z. Rapid detoxification with clonidine for heroin addiction: a comparative study on its efficacy vs. methadone. Chinese J Neurol Psychiat 1993; 26(1): 10–13.
123. Dawe S, Gray J. Craving and drug reward: a comparison of methadone and clonidine in detoxifying opiate addicts. Drug Alcohol Depen 1995; 39(3): 207–12.
124. Howells C, Allen S, Gupta J, Stillwell G, Marsden J, Farrell M. Prison based detoxification for opioid dependence: a randomised double blind controlled trial of lofexidine and methadone. Drug Alcohol Depen 2002; 67(2): 169–76.
125. Bearn J, Gossop M, Strang J. Accelerated lofexidine treatment regimen compared with conventional lofexidine and methadone treatment for in-patient opiate detoxification. Drug Alcohol Depen 1998; 50: 227–32.
126. Washton A, Resnick R. Clonidine in opiate withdrawal: review and appraisal of clinical findings. Pharmacotherapy 1981; 1: 140–6.
127. Washton A, Resnick R. Clonidine versus methadone for opiate detoxification. Lancet 1980; 2(8207): 1297.
128. Rounsaville B, Kosten T, Kleber H. Success and failure at outpatient opioid detoxification: evaluating the process of clonidine and methadone assisted withdrawal. J Nerv Ment Dis 1985; 173(2): 103–10.
129. Benos V. Clonidine in opiate withdrawal syndrome. Fortschr der Medizin 1985; 103(42): 991–5.
130. Gerra G, Marcato A, Caccavari R, et al. Clonidine and opiate receptor antagonists in the treatment of heroin addiction. J Subst Abuse Treat 1995; 12(1): 35–41.
131. Gupta A, Jha B. Clonidine in heroin withdrawal syndrome: a controlled study in India. Brit J Addict 1988; 83(9): 1079–84.
132. Bertschy G, Bryois C, Bondolfi G, et al. The association carbamazepine-mianserin in opiate withdrawal: a double blind pilot study versus clonidine. Pharmacol Res 1997; 35(5): 451–6.
133. O'Connor PG, Kosten TR. Rapid and ultrarapid opiate detoxification techniques. JAMA 1998; 279(3): 229–34.
134. Gowing L, Ali R, White J. Opioid antagonists and adrenergic agonists for the management of opioid withdrawal. Cochrane Database Syst Rev; 2000; 2: CD002021.
135. Streel E, Verbanck P. Ultra-rapid opiate detoxification: from clinical applications to basic science. Addict Biol 2003; 8(2): 141–6.
136. Arnold-Reed DE, Hulse GK. A comparison of rapid (opioid) detoxification with clonidine-assisted detoxification for heroin-dependent persons. J Opioid Manag 2005; 1(1): 17–23.
137. Buntwal N, Bearn J, Gossop M, Strang J. Naltrexone and lofexidine combination treatment compared with conventional lofexidine treatment for in-patient opiate detoxification. Drug Alcohol Depen 2000; 59(2): 183–8.
138. Beswick T, Best D, Bearn J, Gossop M, Rees S, Strang J. The effectiveness of combined naloxone/lofexidine in opiate detoxification: results from a double-blind randomized and placebo-controlled trial. Am J Addict 2003; 12(4): 295–305.

139. Azatian A, Papiasvilli A, Joseph H. A study of the use of clonidine and naltrexone in the treatment of opioid addiction in the former USSR. J Addict Dis 1994; 13(1): 35–52.
140. Bell J, Young M, Masterman S, Morris A, Mattick R, Bammer G. A pilot study of naltrexone-accelerated detoxification in opioid dependence. Med J Australia 1999; 171: 26–30.
141. Seoane A, Carrasco G, Cabré L, et al. Efficacy and safety of two new methods of rapid intravenous detoxification in heroin addicts previously treated without success. Brit J Psychiat 1997; 171: 340–5.
142. Kleber HD, Topazian M, Gaspari J, Riordan CE, Kosten T. Clonidine and naltrexone in the outpatient treatment of heroin withdrawal. Am J Drug Alcohol Ab 1987; 13(1–2): 1–17.
143. Loimer N, Schmid R, Lenz K, Presslich O, Grünberger J. Acute blocking of naloxone-precipitated opiate withdrawal symptoms by methohexitone. Brit J Psychiat 1990; 157: 748–52.
144. Roozen H, de Kan R, van den Brink W, Kerkhof B, Geerlings P. Dangers involved in rapid opioid detoxification while using opioid antagonists: dehydration and renal failure. Addiction 2002; 97(8): 1071–3.
145. Golden S, Sakhrani D. Unexpected delirium during Rapid Opioid Detoxification (ROD). J Addict Dis 2004; 23(1): 65–75.
146. O'Connor PG, Kosten TR. Rapid and ultrarapid opioid detoxification techniques. JAMA 1998; 279(3): 229–34.
147. McGregor C, Ali R, White J, Thomas P, Gowing L. A comparison of antagonist-precipitated withdrawal under anesthesia to standard inpatient withdrawal as a precursor to maintenance naltrexone treatment in heroin users: outcomes at 6 and 12 months. Drug Alcohol Depen 2002; 68(1): 5–14.
148. De Jong C, Laheij R, Krabbe P. General anaesthesia does not improve outcome in opioid antagonist detoxification treatment: a randomized controlled trial. Addiction 2005; 100: 206–15.
149. Saunders JB, Jones R, Dean A, et al. Comparison of rapid opiate detoxification and naltrexone with methadone maintenance in the treatment of opiate dependence: A randomized controlled trial. Drug Alcohol Depen 2002; 66(Suppl 1): S156.
150. Lawental E. Ultra rapid opiate detoxification as compared to 30-day inpatient detoxification program – a retrospective follow-up study. J Subst Ab 2000; 11(2): 173–81.
151. Rabinowitz J, Cohen H, Atias S. Outcomes of naltrexone maintenance following ultra rapid opiate detoxification versus intensive inpatient detoxification. Am J Addict 2002; 11(1): 52–6.
152. Dyer C. Addict died after rapid opiate detoxification. Brit Med J 1998; 17: 170.
153. Pfab R, Hirtl C, Zilker T. Opiate detoxification under anaesthesia: no apparent benefit but suppression of thyroid hormones and risk of pulmonary and renal failure. J Toxicol-Clin Toxicol 1999; 37(1): 43–50.
154. Scherbaum N, Klein S, Kaube H, Kienbaum P, Peters J, Gastpar M. Alternative strategies of opiate detoxification: evaluation of the so-called ultra-rapid detoxification. Pharmacopsychiatry 1998; 31(6): 205–9.

155. Minozzi S, Amato L, Vecchi S, Davoli M, Kirchmayer U, Verster A. Oral naltrexone maintenance treatment for opioid dependence. Cochrane Database Syst Rev 2005; Issue 4 (Art No. CD001333).
156. Sackett D, Richardson W, Rosenberg W, Haynes R. Evidence Based Medicine. New York, New York: Chuchill Livingstone; 1997.

chapter 4

Methadone maintenance treatment

Jeff Ward, Wayne Hall, and Richard P Mattick

Introduction

In any consideration of the effectiveness of pharmacotherapies for opioid dependence, methadone maintenance treatment serves as the treatment with which all other treatments are compared. Over the past 30 years, a voluminous literature has accumulated on the results of research studies and clinical experience with methadone maintenance which it is generally accepted attests to its effectiveness. Despite this evidence, methadone maintenance remains a controversial and contested treatment. Features of the evidence and the debates concerning the acceptability of methadone treatment have influenced the way in which we have approached this chapter. The sheer size of the literature means that we cannot exhaustively review the literature relevant to the question of the effectiveness of methadone maintenance treatment and how it should be delivered. We refer the interested reader to our more comprehensive previous work.[1]

The controversy surrounding methadone maintenance treatment means that we cannot in an objective scientific fashion merely review the literature without addressing the objections of the opponents of methadone treatment. The way in which we have approached our task is as follows. First of all, we provide a history of methadone maintenance treatment and an outline of the basic pharmacology of methadone. Second, we address the criticism that methadone maintenance treatment involves prescribing a drug of dependence to drug-dependent individuals. We then outline our approach to reviewing the literature on methadone treatment. We consider whether methadone maintenance treatment reduces heroin use, crime, drug-related mortality, and HIV and hepatitis infection. We then examine whether variations in treatment practice influence these outcomes. After a consideration of the risks associated with the use of methadone as a maintenance treatment, we then conclude with an analysis of current issues in the use of methadone as a maintenance treatment for opioid dependence.

Methadone

Methadone is a synthetic opioid substance that has effects in human beings similar to heroin. Methadone is easily absorbed from the gut and so can be taken orally, whereas heroin is usually injected. Once absorbed via the gut, methadone has a relatively long elimination half-life (approximately 24–36 hours), making it particularly suitable for managing withdrawal from heroin, which has a much shorter elimination half-life (3–6 hours). As early as 1949, research conducted in the US identified methadone as a useful agent for detoxifying people addicted to heroin.[2] However, it wasn't until Vincent Dole and Marie Nyswander conducted clinical research in New York City in the early 1960s to identify a suitable replacement for heroin that methadone was used for longer-term maintenance treatment.[2,3] After trying various opioid substances as heroin substitutes, Dole and Nyswander discovered that methadone was the most clinically useful drug that suited the purposes of a maintenance treatment program. The long elimination half-life allowed patients to be dispensed methadone once a day, as opposed to several times a day, as was the case with shorter-acting drugs such as morphine and heroin. The oral mode of administration obviated the need for injection and, more importantly, meant that the rapid intoxication experienced after the injection of heroin could be avoided because oral methadone was absorbed slowly into the bloodstream. Furthermore, once the person was stabilized on methadone, they did not seem to experience any significant intoxication. After the successful results of an early case series were published,[4] supported by further reports of treatment success,[5,6] methadone maintenance treatment was adopted widely in the US and soon established in other countries, such as Australia.[7] Methadone maintenance treatment is currently the most commonly used treatment for opioid dependence throughout the world.

Rationale and objectives of methadone maintenance

In their rationale for methadone maintenance treatment, Dole and Nyswander viewed opioid dependence as 'a physiological disease characterised by a permanent metabolic deficiency' which was best treated by administering 'a sufficient amount of drug to stabilise the metabolic deficiency.'[4] Stabilization was achieved by providing high, 'blockade' daily doses of oral methadone which prevented withdrawal symptoms, removed the craving for heroin, and blocked the euphoric effects of heroin if the person injected it. While patients were maintained on methadone, they could also take advantage of the rehabilitative services that were an integral part of the Dole and Nyswander program.[8] The key features of the Dole and Nyswander formulation were long-term treatment, high doses of methadone, and a comprehensive set of psychologic and social services to assist the person to reintegrate into mainstream society.

Once methadone maintenance treatment had been shown to reduce heroin use and criminal activity,[9] it quickly became the most common form of drug replacement therapy for opioid dependence. In the process of this popularization in the US, methadone maintenance underwent a number of important changes that compromised its effectiveness.[10] The treatment goal of many programs shifted from long-term maintenance towards achieving abstinence from all opioid drugs, including methadone, within a period of a few years. The average dose of methadone also declined from the high blockade doses favored by Dole and Nyswander to the much lower doses that were required to avert withdrawal symptoms. Furthermore, under the exigencies of Federal funding cuts for methadone maintenance programs, the extent of ancillary psychosocial services declined. More recently, national surveys of treatment practices in the US[11,12] and literature reviews pertinent to the way methadone treatment is delivered have recommended changes in treatment practice.[10,13,14] In Australia, training programs for medical practitioners involved in providing methadone maintenance treatment have also been developed.[15] Recent evidence suggests that there is a return to the original Dole and Nyswander formulation, in using higher methadone doses and having an orientation toward long- rather than short-term treatment.[16] The question of what level of psychosocial service should be provided is more complicated. It is discussed in detail below.

Controversies about methadone maintenance

Despite the evidence of its effectiveness, there were critics who had strong moral reservations about methadone maintenance treatment. The underlying basis for these moral reservations, and the bearing of research evidence and clinical opinion on them, needs to be briefly discussed. While we accept the Scottish philosopher David Hume's argument that statements about what one ought to do cannot be inferred from statements about what is the case, we nonetheless believe that empirical evidence has a bearing upon the evaluation of moral principles, as do many modern ethicists.[17] This is clearest in the case of the moral justification offered for methadone maintenance by its proponents, who argue, on utilitarian moral grounds, that the benefits of the treatment to both the patients and the community outweigh its costs. They accordingly have an obligation to demonstrate that it achieves its aims of reducing injecting heroin use and crime, while improving the health and well-being of a substantial proportion of its patients, and without incurring greater social harms. Some opponents of methadone maintenance argue that methadone maintenance treatment fails to achieve these goals in that substantial numbers of methadone patients continue to inject illicit drugs and engage in criminal activity. Research evidence on the outcome of methadone maintenance is clearly relevant to an evaluation of these competing claims, and this chapter directly addresses these issues.

A utilitarian appraisal of costs and benefits does not address all the moral objections to methadone maintenance. Some opponents of methadone maintenance treatment, for example, argue that it is unacceptable because it simply 'replaces one drug of dependence with another'. These critics often insist that all methadone treatment entrants should become abstinent from all opioid drugs, including methadone. Empirical evidence is also relevant to the evaluation of this moral objection to methadone maintenance treatment for the reason outlined by the German philosopher Immanuel Kant in the late 18th century – namely, showing that a moral obligation is empirically impossible, or at least extremely difficult to meet, provides a good reason for modifying it. Therefore, research evidence is relevant to an evaluation of the moral claim that abstinence is the only acceptable treatment goal for opioid-dependent people, because this goal presupposes that abstinence can be achieved and sustained by most of those who become dependent upon opioids. This assumption is contradicted by the research evidence on the results of opioid detoxification and drug-free treatment, and the small number of studies of the 'natural history' of opioid dependence.[10,18–20] This evidence indicates that the majority of opioid addicts relapse to heroin use shortly after detoxification. Drug-free treatments attract fewer patients than methadone maintenance, have lower rates of retention in treatment, and lower rates of successful graduation to a sustained drug-free lifestyle, although they do reduce the frequency of injecting drug use and benefit their patients in other ways.[10] The evidence on the natural history of opioid dependence shows that the proportion of people who become and remain abstinent is of the order of 10% within the first year after treatment, and that about 2% per annum achieve abstinence thereafter.[21] While people remain opioid dependent, their annual chances of becoming abstinent are not much higher than their risk of dying prematurely from an opioid overdose or other opioid-related cause.

A related criticism of methadone maintenance treatment is that it prolongs opioid dependence by maintaining people on methadone when they otherwise would become drug-free. It was this criticism that led to a shortening of the duration of treatment during the 1970s and 1980s. Again empirical evidence is relevant to this claim. Long-term follow-up studies have found equivalent rates of abstinence 12 years after entry among untreated individuals and individuals who have been in methadone maintenance treatment.[22,23] The same is true for people who enter methadone maintenance treatment and drug-free treatment.[24] This evidence suggests that methadone maintenance does not prolong opioid dependence or impede eventual abstinence.

The difficulty of achieving abstinence does not preclude abstinence as a viable treatment goal for opioid-dependent people. Drug-free treatments, which aim to achieve abstinence, clearly have a place in the treatment response for those opioid-dependent people who want to become abstinent and find this form of treatment acceptable. However, it is clear from the high failure rate of abstinence-oriented programs that there is no compelling moral reason for insisting that abstinence from all opioids is the *only* acceptable treatment goal for those who are opioid dependent, especially in the case of those who have tried and failed on a number of attempts to achieve abstinence.

The effectiveness of methadone maintenance treatment

Heroin use and crime

In this section, we assess whether methadone maintenance treatment is effective in reducing heroin use and crime. Given the limitations of space, we review the best available evidence, with an emphasis on the most recent evidence. Our coverage of the literature should therefore be seen as indicative rather than comprehensive. The interested reader may refer to our previous work for a more comprehensive review.[1]

The best evidence for the effectiveness of any treatment in modern medicine is a *reproducible* demonstration in a *randomized controlled trial* (RCT) that the treatment produces a superior outcome to a relevant comparison treatment, such as no treatment or minimal treatment. In an RCT people with a condition (e.g. opioid dependence) are randomly assigned to receive either *active* treatment (e.g. methadone maintenance) or a comparison treatment (e.g. drug-free counseling). The evaluation of treatment effectiveness requires a comparison treatment so that we can discover what would have happened if the patient had received a different treatment or no treatment at all. Randomization ensures that the subjects who are allocated to the treatment and comparison conditions are equivalent over a large number of trials in which subjects have been randomly assigned to the treatment and comparison conditions. Only when the two groups have been assigned in this way can we be confident that a difference in treatment outcome is more likely to reflect the effects of the treatment than the pre-existing characteristics of the subjects who were assigned to the different treatments.

Randomized controlled trials of methadone maintenance treatment

When methadone maintenance was introduced,[4] the RCT was not routinely used to evaluate new treatments. By the time that methadone maintenance had become an important part of treatment for opioid dependence in the early 1970s, it was difficult to deny access to people who might have benefited from it. For this reason, there have been few RCTs of methadone maintenance treatment when compared to many other medical treatments. In all there have been nine RCTs in which methadone maintenance has been compared with a non-drug substitution control group for either part or all of the study period.[6,25–33] As can be seen from other chapters in this book, methadone maintenance has also been used as a comparison treatment in RCTs investigating the effectiveness of other pharmacotherapies, but these trials do not bear directly on the assessment of the effectiveness of methadone maintenance treatment.

A detailed description and analysis of the early trials of methadone maintenance treatment can be found in our previous work.[34] Our focus in this chapter, after providing a brief overview of this evidence, is on one of the more recent RCTs which answers a number of important questions pertinent to long-standing debates about methadone treatment.[27] Overall, the RCTs of methadone maintenance have compared methadone maintenance to no-treatment controls, methadone maintenance with ancillary services to a placebo with ancillary services, methadone maintenance with a methadone detoxification control group and 'interim' methadone maintenance (the provision of methadone with few support services) to a waiting list control group. All of these RCTs have found significant differences in favor of the provision of methadone in terms of reductions in heroin use and/or crime. The three earliest trials[6,25,26] together indicate that methadone maintenance retained patients in treatment and led to large reductions in heroin use and the likelihood of reimprisonment when compared with untreated controls. The more recent trials[29–34] have found smaller effects and have followed participating subjects for only short study periods. This smaller effect size is consistent with the findings of a meta-analysis published by Prendergast et al,[35] who reported that the size of the effect in studies of methadone maintenance treatment has diminished over the past three decades. Likely reasons for this diminishing effect size are reductions in the type and amount of ancillary services provided, less adequate implementation of the treatment, and increased patterns of polydrug use among patients being treated.

In this chapter we review in detail an RCT that provides information on a number of the questions being investigated by this review. Sees and colleagues[27] compared 180-day methadone-assisted detoxification with compulsory intensive psychosocial services and aftercare with standard methadone maintenance treatment. The study provides evidence pertinent to questions about the effectiveness of methadone maintenance treatment, about how long it should be provided for, and about the role of intensive psychosocial services in its effectiveness. The latter two questions are addressed in subsequent sections of this chapter.

The question that Sees et al set out to answer was whether, over a 12-month period, equivalent outcomes to methadone maintenance could be achieved in terms of drug use, HIV risk behavior and psychosocial functioning by offering a 6-month methadone detoxification program that included intensive psychosocial services and aftercare for 6 months. After being stratified by sex and ethnicity, participants in the study were randomly assigned to receive either long-term methadone detoxification (n=88) or methadone maintenance (n=91). Both groups were stabilized on an average of approximately 85 mg per day of methadone and, after 4 months of maintenance the methadone detoxification group was detoxified in a gradual fashion over the subsequent 2 months. Participants in the detoxification program were required to attend weekly individual and group psychotherapy and education sessions. If there was evidence of cocaine use, they were also required to attend a weekly therapy group for cocaine users. By contrast, in the methadone maintenance group, participants were required to attend a weekly group for the first 6 months, after which attendance was voluntary. They received monthly individual therapy for the duration of the study. Aftercare for the detoxification group consisted of continued therapy and assistance with criminal, medical, and social service referrals. All participants were assessed at baseline and then monthly for 12 months on all the study outcomes and on their exposure to treatment components received in the previous month.

The analysis of the data for this study was done on an intention-to-treat basis. The first finding was that patients in the detoxification group dropped out of treatment more quickly than those in the methadone group. While approximately 70% of the methadone maintenance group remained in treatment after 1 year, most of the members of the detoxification group left treatment once methadone provision began to be tapered. This shows, as did earlier studies by Newman and Whitehill[26] and Strain et al,[28] that methadone is essential in retaining patients in treatment and that intensive services are not sufficient when methadone is absent.

Heroin use was analyzed in terms of whether there was any evidence of heroin use in the previous month as measured by urine test and the self-reported number of days of heroin use in the previous month. Both of these analyses revealed that there were no differences between the two groups for the first 4 months of the study, but once methadone reduction began in the detoxification group, differences emerged that persisted throughout the follow-up period. These findings for heroin use were confirmed by the findings for HIV risk behavior. Again there was more injection-related risk behavior in the detoxification group after detoxification ended.

Overall, the study by Sees et al suggests that methadone maintenance treatment is more effective than methadone detoxification after 4 months of maintenance, and that the provision of intensive psychosocial services was not sufficient to replace the daily administration of methadone. We can only agree with the authors that: 'the current study does not provide support for diverting resources from methadone maintenance to long-term detoxification, no matter how ideologically attractive the notion of a time limited treatment for opioid abusers is.'

Observational studies of methadone maintenance treatment

There have been numerous observational studies of methadone maintenance treatment that have employed a variety of study designs. The best of these studies have compared the fate of heroin-dependent individuals who have applied for treatment, self-selected into different treatment modalities, and then been followed over time. These studies use statistical adjustment rather than randomization to control for pre-existing differences in study groups that might plausibly account for variations in outcomes after treatment. Statistical adjustment is a weaker form of control than randomization, but observational studies often provide an estimate of the effectiveness of a treatment under treatment-as-usual conditions. The overall findings of these studies suggest that methadone maintenance treatment is superior to short-term detoxification or no treatment at all in terms of reductions in heroin use and crime.[36–41] In this chapter, we review one of the stronger studies using this design.[34] A more comprehensive account can be found in Hall et al.[34]

Bale et al reported one of the best-controlled comparative studies in 1980.[37] In this study, Bale and his colleagues compared methadone maintenance treatment with therapeutic communities and detoxification in terms of outcomes 12 months after treatment. There were several distinctive features of this study. First, subjects who entered methadone and therapeutic communities were very nearly comparable on a comprehensive pretreatment assessment. The main reasons for this were that subjects were recruited from a common pool of potential patients (opioid-addicted veterans in the United States of America Veterans Administration treatment system) by treatment staff who competed for these patients. Secondly, a number of different programs were represented within each treatment modality. Thirdly, 93% of patients were followed up at 6 and 12 months. The results of treatment were therefore available for almost all who entered treatment, regardless of how long they stayed, and not just for the treatment successes. Fourthly, outcomes were assessed by an independent interviewer who was unaware of which treatment the subject had received, and efforts were made to validate self-reported drug use and criminal activity.

The results indicated that the two methadone maintenance programs produced better outcomes than detoxification when measured by reductions in opioid drug use during the month prior to follow-up and the number of convictions recorded during the following year. Moreover, the differences in outcome between methadone maintenance and detoxification persisted after adjustment for 10 patient characteristics that had been shown to predict these outcomes in other studies.

While studies like the ones just described compare groups of patients who self-select into different treatment modalities, another type of study design investigates changes that take place as a result of exposure to treatment. This is often done by either comparing the outcomes of people who dropped out of treatment with the outcomes of people who remained in treatment, or by examining the relationship between length of time spent in treatment and outcome. Conclusions drawn from such pre–post studies are of uncertain value because of the existence of a plausible rival hypothesis – namely that those with the best outcomes (e.g. who were the least dependent on opioids, and the most motivated to discontinue drug use) are more likely to be retained in treatment. The use of statistical adjustment, as described above, can provide a limited evaluation of this rival explanation. First, the hypothesis that patients with a good outcome were more likely to be retained in treatment can be tested by measuring characteristics (e.g. degree of dependence, previous treatment history, and motivation to change) known to predict the outcome interest of those who do and do not remain in treatment. Secondly, statistical methods (e.g. covariate adjustment) can be used to discover whether the relationship between treatment duration and patient outcome persists when such differences in patient characteristics are taken into account.

Overall, the findings of pre–post studies support the findings of the RCTs and the comparative observational studies.[11,42–45] Importantly, some of these studies also suggest that there are significant variations in the effectiveness of methadone clinics, suggesting that variations in treatment practices may be an important factor in any consideration of the effectiveness of methadone maintenance treatment.[11,42,45] We consider in detail three studies that provide the best evidence among the pre–post studies below.

In 1974, Gearing and Schweitzer[43] carried out an independent evaluation of 17,500 patients admitted to Dole and Nyswander's long-term methadone maintenance program in New York City between January 1964 and December 1971. They identified four cohorts by date of admission and assessed outcome by changes in social productivity, arrests for predatory crime, and mortality rates. The demographic characteristics of patients entering the program changed over the period of study. The average age declined from 33 to 29 years; the proportion of women increased from 15% to 23%; and the percentage of whites decreased from 40% to 32%, while the percentage of Hispanics increased from 19% to 26%. Despite these changes in patient characteristics, retention in treatment was high and relatively constant across the first three cohorts, namely, 90% after 1 year, 80% after 2 years, and 75% after 3 years.

Retention in treatment was associated with improved social productivity, reduced crime, and a reduced mortality rate. The percentage who were employed, attending school, or homemakers increased with treatment for all three cohorts, although less so for later cohorts. The three cohorts showed similar decreases in rates of arrest with increasing time in treatment, namely, 6.5% in the first year, 4.6% in the second year, 3.1% in the third year, and 2.9% in the fourth year.

Mortality rates were compared between 3,000 patients in treatment, 850 patients who left methadone, 100 patients entering detoxification in

1965, and the New York population in 1969 to 1970 in the age range 20 to 54 years. The rates among patients while in treatment (7.6 per 1000 population) were not substantially higher than those in the general population (5.6 per 1000 population). The mortality rate among those entering detoxification was almost 11 times higher than that of those in treatment (82.5 per 1000 population), while those who had left treatment had a rate that was almost four times higher than that of those who remained in treatment (28.2 per 1000 population). The percentage of deaths that were judged to be probably or possibly drug-related was 50% among those in treatment, 80% among those who died after leaving treatment, and 100% among those who entered detoxification.

Gearing and Schweitzer's results are noteworthy in replicating the positive results for drug use and crime reported by Dole and Nyswander in their early reports,[4,8] and showing that these positive outcomes were sustained over four cohorts of 17,500 patients admitted to their program over a period of 8 years. The outcomes assessed were relatively objective, and the advantage in favor of methadone maintenance was substantial in the case of mortality where comparative data were available.

In a second large-scale evaluation of methadone maintenance treatment, Ball and colleagues[42,46] evaluated six methadone maintenance clinics, two in each of Baltimore, Philadelphia, and New York, over a 3-year period between 1985 and 1987. During the winter of 1985–86, 633 male patients were interviewed, and 506 were re-interviewed a year later about their drug use history, their last period of injecting drug use, and their past and current criminal activity. The characteristics of the methadone maintenance programs were also extensively assessed to determine if there was any relationship between program characteristics and outcome.

The findings suggested that methadone maintenance had a dramatic impact on injecting drug use and crime among the 388 patients who remained in treatment during the follow-up year: 36% had not injected since the first month on methadone maintenance, 22% had not injected for a year or more, and 13% had not injected in the past one to 11 months. In all, 71% had not injected in the month prior to interview, and the rate of injection among the 29% who had injected in the past month was substantially less than before treatment.

The results also suggested that some programs were more effective at eliminating drug use than others: four of the programs reduced drug use by between 75% and 90%, whereas around 56% of patients in the other two programs were still injecting. Among the 107 patients who had left treatment by the time of follow-up, 68% had relapsed to injecting drug use. The relapse rate was 82% among patients who had been out of treatment for more than 10 months. Those patients who had been in the less successful programs had higher relapse rates after leaving treatment than those who had been in the more successful programs.

The reduction of crime associated with retention in methadone maintenance also appeared impressive. The study sample had an extensive criminal history prior to entering methadone maintenance: a total of 4,723 arrests, with a mean of nine arrests among the 86% of the sample who had ever been arrested. Sixty-six percent of the group had spent some time in jail, 36% for 2 years or more. The sample admitted to 293,308 offences per year during their last period of addiction. Each of these committed 601 crimes per year (range 1 to 3,588), and had done so on 304 days per year during their last addiction period. After entry to methadone maintenance, the number of self-reported offences declined to 50,103 crimes per year and the number of 'crime days' per year decreased from 238 in the year prior to entry to 69 crime days during the early months of methadone maintenance. The number of crime days continued to decline with the number of years spent in treatment. The reduction in the number of crimes committed while in methadone maintenance was 192,000 offences per year.

Ball and colleagues[42,46] found that the more effective programs prescribed higher doses of methadone and had maintenance rather than abstinence as their treatment goal. They also offered better-quality and more intensive counseling services and provided more medical services; retained their patients in treatment, and managed to achieve compliance in terms of regular clinic attendance. They also had close, long-term relationships with their patients and low staff turnover rates. Similar findings have been reported from a study of 17 methadone clinics in New York City.[45] Specifically, the nature of the management, as represented by an assessment of the clinic manager's level of experience and style of management, was associated with less heroin use early on in treatment. Those managers who were more experienced and who would take an active role in treatment activities were more effective. Secondly, more frequent counseling was associated with less cocaine use, suggesting that while methadone might be sufficient to reduce heroin use, additional intervention is required to reduce non-opioid illicit drug use.

In the third pre–post study to be considered here, Kott et al[44] reported on 673 patients randomly selected from 21,889 patients who were enrolled in methadone treatment in New York for between 1 and 6 years of treatment. The total number of subjects comprised five cohorts of patients who had been in treatment continuously for less than 2, 3, 4, 5, and 6 years, respectively. Each of the patients was contacted and interviewed about number of arrests, number of days in prison, number of days in hospital, number of presentations to emergency rooms, and employment status. Each of these variables was assessed for the 6 months prior to entry to treatment and at follow-up for the 6 months before interview. There was a statistically significant reduction in number of self-reported arrests, indicating that after 1 year of methadone treatment there was a reduction in arrest rates, but this did not improve over time. There was also a reduction in number of days spent in hospital but these reductions were quite small because only a small number of subjects had been hospitalized and most of these only briefly. There were no differences between pretreatment and follow-up levels of emergency room use, but again, the usage was so low that there was little to be improved upon. Improvements were seen in employment rates in the 3 to 5 year cohorts, but this was due to their low rates of reported employment at intake rather than improvements over time. In all cohorts the rate of employment remains relatively stable at between 30 and 40%.

A comparison of results: randomized controlled trials and observational studies

The observational studies of the effectiveness of methadone maintenance treatment generally support the results of the RCTs in showing that methadone maintenance reduces heroin use and criminal activity. They also revealed two other things about contemporary methadone maintenance treatment. The first was substantial variation between different programs in treatment retention and rates of heroin use. The second was that the average results of methadone maintenance treatment in recent observational studies are not as impressive as those reported from the early RCTs. For example, the retention rates from the RCTs are usually of the order of

70% or more after 1 year, whereas the retention rate in the observational studies is approximately 50% after 6 months.[11,39] Similarly, the early RCTs reported very little continuing heroin use among those who remained in treatment, whereas the more recent trials and observational studies show much higher rates of heroin use. This is consistent with recent Australian evidence that suggests that approximately half of the patients in methadone treatment continue to use heroin occasionally, while a small proportion (approximately 10%) continue to use heavily.[47] This is also consistent with the findings of the meta-analysis reported by Prendergast et al,[35] who found diminishing effect sizes over the past three decades of studies of methadone maintenance treatment.

HIV infection

As well as reducing heroin use and crime, an important area in which methadone maintenance treatment is expected to be effective is in the reduction of HIV infection among heroin users. Concern has also been raised about the spread of hepatitis C (HCV) in this population. HIV and HCV are the two viruses most often transmitted among injecting drug users as a result of sharing injecting equipment.[48] In this section, we review the evidence for the effectiveness of methadone maintenance treatment in preventing the spread of HIV and HCV.

There are two kinds of evidence relevant to the effectiveness of methadone maintenance programs in reducing the spread of HIV: studies that directly evaluate the protective effect of methadone treatment in terms of HIV seroprevalence rates, and studies that examine whether methadone maintenance treatment reduces behaviors (such as needle sharing) that have been implicated in the spread of HIV among injecting drug users. Recent reviews have consistently concluded that methadone maintenance treatment is effective in reducing the spread of HIV and in reducing the injection-related behaviors known to transmit it.[49–51] The studies reviewed below are indicative of the much larger body of evidence summarized in these reviews.

Initial evidence for the effectiveness of methadone maintenance in preventing HIV infection came from retrospective studies that found an association between length of time in methadone treatment and low rates of HIV seropositivity. For example, patients who entered methadone treatment in New York before 1982 were found to be less likely to be HIV positive than those who had entered treatment after that year.[52] Similarly, Schoenbaum et al[53] found that there was an inverse relationship between total months of methadone treatment since January 1978 and the presence of HIV antibodies among injecting drug users in New York. Further evidence from New York was then published in 1990 by Novick et al[54] reporting no seropositive cases in a group of long-term, stable patients who entered treatment before the spread of HIV in New York. Ninety-one percent of these patients had been exposed to hepatitis B, indicating that nearly all of them had shared injecting equipment at some time in their lives. Two other studies have found that patients in methadone treatment were less likely to be HIV positive than those in detoxification programs[55] and those not yet receiving methadone.[56]

Other evidence suggests that these findings cannot be attributed to the fact that patients who remain in methadone maintenance are less likely to engage in risky behaviors than those who leave methadone treatment early or injecting drug users who do not enter treatment. A Swedish study reported by Blix and Grönbladh[57,58] is of special interest because the way in which patients were accepted into methadone treatment approximated a random selection procedure. In this study, nearly all the patients who entered treatment after 1983 had previously applied and been refused entry because of restricted places in the program. Three percent of patients who entered methadone maintenance before 1983 were found to be HIV positive. This increased to 16% among those who entered treatment between 1984 and 1986 and to 57% among patients who entered treatment after 1987. There had been no seroconversions of any patients who had tested negative for HIV antibodies on entry since 1984.

These findings have been confirmed in two prospective studies conducted in the US. In the first of these studies, Metzger and colleagues[13,59] followed up 255 heroin users in and out of methadone treatment over a period of 36 months and examined changes in HIV seropositivity during the follow-up period. The rate of HIV infection almost doubled during the follow-up period from 21% to 39% among those not in treatment, while those in treatment only increased from 13% to 18%. All of the cases of HIV in the treatment cohort occurred in individuals who had left treatment during the follow-up period.

In the second of these studies from the US, Moss and colleagues[60] followed up 681 heroin users recruited from methadone maintenance clinics and detoxification programs over 5 years from 1985. After adjusting for other major predictors of infection, individuals who spent less than 1 year in methadone treatment in the follow-up period were nearly three times more likely to have seroconverted (hazard ratio = 2.7). Similar findings have been reported from Italy, where it was estimated that the risk of HIV infection was increased by 70% for every 3 months spent out of treatment.[61] This study also found that the risk for HIV infection was reduced by 35% for each 10 mg increase in methadone dose. The latter finding has also been reported from a study in New York City where low methadone doses were also associated with an increased risk of HIV seropositivity.[62]

The studies reviewed so far in this section support the conclusion that methadone maintenance treatment is effective in reducing HIV infection among injecting heroin users. Further support for this comes from studies that have examined whether rates of drug injecting and sharing of injecting equipment are reduced among methadone patients when compared with appropriate comparison groups.[42,52,63–68] For example, Ball and colleagues,[42,46] in the study described earlier in this chapter, found that methadone treatment had a marked effect on both frequency of injecting and on needle sharing among those who did inject. Of the 388 subjects who had remained in methadone maintenance until the end of the study period: 36% had not injected after 1 month of treatment; a further 22% had not injected in the past year; and a further 22% had not injected for between 1 and 11 months. Overall, 71% had not injected in the month prior to being interviewed. Similar results were found for needle sharing. Those who shared during their last period of injecting shared less than those whose last period of drug use occurred before or during the admission phase of treatment. Finally, Ball and colleagues also found that patients on lower methadone doses were more likely to inject. These findings support the finding by Serpelloni et al[61] and Brown and colleagues[62] that lower doses of methadone (<60 mg) may be less effective than higher doses in reducing HIV risk behavior.

Hepatitis C

While the evidence reviewed in the previous section supports the conclusion that methadone maintenance treatment is effective in reducing HIV infection among heroin users, this may not be the case for HCV because HCV is more readily transmitted than HIV. While there are wide variations in prevalence rates of HIV around the world (from nil to 80% or more in places such as Myanmar and China), rates of HCV infection tend to be less variable (between 50 and 95% from different countries around the world).[45,69] In Australia HCV has become a major health issue for injecting drug users.[70] Freeman and colleagues[71] compared rates of HCV infection in cohorts of heroin users from the 1970s and the 1990s. They found that 84% of the 1970s group who had presented for methadone treatment in Sydney, Australia were already HCV antibody positive.

To date, most studies examining the effectiveness of outpatient methadone maintenance in preventing infection with HCV have found no such effect.[72] This is most likely because most entrants to treatment are already infected with HCV. However, a recent Australian trial of methadone maintenance in a prison setting suggests that, at least over the longer term, methadone maintenance may be protective against HCV infection.[73] Dolan and colleagues reported the results of an RCT conducted within a prison methadone program in New South Wales, Australia. While their initial report found reductions in heroin use and drug injection at 5-month follow-up there was no reduction in HCV incidence over this period. However, when the groups were followed up over the next 4 years, within and without the prison environment, they found that retention in methadone maintenance treatment was associated with reduced HCV infection. This is the first study published that has found that heroin users who are HCV negative at baseline and who stayed longer in methadone treatment were less likely to be infected with HCV. More studies are needed that assess exposure to HCV at baseline and follow-up to determine whether and to what extent methadone maintenance is protective in this regard.

Drug-related mortality

Because opioid dependence is associated with a high risk of mortality,[23,74–77] it is an important outcome to consider in evaluating the effectiveness of methadone maintenance treatment. Common causes of death among the opioid dependent are drug overdose, cirrhosis, endocarditis, violence, AIDS-related illnesses, and, more recently, hepatitis-C-related liver disease.[23,74,75,78] Opioid-dependent individuals receiving methadone maintenance have a lower risk of dying than peers who are not in treatment.[43,78–85] As detailed in the previous section, Gearing and Schweitzer,[43] in their evaluation of the New York City methadone program, found that the mortality rate for the methadone maintenance patients was significantly different from their age group in the general population, and was lower than for clients who had left methadone treatment and only received opioid detoxification. Grönbladh and Gunne,[81] in a 6-year follow-up of individuals who participated in a Swedish RCT,[25] reported that untreated control subjects had a death rate 73 times that expected for their age group, while none of the methadone-treated subjects had died. Similarly, in a case-control study of overdose deaths among 4,200 methadone clients in Rome during the period 1980–88, Davoli and colleagues[80] found that individuals who left treatment were eight times more likely to die during the year after they left than clients who stayed. Similarly, in a long-term follow-up of patients admitted to the first methadone program to be established in Sydney, Australia, Caplehorn and colleagues[79] found that remaining in treatment was associated with a threefold reduction in the risk of dying.

More recently, Appel et al[78] reported the results of a study of mortality during and after methadone treatment for a cohort of patients described by Dole and Joseph in 1978.[86] The sample consisted of 1,544 patients admitted to methadone maintenance in two cohorts, one in 1966–67 and the other in 1972. The study conducted in 1981 examined causes of death and death rates for the 10-year period 1966–76. During this time, there were 176 deaths among the 1,544 patients. Of these, 93 deaths occurred during methadone maintenance and 83 after methadone maintenance. The post-treatment death rate among former patients was double that of those still receiving methadone maintenance treatment. Only 2 opiate-related deaths occurred during treatment, while 36 occurred out of treatment. This represented a 51 times greater risk of dying from opiate-related causes after leaving methadone maintenance (15.3 deaths per 1000 years), when compared with those remaining in treatment (0.3 deaths per 1,000 years).

As Desmond and Maddux[82] have observed, the fact that these studies have been conducted in different countries by different researchers increases our confidence that methadone maintenance reduces the high risk of mortality among the heroin dependent. This effect appears to be restricted to mortality from heroin overdose, a conclusion supported by Appel.[78] Finally, van Ameijden et al[87] found a dose–response relationship between daily methadone dose and risk for mortality in The Netherlands. Although lower daily doses of methadone (<55 mg) were effective in reducing mortality, there was a 3-fold greater reduction in mortality for those on higher than those on lower doses. This finding is consistent with other evidence reviewed further in this chapter that higher methadone doses are more effective in reducing heroin use. Higher doses of methadone also induce a higher tolerance to opioids, which is the probable mechanism by which overdose deaths are reduced.

Previous reviews of the effectiveness of methadone maintenance

The literature reviewed in this chapter suggests that methadone maintenance treatment is effective in reducing heroin-use, crime, drug-related mortality, and HIV infection among heroin-dependent individuals. There is one study that suggests that methadone treatment is also effective in lowering the risk of subsequent HCV infection among those who are unexposed when they enter treatment. These conclusions are consistent with more extensive reviews we have conducted[1,14] and with reviews conducted by others.[10,49,50,88] The review reported by Marsch[49] is unique in that, unlike other reviews which were qualitative in nature, a quantitative approach was taken using meta-analysis. Despite inclusion criteria restricting the selection of studies to those that employed fixed dosage schedules irrespective of patients' heroin use, Marsch found that methadone maintenance treatment was successful in reducing heroin use, drug-related and (to a lesser extent) non-drug-related crime, and HIV risk behavior. The strongest effect was the reduction in drug-related crime.

Treatment characteristics associated with the effectiveness of methadone maintenance treatment

As noted above, observational studies of methadone maintenance treatment suggest that some methadone clinics are more effective than others. The key variables that have been identified as possibly the most important are: methadone dose, the duration of treatment, and the extent of psychosocial services, such as counseling and psychotherapy, that are provided as part of the treatment program. In this section, we review the evidence on each of these treatment characteristics. We also review the evidence on the comparative effectiveness of injectable versus oral methadone maintenance.

Methadone dosage

The original formulation for methadone maintenance treatment as devised by Dole and Nyswander[4] included high doses of methadone with the aim of long-term maintenance during which extensive adjunctive psychosocial treatment services would be provided. In this and the next two sections, we examine whether variations in this formulation compromise the effectiveness of methadone maintenance treatment or not.

The use of high maintenance doses of methadone (>60 mg per day) was originally meant to achieve three purposes: to prevent withdrawal symptoms, to induce a sufficient cross-tolerance to heroin to prevent intoxication, and to prevent craving for heroin. However, in many clinics lower doses have been prescribed, and as Leavitt and colleagues[89] have observed, this is more for philosophical, psychologic, and moral reasons than empirical evidence. The evidence, which consists of both RCTs and observational studies, clearly shows that, on average, higher doses of methadone lead to longer stays in treatment and less heroin use.[28,90–95] In a recent study, Preston et al[96] found that increasing methadone dose in response to ongoing heroin use was as effective as paying patients not to use heroin. However, a study by Trafton et al[97] published in 2005 suggests that some patients may require higher doses than others to achieve reductions in heroin use. They found a number of patient characteristics that were associated with heroin abstinence and higher doses of methadone in a cohort of 222 US war veterans. Patients with a diagnosis of post-traumatic stress disorder or depression, who were in treatment longer, and who had more previous opioid detoxifications in the past were more likely to require higher doses. This study suggests that the picture might be somewhat more complex than the RCTs comparing fixed high and low doses suggest. However, at this time, there is little other research to inform methadone dosage guidelines. A more extensive review of this literature can be found in Ward et al.[98]

Duration of treatment

There is substantial evidence that longer stays in methadone maintenance treatment are associated with better treatment outcomes in terms of less heroin use and crime.[35,99,100] An important question is whether varying the length of treatment as originally formulated by Dole and Nyswander improves or reduces the effectiveness of methadone maintenance treatment. The evidence clearly suggests that arbitrarily restricting the length of treatment leads to poor post-treatment outcomes for most patients.[101-103] More light is shed on this issue when we consider the evidence on reasons for leaving treatment and post-treatment success. Some individuals leave treatment before they have shown the relevant prognostic indicators of post-treatment success, such as cessation of heroin use and psychosocial stabilization. These individuals are more likely to return to regular heroin use than those who show these signs.[104–106] However, the accumulated evidence suggests that few patients show such signs and most who leave treatment do so when it would be better for them to remain in treatment.[100] Considered as a whole, this evidence suggests that methadone treatment with an orientation toward long-term maintenance, as originally formulated by Dole and Nyswander, is the most appropriate orientation for the majority of patients who enter it.

Ancillary services

Given the high levels of medical, psychiatric, and social problems found among dependent opioid users,[107–109] there is an obvious case for the provision of medical and psychosocial services as an integral part of effective methadone maintenance treatment. From a number of different theoretic perspectives, drug abuse and dependence are motivated in part by alleviating distress caused by psychologic disorder and social deprivation that good treatment should address. Such services were part of the original Dole and Nyswander formulation.

While the rationale for these services seems compelling, the question remains whether the effectiveness of methadone maintenance treatment is improved by providing services such as medical treatment, addiction counseling, psychotherapy, and so on. Because these services are often the most expensive components of a methadone treatment program it is important to ask how much more effective treatment becomes when these services are provided and how much it costs to provide them. In this section we address this question in the light of the available literature, focusing on the best and the most recent studies. A more comprehensive review can be found in Mattick et al.[110]

There is evidence that drug counseling,[42,45,111,112] psychotherapy for comorbid psychiatric problems,[113,114] and primary health care services[42,115,116] improve outcomes from methadone maintenance treatment. Another way in which this question has been examined has been to question whether varying the intensity of ancillary services results in variations in the effectiveness of treatment. In one of the best studies designed to address this issue McLellan and colleagues[111] randomized 92 male war veterans to minimal, standard, or enhanced methadone maintenance treatment. They found increasing improvements in outcome across the three levels of service.

In 1997, Kraft and colleagues[117] examined the costs associated with the three levels of services in relation to the outcomes achieved. The authors concluded that there is a level of service provision below which methadone maintenance treatment becomes more rather than less cost-effective. The results suggest that the provision of counseling services in addition to daily methadone was the most cost-effective. The addition of psychotherapy, vocational counseling, and so on led to only marginal improvements in outcome at much greater cost.

More recently, Avants et al[118] randomized 291 patients to receive 12 weeks of either 2 hours per week of cognitive behavioral therapy, or a 5-hour per day intensive program of group psychotherapy that addressed a range of issues, including drug use, health issues, living skills, and social skills. Outcome was assessed on a range of self-report indicators measured by the Addiction Severity Index. Drug use was validated in the case of heroin and cocaine use by urine testing. Overall, both groups showed improvement at the end of the 3-month study period and at 6-month follow-up after program completion, but there were no differences between the two groups at any time. The only differences were in patients who were new to methadone maintenance, among whom participation in the lower-intensity program led to better retention and higher rates of abstinence at 6-month follow-up. When asked prior to the study which program participants preferred, the majority (78%) nominated the low-intensity program. This study guarded against the problem of patients not attending by ensuring compliance but, as the authors note, participants received services regardless of whether they needed them, so the question of which services were appropriate for which patient was not directly addressed.

Another recent RCT that included both a standard and minimal counseling condition has been reported by Gruber and colleagues.[119] They compared methadone maintenance with standard and minimal counseling conditions to a 21-day methadone detoxification group over a 6-month period. While methadone maintenance was more effective than the 21-day detoxification group, there were no differences between the two counseling groups on any of the outcome measures.

At this time, the evidence suggests that offering counseling and medical care improves outcomes from methadone maintenance treatment. However, providing high-intensity programs does not seem to improve outcome over and above what is achievable with a minimal level of service. Small improvements may be observed, but given the ever-increasing demand for treatment, the resources required would be better spent in providing more treatment places with lower levels of services than more intensive services for fewer patients.

Mode of administration

Methadone can be dispensed as either an oral or an injectable preparation. Injectable methadone is prescribed routinely in the UK but is not available within Australia. The main rationale for the provision of injectable methadone is that it will attract into treatment individuals who would not present for oral methadone. This assumption has yet to be tested empirically and, given the added risks associated with injecting rather than orally ingesting methadone, it is worthy of investigation. However, assuming that injectable methadone maintenance is a viable alternative to an oral regimen, the question arises as to whether one mode of administration is more effective than the other.

Strang and colleagues[120] reported the findings of an RCT in which 40 applicants for methadone treatment were assigned to receive supervised oral methadone or supervised injectable methadone. The practice of supervised injecting is unusual for the UK, where methadone ampoules are usually dispensed at a pharmacy for use at home. This trial was prompted by the Swiss experience in running supervised injectable methadone clinics. The study found no differences between the two groups in retention, in treatment, or in heroin or other drug use 6 months after treatment commenced. However, patients assigned to the supervised injectable condition reported being more satisfied with treatment than those assigned to the oral methadone group. Strang and colleagues also assessed the comparative cost of the two services and found that the cost of the injectable methadone program was approximately 4 to 5 times higher than the oral methadone program. On the basis of these findings, injectable methadone appears to be as effective as oral methadone and leads to greater patient satisfaction, but at a much higher cost. Longer-term studies are needed to assess whether the increased satisfaction translates into better longer-term retention and treatment outcomes.

Risks associated with methadone maintenance treatment

As with most other pharmacotherapies employed in modern medicine, there are risks associated with the prolonged use of methadone that have to be considered in arriving at definitive conclusions about its risks and benefits. Nies[121] summarizes the nature of such decision making as follows: 'The utility of a regimen can be defined as the benefit it produces plus the dangers of not treating the disease minus the sum of the adverse effects of therapy'. In this section, we consider the safety of the long-term administration of therapy, mortality associated with the induction phase of treatment, and problems created by the diversion of methadone from those to whom it has been prescribed.

Safety of long-term methadone administration

The main side-effects of taking methadone on a daily basis are increased perspiration and constipation.[2] An investigation of the consequences of long-term methadone administration among a cohort of patients in New York City who had been in treatment for 10 years or more found no adverse effects as a result of treatment.[122]

Mortality in induction phase of treatment

The first 2 weeks of methadone treatment are a time when there is an increase in death from methadone overdose.[123] In Australia, most of these deaths are associated with the concomitant use of other central nervous system depressants, but rapid escalation of methadone dose during the first days of treatment is also implicated in cumulative methadone toxicity. The risks of these deaths can be substantially reduced by the proper training of medical practitioners involved in methadone prescribing and by educating drug users about the safe use of methadone during induction.[124]

Diversion of methadone

Another risk of methadone maintenance treatment is its diversion to persons other than the patient in treatment. Methadone, if dispensed in a take-home manner, can be given away or sold to other people for their own non-medical use. The main risk associated with the use of diverted methadone is death by overdose. For example, an increase in the availability of methadone in Manchester led to a parallel increase in deaths attributed to diverted methadone.[125] Similar results have been reported elsewhere.[31,126] However, as Bell and Zador[47] have observed, this risk varies with the extent to which take-home methadone is made available. For example, heroin use is the major cause of opioid-related death in Australia where take-home methadone is relatively restricted, whereas in the UK, which has had a more liberal take-home dispensing policy, methadone accounted for about half of all opioid-related deaths.[47] As Bell[15] has also observed, methadone programs that allow overly liberal take-away methadone will ultimately threaten methadone maintenance as a viable treatment modality. We agree with the United States Institute of Medicine[13] that methadone diversion is a serious concern, but not one that warrants restricting the availability of an effective treatment to those in need of it. Take-home methadone for stable patients is a necessary part of good treatment for individuals who find it difficult to attend on a daily basis for supervised dispensing (e.g. mothers of young children, employed patients, the chronically ill). This privilege needs to be used in ways that reduce the risk of diversion.

Conclusions

The literature on the effectiveness of methadone maintenance treatment suggests that it is effective in reducing heroin use, crime, drug-related mortality, and HIV. There is also suggestive evidence from one study that it might be effective in preventing HCV infection among opioid users who have not been previously exposed to the virus. The formulation of methadone maintenance developed by Dole and Nyswander – high-dose, long-term maintenance with ancillary services – is best supported by the available evidence. The evidence clearly indicates that higher rather than lower doses of methadone and longer rather than shorter periods of treatment are more effective in reducing heroin use and crime. The role of ancillary services is less clear, although, on the available evidence, comprehensive ancillary services are not warranted as a routine part of methadone maintenance treatment. Drug counseling, treatment for comorbid psychiatric disorders, and primary health care services do appear to improve treatment effectiveness.

Methadone is generally safe when used as a long-term maintenance medication. There is an increased risk of overdose death during the first 2 weeks of treatment and diverted methadone can increase the risk of deaths from methadone overdose. These risks are smaller than the benefits of making the treatment available and can be minimized by training the medical practitioners and restricting take-home methadone doses to patients who are managing their medication responsibly. Education of patients and illicit drug users about the safe use of methadone would also help with both these problems. In conclusion, the results of more than four decades of research suggest that methadone maintenance treatment is an effective treatment for opioid dependence, whose widespread global use provides a good example of an evidence-based intervention for the treatment of opioid dependence.

References

1. Ward J, Mattick RP, Hall W, eds. Methadone Maintenance Treatment and Other Opioid Replacement Therapies. Amsterdam: Harwood Academic; 1998.
2. Joseph H, Stancliff S, Langrod J. Methadone maintenance treatment (MMT): A review of historical and clinical issues. Mt Sinai J Med 2000; 67: 347–64.

3. Courtwright D, Joseph H, Des Jarlais D. Addicts who survived: an oral history of narcotic use in America 1923–1965. USA: University of Tennessee Press; 1989.
4. Dole VP, Nyswander M. A medical treatment for diacetylmorphine (heroin) addiction: A clinical trial with methadone hydrochloride. J Am Med Assn 1965; 193: 80–4.
5. Dole VP, Nyswander M, Warner A. Successful treatment of 750 criminal addicts. JAMA 1968; 206: 2708–11.
6. Dole VP, Robinson JW, Orraca J, Towns E, Searcy P, Caine E. Methadone treatment of randomly selected criminal addicts. New Engl J Med 1969; 280: 1372–5.
7. Caplehorn JRM, Batey RG. Methadone maintenance in Australia. J Drug Issues 1992; 22: 661–78.
8. Dole VP, Nyswander M. Heroin addiction: a metabolic disease. Arch Intern Med 1967; 120: 19–24.
9. Dole VP, Nyswander M. Methadone maintenance treatment: a ten-year perspective. JAMA 1976; 235: 2117–19.
10. Gerstein DR, Harwood HJ, eds. Treating Drug Problems, Vol. I. A Study of the Evolution, Effectiveness, and Financing of Public and Private Drug Treatment Systems. Washington: National Academy Press; 1990.
11. General Accounting Office. Methadone Maintenance: Some Treatment Programs are not Effective: Greater Federal Oversight Needed. Washington, DC.: General Accounting Office; 1990.
12. D'Aunno T, Vaughn TE. Variations in methadone treatment practices: Results from a national study. JAMA 1992; 267: 253–8.
13. Institute of Medicine. Federal Regulation of Methadone Treatment. Washington: National Academy Press; 1995.
14. Ward J, Mattick RP, Hall W. Key Issues in Methadone Maintenance Treatment. Sydney: New South Wales University Press; 1992.
15. Bell J. Quality improvement for methadone maintenance treatment. Subst Use Misuse 2000; 35: 1735–56.
16. D'Aunno T, Folz-Murphy N, Lin X. Changes in methadone treatment practices: results from a panel study, 1988–1995. Am J Drug Alcohol Ab 1999; 25: 681–99.
17. Rachels J. The Elements of Moral Philosophy. Philadelphia: Temple University Press; 1986.
18. Thorley A. Longitudinal studies of drug dependence. In: Edwards G, Rush C, eds. Drug Problems in Britain: A Review of Ten Years. London: Academic Press; 1980.
19. Vaillant GE. A twelve-year follow-up of New York narcotic addicts: I. The relation of treatment to outcome. Am J Psychiat 1966; 122: 727–37.
20. Vaillant GE. A 20 year follow-up of New York narcotic addicts. Arch Gen Psychiat 1973; 29: 237–41.
21. Wodak A. The treatment of heroin dependence: an overview. Proc Inst Criminol 1985; 65: 27–44.
22. Goldstein A, Herrera J. Heroin addicts and methadone treatment in Albuquerque: a 22-year follow-up. Drug Alcohol Depen 1995; 40: 139–50.

23. Hser Y, Anglin MD, Powers K. A 24-year follow-up of California narcotics addicts. Arch Gen Psychiat 1993; 50: 577–84.
24. Maddux JF, Desmond DP. Methadone maintenance and recovery from opioid dependence. Am J Drug Alcohol Ab 1992; 18: 63–74.
25. Gunne L-M, Grönbladh L. The Swedish methadone maintenance program: A controlled study. Drug Alcohol Depen 1981; 7: 249–56.
26. Newman RG, Whitehill WB. Double-blind comparison of methadone and placebo maintenance treatments of narcotic addicts in Hong Kong. Lancet 1979; 2: 485–8.
27. Sees KL, Delucchi KL, Masson C, et al. Methadone maintenance vs 180-day psychosocially enriched detoxification for treatment of opioid dependence. JAMA 2000; 283: 1303–10.
28. Strain EC, Stitzer ML, Liebson IA, Bigelow GE. Dose–response effects of methadone in the treatment of opioid dependence. Ann Intern Med 1993; 119: 23–7.
29. Vanichseni S, Wongsuwan B, Staff of the BMA Narcotics Clinic No. 6, Choopanya K, Wongpanich K. A controlled trial of methadone maintenance in a population of intravenous drug users in Bangkok: implications for prevention of HIV. Int J Addict 1991; 26: 1313–20.
30. Yancovitz SR, Des Jarlais DC, Peyser NP, et al. A randomised trial of an interim methadone maintenance clinic. Am J Public Health 1991; 81: 1185–91.
31. Perret G, Déglon J, Kreek MJ, Ho A, Harpe RL. Lethal methadone intoxications in Geneva, Switzerland, from 1994 to 1998. Addiction 2000; 95: 1647–53.
32. Schwartz RP, Highfield DA, Jaffe JH, et al. A randomized controlled trial of interim methadone maintenance. Arch Gen Psychiat 2006; 63:102–9.
33. Schwartz RP, Jaffe JH, Highfield DA, Callaman JM, O'Grady KE. A randomized controlled trial of interim methadone maintenance: 10-month follow-up. Drug Alcohol Depen 2007; 86: 30–6.
34. Hall W, Ward J, Mattick RP. The effectiveness of methadone maintenance treatment 1: heroin use and crime. In: Ward J, Mattick RP, Hall W, eds. Methadone Maintenance Treatment and Other Opioid Replacement Therapies. Amsterdam: Harwood Academic; 1998; 17–58.
35. Prendergast ML, Podus D, Chang E. Program factors and treatment outcomes in drug dependence treatment: an examination using meta-analysis. Subst Use Misuse 2000; 35: 1931–65.
36. Anglin MD, McGlothlin WH. Outcome of narcotic addict treatment in California. In: Tims FM, Ludford JP, eds. Drug abuse treatment evaluation: Strategies, progress, and prospects. NIDA Research Monograph, 51. Maryland: National Institute on Drug Abuse; 1984; 106–28.
37. Bale RN, Van Stone WW, Kuldau JM, Engelsing TMJ, Elashoff RM, Zarcone VP. Therapeutic communities vs methadone maintenance. A prospective controlled study of narcotic addiction treatment: Design and one-year follow-up. Arch Gen Psychiat 1980; 37: 179–93.
38. Hubbard RL, Marsden ME, Rachal JV, Harwood HJ, Cavanagh ER, Ginzburg HM. Drug Abuse Treatment: A National Study of Effectiveness. USA: University of North Carolina Press; 1989.
39. Simpson DD, Sells SB. Effectiveness of treatment for drug abuse: an overview of the DARP research program. Advan Alcohol Subst Ab 1982; 2: 7–29.

40. Gossop M, Marsden J, Stewart D, Rolfe A. Patterns of improvement after methadone treatment: 1 year follow-up results from the National Treatment Outcome Research Study (NTORS). Drug Alcohol Depen 2000; 60: 275–86.
41. Hubbard RL, Craddock G, Flynn PM, Anderson J, Etheridge RM. Overview of 1-year follow-up outcomes in the drug abuse treatment outcome study (DATOS). Psychol Addict Behav 1997; 11: 261–78.
42. Ball JC, Ross A. The effectiveness of methadone maintenance treatment: Patients, programs, services, and outcome. New York: Springer-Verlag; 1991.
43. Gearing FR, Schweitzer MD. An epidemiologic evaluation of long-term methadone maintenance treatment for heroin addiction. Am J Epidemiol 1974; 100: 101–12.
44. Kott A, Habel E, Nottingham W. Analysis of behavioural patterns in five cohorts of patients retained in methadone maintenance programs. Mt Sinai J Med 2001; 68: 46–54.
45. Magura S, Nwakeze PC, Sung-Yeon K, Demsky S. Program quality effects on patient outcomes during methadone maintenance: A study of 17 clinics. Subst Use Misuse 1999; 34: 1299–324.
46. Ball JC, Lange WR, Myers CP, Friedman SR. Reducing the risk of AIDS through methadone maintenance treatment. J Health Soc Behav 1988; 29: 214–26.
47. Bell J, Zador D. A risk-benefit analysis of methadone maintenance treatment. Drug Safety 2000; 22: 179–90.
48. Hagan H, Des Jarlais DC. HIV and HCV infection among injecting drug users. Mt Sinai J Med 2000; 67: 423–8.
49. Marsch LA. The efficacy of methadone maintenance interventions in reducing illicit opiate use, HIV risk behaviour and criminality: a meta-analysis. Addiction 1998; 93: 515–32.
50. Sorensen JL, Copeland AL. Drug abuse treatment as an HIV prevention strategy: a review. Drug Alcohol Depen 2000; 59: 17–31.
51. Ward J, Mattick RP, Hall W. The effectiveness of methadone maintenance treatment 2: HIV and infectious hepatitis. In: Ward J, Mattick RP, Hall W, eds. Methadone Maintenance Treatment and Other Opioid Replacement Therapies. Amsterdam: Harwood Academic; 1998; 59–74.
52. Abdul-Quader AS, Friedman SR, Des Jarlais D, Marmor MM, Maslansky R, Bartelme S. Methadone maintenance and behaviour by intravenous drug users that can transmit HIV. Contemp Drug Prob 1987; 14: 425–34.
53. Schoenbaum EE, Hartel D, Selwyn PA, et al. Risk factors for human immunodeficiency virus infection in intravenous drug users. New Engl J Med 1989; 321: 874–9.
54. Novick DM, Joseph H, Croxson TS, et al. Absence of antibody to human immunodeficiency virus in long-term, socially rehabilitated methadone maintenance patients. Arch Intern Med 1990; 150: 97–9.
55. Marmor M, Des Jarlais DC, Cohen H, et al. Risk factors for infection with human immunodeficiency virus among intravenous drug abusers in New York City. AIDS 1987; 1: 39–44.

56. Chaisson RE, Bacchetti P, Osmond D, Brodie B, Sande MA, Moss AR. Cocaine use and HIV infection in intravenous drug users in San Francisco. J Am Med Assn 1989; 261: 561–5.
57. Blix O, Grönbladh L. AIDS and IV Heroin Addicts: The Preventive Effect of Methadone Maintenance in Sweden. Paper presented to 4th International Conference on AIDS, Stockholm, 1988.
58. Des Jarlais DC. The first and second decades of AIDS among injecting drug users. Brit J Addict 1992; 87: 347–53.
59. Metzger DS, Woody GE, McLellan AT, et al. Human immunodeficiency virus seroconversion among intravenous drug users in- and out-of-treatment: an 18-month prospective follow-up. J Acq Immun Def Synd 1993; 6: 1049–55.
60. Moss AR, Vranizan K, Gorter R, Bacchetti P, Watters J, Osmond D. HIV seroconversion in intravenous drug users in San Francisco 1985–1990. AIDS 1994; 8: 223–31.
61. Serpelloni G, Carrieri MP, Rezza G, Morganti S, Gomma M, Binkin N. Methadone treatment as a determinant of HIV risk reduction among injecting drug users: a nested case control study. AIDS Care 1994; 16: 215–20.
62. Brown LS, Chu A, Nemoto T, Ajuluchukwu D, Primm BJ. Human immunodeficiency virus infection in a cohort of intravenous drug users in New York City: demographic, behavioural, and clinical features. New York State J Med 1989; 89: 506–10.
63. Darke S, Hall W, Carless J. Drug use, injecting practices and sexual behaviour of opioid users in Sydney, Australia. Brit J Addict 1990; 85: 1603–9.
64. Longshore D, Hsieh S, Danila B, Anglin MD. Methadone maintenance and needle/syringe sharing. Int J Addict 1993; 28: 983–96.
65. Selwyn PA, Feiner C, Cox CP, Lipshutz C, Cohen RL. Knowledge about AIDS and high-risk behaviour among intravenous drug users in New York City. AIDS 1987; 1: 247–54.
66. Klee H, Faugier J, Hayes C, Morris J. The sharing of injecting equipment among drug users attending prescribing clinics and those using needle-exchanges. Brit J Addict 1991; 86: 217–33.
67. Stark K, Müller R. HIV prevalence and risk behaviour in injecting drug users in Berlin. Forensic Sci Intern 1993; 62: 73–81.
68. Caplehorn JRM, Ross M. Methadone maintenance and the likelihood of risky needle sharing. Int J Addict 1995; 30: 685–98.
69. Crofts N, Thompson S, Kaldor J. Epidemiology of Hepatitis C Virus. Canberra: Commonwealth of Australia; 1999.
70. Novick DM. The impact of hepatitis C virus infection on methadone maintenance treatment. Mt Sinai J Med 2000; 67: 437–43.
71. Freeman AJ, Zekry A, Whybin LR, et al. Hepatitis C prevalence among Australian injecting drug users in the 1970s and profiles of virus genotypes in the 1970s and 1990s. Med J Australia 2000; 172: 588–91.
72. Crofts N, Nigro L, OMan K, Stevenson E, Sherman J. Methadone maintenance and hepatitis C virus among injecting drug users. Addiction 1997; 92: 999–1005.
73. Dolan KA, Shearer J, White B, Zhou J, Kaldor J, Wodak AD. Four-year follow-up of imprisoned male heroin users and methadone treatment: Mortality, re-incarceration and hepatitis C infection. Addiction 2005; 100: 820–8.

74. Haastrup S, Jepsen PW. Seven year follow-up of 300 young drug abusers. Acta Psychiat Scand 1984; 70: 503–9.
75. Joe JW, Simpson DD. Mortality rates among opioid addicts in a longitudinal study. Am J Public Health 1987; 77: 347–8.
76. Perucci CA, Davoli M, Rapiti E, Abeni DD, Forastiere F. Mortality of intravenous drug users in Rome: a cohort study. Am J Public Health 1991; 81: 1307–10.
77. Perucci CA, Forastiere F, Rapiti E, Davoli M, Abeni DD. The impact of intravenous drug use on mortality of young adults in Rome, Italy. Brit J Addict 1992; 87: 1637–41.
78. Appel PW, Joseph H, Richman BL. Causes and rates of death among methadone maintenance patients before and after the onset of the HIV/AIDS epidemic. Mt Sinai J Med 2000; 67: 444–51.
79. Caplehorn JRM, Dalton MSYN, Cluff MC, Petrenas A. Retention in methadone maintenance and heroin addicts' risk of death. Addiction 1994; 89: 203–7.
80. Davoli M, Perucci CA, Forastiere F, et al. Risk factors for overdose mortality: a case-control study within a cohort of intravenous drug users. Int J Epidemiol 1993; 22: 273–7.
81. Grönbladh L, Öhlund LS, Gunne LM. Mortality in heroin addiction: impact of methadone treatment. Acta Psychiat Scand 1990; 82: 223–7.
82. Desmond DP, Maddux JF. Deaths among heroin users in and out of methadone treatment. J Maint Addict 2000; 1: 45–61.
83. Esteban J, Gimeno C, Aragones A, Climent JM, de la Cruz Pellin M. Survival study of opioid addicts in relation to its adherence to methadone maintenance treatment. Drug Alcohol Depen 2003; 70: 193–200.
84. Bauer SM, Loipl R, Jagsch R, et al. Mortality in opioid-maintained patients after release from an addiction clinic. Eur Addict Res 2008; 14: 82–91.
85. Clausen T, Anchersen K, Waal H. Mortality prior to, during and after opioid maintenance treatment (OMT): a national prospective cross-registry study. Drug Alcohol Depen 2008; 94: 151–7.
86. Dole VP, Joseph HJ. Long-term outcome of patients treated with methadone maintenance. Ann NY Acad Sci 1978; 311: 181–9.
87. van Ameijden EJC, Langendam MW, Coutinho RA. Dose–effect relationship between overdose mortality and prescribed methadone dosage in low-threshold maintenance programs. Addict Behav 1999; 24: 559–63.
88. Des Jarlais DC. Cross-national studies of AIDS among injecting drug users. Addict 1994; 89: 383–92.
89. Leavitt SB, Shinderman M, Maxwell S, Paris P. When 'enough' is not enough: new perspectives on optimal methadone maintenance dose. Mt Sinai J Med 2000; 67: 404–11.
90. Strain EC, Bigelow GE, Liebson IA, Stitzer ML. Moderate- vs high-dose methadone in the treatment of opioid dependence. JAMA 1999; 281: 1000–5.
91. Maddux JF, Prihoda TJ, Vogtsberger KN. The relationship of methadone dose and other variables to outcome of methadone maintenance. Am J Addict 1997; 6: 246–55.

92. Hartel DM, Shoenbaum EE, Selwyn PA, Kline J, Davenny K, Klein RS, et al. Heroin use during methadone maintenance treatment: The importance of methadone dose and cocaine use. Am J Public Health 1995; 85: 83–8.
93. Banys P, Tusel DJ, Sees KL, Reilly PM, Delucchi KL. Low (40 mg) versus high (80 mg) dose methadone in a 180-day heroin detoxification program. J Subst Abuse Treat 1994; 11: 225–32.
94. Caplehorn JRM, Bell J, Klein DG, Gebski VJ. Methadone dose and heroin use during maintenance treatment. Addiction 1993; 88: 119–24.
95. Magura S, Nwakeze PC, Demsky S. Pre- and in-treatment predictors of retention in methadone treatment using survival analysis. Addiction 1998; 93: 51–60.
96. Preston KL, Umbricht A, Epstein DH. Methadone dose increase and abstinence reinforcement for treatment of continued heroin use during methadone maintenance. Arch Gen Psychiat 2000; 57: 395–404.
97. Trafton JA, Minkel J, Humphreys K. Determining effective methadone doses for individual opioid-dependent patients. PLoS Medicine 2005; 3: 380–7.
98. Ward J, Mattick RP, Hall W. The use of methadone during maintenance treatment: pharmacology, dosage and treatment outcome. In: Ward J, Mattick RP, Hall W, eds. Methadone Maintenance Treatment and Other Opioid Replacement Therapies. Amsterdam: Harwood Academic; 1998; 205–38.
99. Ward J, Mattick RP, Hall W. How long is long enough? Answers to questions about the duration of methadone maintenance treatment. In: Ward J, Mattick RP, Hall W, eds. Methadone Maintenance Treatment and Other Opioid Replacement Therapies. Amsterdam: Harwood Academic; 1998; 305–6.
100. Magura S, Rosenblum A. Leaving methadone treatment: lessons learned, lessons forgotten, lessons ignored. Mt Sinai J Med 2001; 68: 62–74.
101. Anglin MD, Speckart GR, Booth MW, Ryan TM. Consequences and costs of shutting off methadone. Addict Behav 1989; 14: 307–26.
102. McGlothlin WH, Anglin MD. Shutting off methadone: costs and benefits. Arch Gen Psychiat 1981; 38: 885–92.
103. Rosenbaum M, Irwin J, Murphy S. De facto destabilization as policy: The impact of short-term methadone maintenance. Contemp Drug Prob 1988; 15: 491–517.
104. Cushman P. Abstinence following detoxification and methadone maintenance treatment. Am J Med 1978; 65: 46–52.
105. Stimmel B, Goldberg J, Cohen M, Rotkopf E. Detoxification from methadone maintenance: risk factors associated with relapse to narcotic use. Ann NY Acad Sci 1978; 311: 173–80.
106. Simpson DD. Treatment for drug abuse: follow-up outcomes and length of time spent. Arch Gen Psychiat 1981; 38: 875–80.
107. Callaly T, Trauer T, Munro L, Whelan G. Prevalence of psychiatric disorder in a methadone maintenance population. Aust Nz J Psychiat 2001; 35: 601–5.
108. Darke S. The effectiveness of methadone maintenance treatment 3: Moderators of treatment outcome. In: Ward J, Mattick RP, Hall W, eds. Methadone Maintenance Treatment and Other Opioid Replacement Therapies. Amsterdam: Harwood Academic; 1998; 75–90.

109. Ward J, Mattick RP, Hall W. Psychiatric comorbidity among the opioid dependent. In: Ward J, Mattick RP, Hall W, eds. Methadone Maintenance Treatment and Other Opioid Replacement Therapies. Amsterdam: Harwood Academic; 1998; 419–40.
110. Mattick RP, Ward J, Hall W. The role of counselling and psychological therapy. In: Ward J, Mattick RP, Hall W, eds. Methadone Maintenance Treatment and Other Opioid Replacement Therapies. Amsterdam: Harwood Academic; 1998. 265–304.
111. McLellan AT, Arndt IO, Metzger DS, Woody GE, O'Brien CP. The effects of psychosocial services in substance abuse treatment. J Am Med Assn 1993; 269: 1953–9.
112. McLellan AT, Woody GE, Luborsky L, Goehl L. Is the counselor an 'active ingredient' in substance abuse rehabilitation? An examination of treatment success among four counselors. J Nerv Ment Dis 1988; 176: 423–30.
113. Woody GE, McLellan AT, Luborsky L, et al. Severity of psychiatric symptoms as a predictor of benefits from psychotherapy: The Veterans Administration-Penn study. Am J Psychiat 1984; 141: 1172–7.
114. Woody GE, McLellan AT, Luborsky L, O'Brien CP. Psychotherapy in community methadone programs: a validation study. Am J Psychiat 1995; 152: 1302–8.
115. Umbricht-Schneiter A, Ginn DH, Pabst KM, Bigelow GE. Providing medical care to methadone clinic patients: Referral vs on-site care. Am J Public Health 1994; 84: 207–10.
116. McLellan AT, Alterman AI, Metzger DS, et al. Similarity of outcome predictors across opiate, cocaine, and alcohol treatments: role of treatment services. J Consult Clin Psychol 1994; 62: 1141–58.
117. Kraft MK, Rothbard AB, Hadley TR, McLellan AT, Asch DA. Are supplementary services provided during methadone maintenance really cost-effective? Am J Psychiat 1997; 154: 1214–19.
118. Avants SK, Margolin A, Sindelar JL, et al. Day treatment versus enhanced standard methadone services for opioid-dependent patients: A comparison of clinical efficacy and cost. Am J Psychiat 1999; 156: 27–33.
119. Gruber VA, Delucchi KL, Kielstein A, Batki SL. A randomized trial of 6-month methadone maintenance with standard or minimal counselling versus 21-day methadone detoxification. Drug Alcohol Depen 2008; 94: 199–206.
120. Strang J, Marsen J, Cummins M, et al. Randomised trial of supervised injectable versus oral methadone maintenance: report of feasibility and 6-month outcome. Addict 2000; 95: 1631–45.
121. Nies AS. Principles of therapeutics. In: Gilman AG, Rall TW, Nies AS, Taylor P, eds. The Pharmacological Basis of Therapeutics. 7th ed. USA: Pergamon; 1990; 62–83.
122. Novick DM, Richman BL, Friedman JM, et al. The medical status of methadone maintenance patients in treatment for 11–18 years. Drug Alcohol Depen 1993; 33: 235–45.
123. Humeniuk R, Ali R, White J, Hall W, Farrell M. Proceedings of Expert Workshop on the Induction and Stabilisation of Patients onto Methadone. Canberra: Commonwealth of Australia; 2000.

124. Ali RL, Quigley AJ. Accidental drug toxicity associated with methadone maintenance treatment. Med J Australia 1999; 170: 100–1.
125. Cairns A, Roberts ISD, Benbow E. Characteristics of fatal methadone overdose in Manchester, 1985–94. Brit Med J 1996; 313: 264–5.
126. Heinemann A, Iwersen-Bergmann S, Stein S, Schmoldt A, Püschel K. Methadone-related fatalities in Hamburg 1990–1999: Implications for quality standards in maintenance treatment? Forensic Science International 2000; 113: 449–55.

chapter 5

LAAM in the treatment of opioid dependence: A systematic review

Nicolas Clark, Alan Gijsbers, and Jason M White

Levo-alpha-acetylmethadol (LAAM) is a synthetic, long-acting, full μ opioid agonist that has been used for the treatment of opioid dependence since 1971. The long duration of action has enabled LAAM to be used on alternate days or three times a week. Although it performed well in clinical trials, LAAM's uptake in the US was slow. Concerns about LAAM's potential to cause life-threatening cardiac arrhythmias in 2001 led to its withdrawal in Europe and its use as a second-line agent in the US. The poor commercial outlook for LAAM led to the cessation of its production in 2003, just as evidence was beginning to emerge of the superior efficacy of LAAM over methadone and buprenorphine for the treatment of opioid dependence.

History of LAAM

LAAM was first synthesized by German scientists around the time of World War II. In the late 1940s, a number of researchers began to explore the pharmacology of methadone and related compounds.[1–5] In the early 1950s, Keats and Beacher[6] examined the efficacy of LAAM as a post-operative analgesic. Injections of LAAM provided effective analgesia for 12 hours, but repeated doses led to significant sedation and coma in a number of patients. In a series of experiments in opioid users, Fraser and Isbell[7] discovered that

LAAM, its isomer DAAM (dextro-alpha-acetylmethadol), and the racemic mixture DLAAM (dextro-levo-alpha-acetylmethadol) were all long acting, capable of producing opiate effects and relieving opioid withdrawal symptoms for up to 72 hours. Subsequently it was discovered that the long duration of action of LAAM was due to the active metabolites nor-LAAM and dinor-LAAM.[8] Fraser and Isbell observed that the effects of LAAM were first apparent 2 hours after dosing, peaking at approximately 4 hours, and that miosis was still apparent at 24 hours. LAAM appeared to have a more rapid rate of onset when taken orally than when injected subcutaneously or intravenously, which may reduce its potential for abuse. By trial and error, it was estimated that the potency of oral LAAM given once daily was such that 1 mg LAAM would approximate 6–8 mg parenteral morphine. In a series of five participants dosed over 8 weeks, Fraser and colleagues determined that, by increasing the dose of LAAM from 40 to 60 mg, the dosing interval could be extended to 48 or 72 hours without difficulty, but not 96 hours.[9–10]

It was realized that the extremely long duration of action of LAAM made it inappropriate for use in the management of acute pain. Although there was some experimentation with DLAAM for chronic pain,[11] it was not until Dole and Nyswander[12] announced the benefits of methadone in the medical treatment of heroin addiction, that clinical research into LAAM as a treatment for opioid dependence began in earnest. Dole and Nyswander's work was particularly significant because it had been illegal to prescribe opiates to drug addicts without a government permit, since the Harrison Narcotics Act of 1914. Such permits were rarely given and a number of doctors had been prosecuted for prescribing opioids to addicts without a permit. The use of long-acting opioids with supervised administration created a new model for the prescription of opioids to heroin addicts that might be more palatable to authorities.

In the late 1960s America was in the midst of a heroin epidemic. Methadone substitution programs began to develop in several states, but were struggling to keep up with demand. Clinics had to comply with federal, state, and county regulations, thus methadone was not available in all states. Where it was available its dispensing was tightly controlled for fear of finding illicit methadone on the streets. Many clinics did not open on Sundays, so patients had to be given take-home doses regardless of the likelihood of them selling or injecting them. The development of LAAM became a priority for the Division of Narcotic Addiction and Drug Abuse (DNADA) under the direction of Jerome Jaffe, as the long action of LAAM could reduce the need for patients to attend clinics daily and reduce the need for take-home doses.

The federal authorities through DNADA contracted a supply of LAAM and DLAAM and arranged for a series of clinical trials to be conducted,[13–20] and later commissioned research through the Special Action Office for Drug Abuse Prevention (SAODAP) to gather the necessary preclinical and clinical data for registration of LAAM.

The first large-scale study was conducted in Veterans Administration (VA) hospitals (the VA Cooperative study).[21] In a double-blind randomized controlled trial (RCT), LAAM (80 mg three times a week) was compared to 50 mg methadone and 100 mg methadone in 430 heroin addicts. It demonstrated that LAAM was more effective than 50 mg methadone, although not more effective than 100 mg methadone. It was noticed that there were more people in the LAAM group who withdrew from the study early and this was thought to be due to the slow rate of induction onto LAAM.

The SAODAP study was a separate open label RCT conducted using flexible dosing with LAAM and methadone in 636 methadone patients.[22] There were still more people who ceased LAAM than methadone, however there was also less heroin use with LAAM. In addition, most participants who had experienced both LAAM and methadone treatment preferred LAAM.[23]

In collaboration with John Whysner and associates, a further series of trials was conducted, including a methadone compared with LAAM RCT of over 1300 people, a LAAM cohort of approximately 2000 patients and studies of alternate induction schedules from methadone and heroin.[24,25] These studies have never been published in their entirety.

Following failed attempts to gain approval for the marketing of LAAM in the US in 1981 and 1983, NIDA then turned its main focus on research into medications for stimulant abuse and dependence. Returning to LAAM in 1990, a Medications Development Division (MDD) was created at NIDA, with one of its principal aims being to make LAAM available for clinical use. Under a partnership with the Biometrics Research Institute to manufacture and market LAAM, a submission for registration was prepared. Two further studies were conducted, a pharmacokinetic study[26] and a labeling assessment study.[27] The registration of LAAM was eventually approved in 1993, 18 days after resubmission.

Following its registration, uptake of LAAM was slow due to a variety of factors. Firstly, the use of LAAM was subject to a range of bureaucratic red tape as the scheduling of LAAM needed to be changed in individual states, and the regulations governing methadone treatment clinics revised to include LAAM. Secondly, some clinics in the US were reluctant to make LAAM treatment available as it was anticipated that alternate-day dosing would be used as a premise for a funding cut. Thirdly, patients or clinics needed to pay the additional cost of the LAAM itself. Fourthly, LAAM was not considered safe for use in pregnancy – a barrier to its use by women of child-bearing potential. Finally, LAAM take-away doses were not available in line with registration requirements, whereas take-home doses of methadone were available up to 6 days a week in some circumstances. One of the conditions of LAAM's registration was that there would be no take-aways. The titles of some of the early research papers reveal this agenda; for example, 'Can the community be protected against the dangers of take-home methadone.'[28]

Within 2 years of registration, approximately 2000 patients were taking LAAM, 10% of the expected number, and in January 1995 the marketing and distributing rights for LAAM were sold to Roxane Laboratories. Approval for take-home doses of LAAM was given in 2001, however less than 500 out of an estimated 9000 opiate treatment programs were dispensing LAAM, with a maximum of only approximately 5000 patients taking LAAM at any one time.[29]

Meanwhile, there was interest in the use of LAAM in Europe and Australia. Boeringher-Ingelheim (BI) pursued LAAM registration in Europe in 1997, and a number of clinical trials were conducted in Australia. Shortly after LAAM was registered in Europe, a number of life-threatening arrhythmias were reported in people taking LAAM and registration in Europe was suspended pending further investigation.[30,31] In the US, LAAM was then limited for use in those who had not responded to methadone. Subsequent studies have confirmed that LAAM does cause some QT prolongation,[32] although the extent of this risk was not quantified. At the time, the assessment was made by the European Medicines Agency (EMEA) that LAAM was not more effective than methadone, and thus there were no definable groups in whom the benefits of LAAM would outweigh the risks, marketing approval for LAAM was withdrawn in Europe, and later voluntarily withdrawn by the pharmaceutical company worldwide. Subsequent data indicating increased efficacy of LAAM over methadone[33,34] has thus far not prompted a reevaluation of this situation.

Review methods

This chapter is based on a systematic review of published human clinical data on LAAM. The search strategy is outlined in Table 5.1. The results of the review are divided into pharmacologic studies and clinical treatment studies. The titles and abstracts of these 337 references were screened and all relevant articles retrieved in full. Abstracts from the College on Problems of Drug Dependence (CPDD) to 2001 were hand searched. Reference lists of included studies were screened. All RCTs, controlled clinical trials (CCTs) and significant cohort studies were selected for inclusion in the review. The quality of studies was assessed using the quality scoring system developed by the Cochrane Collaboration Drug & Alcohol Review Group. Topics of clinical importance were selected and all identified papers were screened for relevance to any of these topics.

To compare efficacy between treatments, heroin use and retention in treatment were selected as end-points. Heroin use was defined dichotomously as heroin use or no heroin use over a given period, or by the proportion of urine tests positive for heroin use. Retention in treatment was taken to mean retention in any opioid substitution treatment, although retention in allocated treatment was also considered. Where available, 'intention to treat' analyses, where all participants identified at the start

Table 5.1 Search strategy for LAAM review

(Medline – OVID) 1966 to September 2004	*Hits*
1. exp Methadyl Acetate/ or LAAM.mp.	434
2. 1 or (methadyl and acetate).mp. or (methadol and (alpha or acetyl)).mp. or methadylacetate$.mp. or acetylmethadol.mp [mp=title, abstract, registry number word, mesh subject heading]	474
3. limit 2 to animal	191
4. limit 3 to human	54
5. 2 not (3 not 4)	337

of the trial were included in the analysis, were seen as more valid than 'in treatment' samples.

A qualitative review of studies was performed. Levels of evidence were taken from NHMRC guidelines.[35] All identified meta-analyses, RCTs, controlled prospective studies, and larger cohort studies are included in this review.

Pharmacology and metabolism – pharmacokinetics

LAAM is commercially available as ORLAAM, a clear solution with 10 mg LAAM per ml. It is well absorbed orally, with 50% bioavailability.[26] Peak LAAM levels occur within 2.6 hours.[26] LAAM pharmacokinetics follows a multicompartmental model. LAAM is metabolized by hepatic P450 enzymes 3A4, 2B6, 2C8, and 2C18 to its active metabolite nor-LAAM.[36–40] The half-lives of LAAM and its metabolites have been measured in six studies using a total of 64 participants. The terminal half-life of LAAM is approximately 2.5 days (range 8 hours to 3 days). Nor-LAAM has a half-life of approximately 2 days (range 13 hours to 3 days) and is further metabolized to dinor-LAAM which is also active and has a half-life of approximately 4 days (range 30 hours to more than a week).[8,26,36,41–44] Nor-LAAM and dinor-LAAM appear to be at least as potent as LAAM itself.[41]

Chiang[45] studied the PK of LAAM in 25 patients following 15 days of treatment. LAAM peaked at 2 hours, nor-LAAM peaked at 3 hours, and dinor-LAAM peaked at 8 hours. The terminal half-lives of LAAM and nor-LAAM were both 2–3 days, with a parallel decline in LAAM and nor-LAAM levels due to the slow rate of conversion of LAAM to nor-LAAM. Nor-LAAM itself is eliminated at a faster rate (0.7 days). Dinor-LAAM has a very long half-life (greater than a week in some cases) due to its slow elimination.

In the different studies there has been considerable variablility in estimates of terminal elimination half-lives of LAAM, nor-LAAM, and dinor-LAAM. To some extent these may represent differences in method (acute versus chronic dosing, high versus low doses), however even within individual studies there was considerable variability between subjects.[42,43]

Drug interactions

Drugs which induce or inhibit P450 3A4, and to a lesser extent 2B6, 2C6, and 2C18, may interfere with the metabolism of LAAM.[36–40,46] Agents, such as rifampsin, which increase the rate of metabolism of LAAM lead to more rapid breakdown of LAAM to its active metabolites nor-LAAM and dinor-LAAM, and to a more rapid breakdown of these active metabilites to inactive metabolites, resulting in less overall clinical effect.[46] Agents that inhibit the metabolism of LAAM, such as erythromycin, cimetidine, antidepressants, and antifungals (such as ketoconazole), may increase the peak effects of LAAM, slow the onset and increase the duration of action of LAAM.[40,47] Antiretroviral medication can alter the metabolism of LAAM, although these interactions appears to make little difference to overall opiate effects clinically.[48–50]

Other sedative medications interact with LAAM on a pharmacodynamic level, adding to its sedative effects. It appears that alcohol may have both a pharmacokinetic and pharmacodynamic interaction with LAAM, with breath alcohol levels of ethanol lower in subjects taking LAAM.[51,52]

Since LAAM can prolong the QT interval, other drugs that also prolong the QT interval will interact to further prolong the QT interval.

Pharmacology – pharmacodynamics

Dose equivalence with methadone

LAAM product information indicates that it is less potent than methadone and recommends a conversion ratio of 1.2 to 1.3 times the methadone dose for a 48-hour LAAM dose. The evidence for this recommendation appears to be based on a series of small studies in which patients were converted from other opiates to LAAM. Fraser and Isbell found in 17 patients that 1 mg/kg/day oral LAAM, substituted for 6–8 mg/kg/day s/c morphine.[7] In a study in 1971,[53] 23 patients transferred from methadone to LAAM (at one sixth of the dose), with 22/23 dropping out within the first week. Fifty-one patients were then transferred at the same dose and only 27 dropped out.

One study by Resnick et al[54] observed what LAAM dose 60 patients stabilized on when transferring from methadone. There appeared to be a non-linear ratio between methadone and LAAM stabilization doses, with patients on lower methadone doses requiring proportionally more LAAM to stabilize. Low-dose methadone patients (mean 33 mg) stabilized on 52 mg LAAM. Moderate-dose patients (mean 58 mg) stabilised on 55 mg LAAM. High-dose methadone patients (mean 79 mg) stabilized on 85 mg. This study may represent the variability of methadone and LAAM metabolism between individuals, or the need for a minimal LAAM dose to last 48 hours comfortably.

In the study by Eissenberg et al,[55] it was estimated that the conversion ratio from a 48-hour LAAM dose to a 24-hour methadone dose should be 1.0:1 to 1.4:1. In this study 5 participants were given single doses of placebo, LAAM, or methadone (15, 30, or 60 mg/70 kg) and effects were observed over 12 hours. In some measures LAAM was significantly more potent than methadone and three participants had to be withdrawn from the study after 60 mg/70 kg doses of LAAM induced respiratory depression; 1 mg/70 kg naloxone only partially reversed the papillary constriction on LAAM (as opposed to methadone). The range of relative potency estimates is 1–1.4:1.0 (in favor of LAAM). This is consistent with the earlier study of Fraser,[9] in which 40 mg methadone produced less papillary constriction than 40 mg LAAM. One limitation of this study is that it only compared LAAM and methadone during the first 12 hours of LAAM treatment. On the second day of LAAM (during second-daily dosing), LAAM exerted less opiate effects.

Relative potency of metabolites

Billings et al examined plasma levels and urine levels of nor-LAAM and dinor-LAAM in 3 patients being transferred from 80 mg methadone to 100 mg LAAM. Following a single dose of LAAM, the active metabolites were at low plasma levels, but after 40 days they increased 5- to 10-fold and urinary excretion increased 6–8-fold.[8]

In animal studies, the potency of nor-LAAM is estimated at 5–10 times that of methadone and dinor LAAM 1–4 times more potent.[56,57] In humans, clinical effects are most closely related to nor-LAAM concentrations.[46,58]

Action over the interdosing interval compared with methadone and buprenorphine

LAAM is a μ opioid agonist with similar potency to methadone.[55] Following oral intake, effects of a single dose of LAAM begin to be felt 2 hours after the dose, with miosis peaking at 8 hours and lasting up to 48 hours.[58] The duration of effects is not well correlated with LAAM levels, which peak at 2.6 hours. The decay of miosis is slower than the decline in LAAM levels but approximates the decline in nor-LAAM levels.

Biphasic effects were observed for LAAM (and to a lesser extent methadone) in a study in which 28 volunteers were given single doses of LAAM and methadone (0.1–0.2 mg/kg).[53,59] The first phase, which lasted roughly the first 12 hours after the medication was taken and included features of activation, mood elevation, and a liking for the drug, was followed by the second phase, which was characterized by lethargy lasting until the next dose. The division between the two phases corresponded to the point at which peak effects of LAAM were experienced (8–12 hours).[53] Methadone, on the other hand, appeared more of a depressant with reduced arousal, reduced psychomotor activity, and worsened mood at time of peak effects compared to LAAM.

Crowley et al[60] examined physical activity in 12 LAAM patients and found that they were 50% more physically active on dosing days than non-dosing days ($p=0.001$). They subsequently confirmed these findings in an unblended cross-over comparison with methadone in which LAAM participants were required to attend the clinic daily and given placebo on non-dosing days.[61] In this study of 8 participants, LAAM patients' overall activity in the 14 hours after 7 am dosing was again 50% more on LAAM days than placebo days. The difference peaked at 6–8 hours after dosing (2–4 pm). Activity at this time of day was twice as much on LAAM dosing days as on non-dosing days. Patients reported more fatigue on placebo days, fewer ejaculations, and less vigor on the Profile of Mood Status (POMS). In other areas, mood disturbance was subtly (but statistically) higher with methadone than LAAM (on dosing or placebo days). Patients accurately guessed which days were active days but attended for dosing anyway to meet the requirements for the study (including a significant cash payment for completion of the study). Participants did not notice the difference in activity on dosing or non-dosing days. Marcovici et al[62] also reported that LAAM patients felt a stimulatory effect on the day of dosing and felt sluggish for the next 1 or 2 days.

A study by Newcombe et al[63] demonstrated that patients who metabolize methadone quickly, with resulting withdrawal symptoms between daily methadone doses, experience more stable opioid concentrations and less opioid withdrawal between doses with LAAM.

Withdrawal symptoms following cessation of LAAM

Following 14 days of LAAM in 10 subjects, abrupt cessation led to a mild withdrawal syndrome[7] similar to methadone withdrawal, peaking at 2 weeks after the last dose. Gradual reduction of LAAM in the following 4 patients did not reduce the severity of opiate withdrawal symptoms.

Blocking effects

LAAM produces dose-dependent blockade of hydromorphone. Twenty-five milligrams LAAM only partially blocked the effects of 12 mg hydromorphone whereas 75 mg LAAM effective blocked 12 mg hydromorphone for up to 96 hours.[64] Zaks and Feldman[65] found that 80 mg LAAM effectively blocked 50 mg heroin in 5 patients 24 hours after the LAAM dose (as did 100 mg methadone), whereas 30–40 mg doses of LAAM only blocked 50 mg heroin in 1 out of 4 patients. Levine et al[66] observed that 70–100 mg LAAM completely blocked 25 mg heroin in 6 patients at 72 hours after the last dose; at 50 mg patients did not perceive any effect from heroin but there was a small change in pupil diameter; at 30 mg LAAM 4 out of 6 felt the effects of heroin. Zaks et al[19] found that 9 subjects on LAAM were able to distinguish 30 mg morphine sulfate from placebo, particularly when it was administered 3–8 hours or 52–54 hours after the LAAM dose.

Acute and chronic pain

There is little experience with LAAM in chronic pain. Tennant[67] reported 4 cases in which LAAM was effective in managing chronic pain.

Potential for abuse

Initial reports by Fraser and Isbell suggested that intravenous LAAM produced no immediate reinforcing effects. At the same time that Fraser and Isbell were conducting their research, Keats and Beecher[6] were using subcutaneous LAAM (5–20 mg) 4 hourly. LAAM was providing effective immediate action analgesia, but caused significant respiratory depression in those who received enough doses. More recent work by Walsh[26] indicates that intravenous LAAM (20 and 40 mg) produces acute effects experienced within 5 minutes of administration and lasting as long as orally administered LAAM. Orally administered, 20 mg LAAM had a minimal effect, while 40 mg oral LAAM produced a measurable opiate effect which, after the first 4–6 hours, was of similar magnitude to that induced by 40 mg iv LAAM. The peak concentration of orally administered LAAM was at 3 hours post-administration, at which time levels were similar to those post iv administration. Initial concentrations by intravenous administration were 5- and 12-fold higher for 20 mg and 40 mg LAAM, respectively.

Dosing considerations

Induction from heroin

Induction from heroin is complicated by the long half-life of LAAM. Steady state is not achieved until 14 days after each dose adjustment. Initial doses greater than 40 mg have resulted in oversedation, and a non-prescribed dose of 75 mg was nearly fatal in one heroin user.[68] On the other hand, very cautious induction schedules have resulted in increased numbers of drop-outs early in treatment when compared with methadone. Some clinical trials have commenced heroin users on methadone first, others have started directly on LAAM using doses ranging from 10 to 60 mg.

Two RCTs have compared induction protocols (see Table 5.2), however they do not provide clear evidence of the best way of commencing LAAM. Ling et al[69] found that there was no advantage in routinely commencing with daily LAAM dosing or using methadone on non-dosing days during LAAM induction. Commencing with LAAM alone resulted in more drop-outs due to underdosing, but daily LAAM and LAAM plus methadone resulted in more drop-outs due to overmedication. They concluded that patients should be offered supplementary methadone or LAAM doses on non-dosing days during induction, but that these need not be routine. Jones et al[70] examined the rate of dose increases during induction. They found that starting at 30 mg and increasing each dose by 10 mg up to 100 mg resulted in a higher drop-out rate due to feelings of overmedication than starting at a stable 25 mg or starting at 30 mg and increasing each dose by 10 mg up to 50 mg. They concluded that dose increases should be individualized.

Judson and Goldstein[71] conducted a non-randomized comparison of a slow and a more rapid induction schedule. They found that the rapid induction schedule (commencing on 20 mg and increasing by 10 mg on most dosing days, i.e. alternate days up to 50 mg) did not result in over-sedation but retention in treatment was no better than a slower induction schedule.

Table 5.2 Studies examining induction from heroin

Study	*Methods*	*Participants*	*Interventions*	*Outcomes*	*Results*	*Notes*
Jones 1998[70]	Double-blind, RCT	180 opioid-dependent patients seeking maintenance treatment	3 different induction regimens, alternate daily dosing for 2 weeks then tiw for 2 weeks with the 3-day dose at 1.4 times the 2-day dose: (1) LAAM 25 mg; (2) LAAM 25 mg increasing by 5 mg every dose to 50 mg; (3) LAAM 25 mg, 30 mg then increasing by 10 mg every dose to 100 mg	Heroin use, withdrawal symptoms, retention, attendance for counseling, intoxication	High-dose group had higher drop-out rates	Same study as Eissenberg 1997
Ling 1984[69]	Double-blind, parallel group RCT	255 heroin addicts seeking maintenance treatment	4-week LAAM induction: (1) LAAM tiw commencing at 30 mg and increasing by 10 mg per week with each 3-day dose to 60 mg tiw with placebos on non-dosing ;or (2) same LAAM regimen but with 3 supplementary doses of LAAM each week, 20 mg week one, 10 mg week two and 5 mg week three; or (3) same tiw LAAM regimen as in (1) but with supplementary doses as with (2) but with methadone instead of LAAM	Heroin use, withdrawal symptoms, global evaluation by physicians	No difference between the groups	Two studies – one paper

(Continued)

Table 5.2 (*Continued*)

Study	*Methods*	*Participants*	*Interventions*	*Outcomes*	*Results*	*Notes*
Judson 1979[71]	Cohort study	179 street heroin addicts	Flexible induction with LAAM commencing with (1) a slow regimen ($n = 92$) starting with 20 mg and increasing by 10 mg every second dose to 75 mg; or (2) a faster regimen of 20, 30, 40, 40, 50 mg	Heroin use (urinalysis), actual doses received	55% of patients on the slow regimen requested more rapid dose induction	
Fudala 1997[27]	Cohort study	623 opioid-dependent patients, 439 on methadone for at least 30	Flexible induction according to proposed product label. For heroin users ($n = 93$) LAAM commenced at 20–30 mg increasing by 5–10 mg each dose. For methadone users ($n = 530$), LAAM commenced at 1.2	Retention, doses consumed	4% drop-out per week in first 4 weeks. Heroin induction dose increased to	

		days, 93 heroin users and 91 on methadone for less than 30 days	to 1.3 times the daily methadone dose, up to 100 mg		30–40 mg, initial maximum LAAM dose of 100 mg abandoned. Option to commence LAAM via methadone also added
Tennant 1986[72]	Cohort study	429 methadone patients, 429 street heroin users and 39 propoxyphene napsylate users	Flexible induction commencing with 20–25 mg LAAM increasing by 2–5 mg with each dose	Retention, side-effects	25% drop-out at 1 month. 2 deaths, 1 coma, and 1 footdrop during induction due to illicit drug use

tiw, three times weekly

Tennant et al[72] commenced 429 street heroin users on 20–25 mg LAAM, increasing by 2–5 mg each dose. It was the authors' impression that patients suffered significant withdrawal symptoms during this time and were regularly prescribed clonidine or guanabenz acetate. Four subjects overdosed during the first week of treatment from abuse of non-prescribed drugs. Two were commencing LAAM from heroin use and two from short-term methadone. Two subjects died and a third became comatose. Tennant concluded that withdrawal symptoms during the transfer increased the risk of non-prescribed drug use and subsequent overdose.

In the labeling assessment study[27] patients either commenced on methadone first or on 30–40 mg LAAM, increasing in 5–10 mg increments. This appeared well tolerated with no higher rate of drop-out occurring in the initial weeks of treatment.

LAAM product information suggests a starting dose of between 20 and 40 mg depending on the level of neuroadaptation, a second day dosing interval, and an individualized dose adjustment of 5–10 mg each dosing day. The evidence from published studies indicates that there is variability in the response to LAAM during induction and that fixed protocols will result in some patients dropping out due to over- or undermedication. Whether commencing LAAM straight from heroin or from heroin via methadone, flexible dosing with frequent review is likely to be the most effective approach.

Transfer from methadone

Two RCTs have specifically addressed patient transfer from methadone to LAAM. Ling et al[69] compared a straight transfer with one that included supplemental LAAM doses on non-dosing days and one that included supplemental methadone on non-dosing days during the first 3 weeks (see Table 5.3). The supplementation offered no advantage; rather, there were higher drop-out rates in the group with supplemental LAAM doses. In contrast, Whysner and Levine[73] found that LAAM supplementation was superior. It is difficult to interpret the results of these transfer studies as they used protocols in which doses were fixed for 2 to 3 weeks. In reality there are wide variations in the metabolism of both LAAM and methadone and frequent medical review and cautious dose adjustment is likely to be the most important factor in enabling smooth

Table 5.3 Studies examining transfer to LAAM from methadone

Study	*Methods*	*Participants*	*Interventions*	*Outcomes*	*Results*	*Notes*
Ling 1984[69]	Double-blind, parallel group, multicenter RCT	310 patients on various doses of methadone	Basic LAAM dose (BLD) was 1.0–1.2 × methadone dose but not exceeding 80 mg. (1) BLD was given tiw for 4 weeks; (2) BLD with supplementary LAAM dosing on BLD days of 20 mg in week 1, 15 mg in week 2 and 10 mg in week 3; or (3) BLD with supplementary methadone dosing on the day prior to BLD days of 20 mg in week 1, 15 mg in week 2, 10 mg in week 3	Retention, heroin use, symptoms	More drop-outs in group 2, slightly less heroin use in group 3	
Whysner 1978 Protocol III[73]	Parallel, 3 group RCT	424 patients on methadone	3 regimens consisting of various combinations of LAAM and methadone or LAAM alone	Retention, dose adjustments required	Not analyzed	Unpublished

transition between LAAM and methadone, avoiding the risk of over or under dosing.

Abrupt transfer from methadone to LAAM at 1:1 dose conversion with minimal dose adjustment in the SAODAP study was found to induce opiate withdrawal symptoms,[69] particularly on non-dosing days. This would be consistent with the low levels of active metabolites at this time, particularly nor-LAAM.

The labeling assessment study[27] used direct transfers from methadone to LAAM in 439 patients with a dose conversion of 1:1.2–1.3 and dose adjustments as necessary. They found that most patients on less than 40 mg methadone stabilized on a LAAM dose more than 1.3 times the methadone dose, while patients on methadone doses of more than 80 mg stabilized on LAAM doses less than 1.2 times the methadone dose. Methadone patients on 40–80 mg stabilized on LAAM doses 1.2–1.3 times the methadone dose.

Frequency of dosing

LAAM has been used on a daily, second-daily, three times a week, third-daily, and twice a week basis. Less frequent dosing has the advantage of less frequent attendance,[74] and the disadvantage of greater fluctuation in opiate levels between doses. Optimal dosing frequency is a balance between these two. Controlled trials of dosing frequency have been conducted. Karp-Gelernter et al[74] compared methadone and LAAM, with daily or second-daily attendance requirements. The study was double blind and methadone patients received take-home doses if attending second daily. In both the methadone and LAAM groups, there was a trend for better retention in the group attending less frequently.

Casadonte[75,76] offered twice-weekly dosing to patients maintained on LAAM. Of those who had requested twice-weekly LAAM and could be contacted 2 months later, 63% had elected to stay on twice-weekly dosing. Twice-weekly LAAM was compared to thrice-weekly LAAM in one randomized cross-over trial (see Table 5.4), however only a few patients completed the study. While this may have been due to the poor performance of twice-weekly LAAM, the investigators report the study being effectively sabotaged by the patients who saw LAAM as a threat to methadone take-away doses.

Table 5.4 Studies examining LAAM dosing frequency

Study	*Methods*	*Participants*	*Interventions*	*Outcomes*	*Notes*
Segal 1976[77]	Open label randomized cross-over design	9 methadone-maintained patients	(1) LAAM tiw @ 1 × meth dose and 1.3 × meth dose for Fridays; (2) LAAM twice weekly @ 1.3 × meth dose. Doses were adjusted if necessary	Retention, heroin use, withdrawal symptoms	Only one subject completed the study. Most withdrew complaining of withdrawal symptoms, although the authors suggest that the participants withdrew as they saw LAAM as a threat to methadone take-aways

Pharmacologic principles would suggest that more LAAM would be required for a 3-day dose than a 2-day dose. This is supported by initial studies that did not increase the Friday (3-day) dose and found that many participants found the 3-day dosing interval difficult. Subsequent studies gave 3-day doses of up to 50% greater than the 2-day dose.[33,78] In addition, the ability of LAAM doses to last for longer periods of time appears to be dose dependent. Houtsmuller et al[64] found that people on 75 mg LAAM were more likely to be able to tolerate 96 hours without dosing than people maintained on 25 mg.

A study by Newcombe et al[63] demonstrated that, for people who feel that methadone does not hold them for 24 hours, LAAM provides more stable opiate effects over 48 hours than methadone does over 24 hours.

Optimal maintenance doses

Three RCTs have compared different doses of LAAM (see Table 5.5). Eissenberg[79,80] compared Monday, Wednesday, and Friday doses of 25/25/35 mg, 50/50/70 mg, and 100/100/140 mg in 180 initiates to opioid-dependent substitution treatment using a double-blind, randomized parallel group design over 17 weeks. The higher LAAM doses resulted in fewer days of heroin use and higher rates of abstinence per month compared with the medium and low doses of LAAM.

Olivetto et al[81] compared 50/50/65 mg to 100/100/130 mg in 9 individuals using a double-blind, randomized cross-over design allowing 4 weeks for dose stabilization and 4 weeks for evaluation of each treatment. Participants in the high-dose LAAM group had fewer urine samples positive for opioids.

Naturalistic studies have also found that patients on higher LAAM doses use less heroin.[72,82] Valdivia et al[82] found that 63% of patients on doses above 96 mg were abstinent from heroin compared with 37% of those on less than 96 mg.

One of the reasons for the greater efficacy of higher doses may be the ability of higher doses of LAAM to more effectively block the effects of heroin use. Four studies have assessed the ability of LAAM to block heroin and other opiates. As expected, the ability to block the effect of opiates is dose dependent,[19,64,66] as has been described in the section on blocking effects.

Table 5.5 Studies comparing high-dose LAAM versus low-dose LAAM

Study	*Methods*	*Participants*	*Interventions*	*Outcomes*
Eissenberg 1997[79]	Double-blind, parallel group RCT	180 opioid-dependent volunteers seeking treatment	17 weeks of thrice weekly LAAM at (1) 25/25/35 mg; (2) 50/50/70 mg; (3) 100/100/140 mg	Retention, heroin use
Houtsmuller 1998[64]	Residential behavioral laboratory study, open label LAAM, blind hydromorphone challenges	16 dependent street heroin users	6 weeks outpatient LAAM dosing at (1) 25 mg alternate days or (2) 75 mg alternate days followed by 5 weeks inpatient at the same doses for hydromorphone challenges	Responses to hydromorphone challenges
Olivetto 1998[81]	Double-blind cross-over RCT	9 methadone-maintained patients	8 weeks of (1) LAAM 165 mg/week or (2) LAAM 330 mg/week then reverse	Heroin use and withdrawal symptoms in the second 4 weeks of each treatment cycle

Withdrawal from LAAM maintenance

Given the long terminal elimination half-life of LAAM and its active metabolites, it might be expected that LAAM withdrawal would be milder than withdrawal from heroin or methadone. It might also be expected that withdrawal symptoms would last for a longer period of time. No studies have directly compared the withdrawal syndromes from methadone, heroin, and LAAM in this way. One study has examined the withdrawal syndrome following LAAM maintenance therapy (50/50/65 mg dose)[83] (see Table 5.6). A randomized double-blind comparison of a gradual 15-week reduction of 4 mg per week with a sudden cessation of LAAM treatment in the final week in preparation to commence naltrexone was used.[83] Participants (n = 107) in both groups were given placebo when the LAAM dose reached zero. As would be expected, the gradual-reduction group experienced an increase in opiate withdrawal before the sudden-cessation group, although there was no difference in peak severity of opiate withdrawal or heroin use between the two groups. The peak severity of withdrawal during LAAM cessation in both groups was fairly mild, about the same as that measured during the first week of LAAM induction from heroin. A higher rate of transition to naltrexone (46% vs 24%, $p > 0.05$) with the abrupt-transition group was reported. In spite of this, at 12-month follow-up, 42% of each group had not used heroin in the previous month.

Table 5.6 Study comparing gradual versus rapid detoxification from LAAM maintenance

Study	*Methods*	*Participants*	*Interventions*	*Outcomes*
Judson 1983[83]	Double-blind parallel group RCT	119 patients in a 'pre-naltrexone detoxification program'	(1) 23 weeks LAAM 50/50/65 mg followed by 4 weeks placebo; (2) 4 weeks of LAAM 50/50/65 mg gradually reducing over the next 19 weeks then 4 weeks placebo	Retention, withdrawal symptoms, depression, transition to naltrexone, heroin use 1 year later

Efficacy of LAAM

Comparison with placebo, detoxification, or no treatment

There has been only one study comparing LAAM with no treatment. Conducted in a prison setting, Kinlock et al[84] conducted a study in which patients were randomly allocated to LAAM treatment pre-release or the control intervention of advice to take up opioid agonist treatment on leaving prison. Of 33 participants who were randomly allocated to LAAM, 20 commenced LAAM, and 19 entered community-based agonist maintenance treatment, compared to 3 of 31 controls. Although there were clinically significant reductions in heroin use and crime in the LAAM group, the differences were not statistically significant for this sample size.

Comparison with methadone

Most studies comparing methadone and LAAM have been small and unable to demonstrate a statistically significant difference between the two treatments (see Tables 5.7–5.10). The more important studies of LAAM are discussed below in detail, followed by a review of meta-analyses and other studies. Initial clinical trials used DAAM which, although also a long-lasting opioid, has a different pharmacologic profile and the results are not discussed here.

The VA Cooperative study was the first multisite study using LAAM.[21] It was a double-blind RCT comparing fixed doses of methadone, 50 mg and 100 mg daily, with 80 mg LAAM (Monday, Wednesday, and Friday) in 430 dependent street heroin users at Veterans' Affairs hospitals. All groups started at 30 mg LAAM or methadone and increased by 10 mg each week to their allocated dose. Being a double-blind study, participants attended each day for dosing even if they were in the LAAM group, although, at the physician's discretion, both groups were able to receive take-home doses, with placebo doses for the LAAM group after week 12 of treatment. Unfortunately, the ability of patients to determine which treatment group they were in was not reported.

The study found more people dropped out of the LAAM 80 mg group than the methadone 100 mg group (69% vs 48%, $p<0.05$) and that the LAAM 80 mg and methadone 100 mg groups were more effective in controlling heroin use than the methadone 50 mg group. The methadone

Table 5.7 Methadone versus LAAM fixed-dose RCTs

Study	*Methods*	*Participants*	*Interventions*	*Outcomes*	*Safety*	*Notes*
Goldstein 1974[20]	Mixed open/ blind parallel group RCT	80 male and 20 female outpatients (although the female participants were subsequently withdrawn) in a methadone clinic	13 weeks: (1) methadone (6 days per week) 50 mg daily, or (2) LAAM tiw (open and blind groups) at 75 mg MWF, later 100 mg on Friday	Retention, heroin use, side-effects		Quality score = 6; incomparable LAAM and methadone dosing schedule
Ling 1976[21]	Double-blind, parallel group RCT	430 street-heroin-dependent outpatients	40 weeks: (1) 50 mg methadone, (2) 100 mg methadone, (3) 80 mg LAAM 3 × per week, with placebo on intervening days, take-aways according to US policy	Retention, heroin use, drug safety (biochemical markers), side-effects	No LAAM deaths. 8 LAAM patients ceased due to side-effects, one with fatigue and chest pains	Quality score = 6; not included in the analysis; incomparable LAAM and methadone dosing schedule

MWF, Monday, Wednesday, Friday

Table 5.8 Methadone versus LAAM flexible dose studies

Study	*Methods*	*Participants*	*Interventions*	*Outcomes*	*Notes*
Freedman 1981[88]	Single-blind parallel group RCT	48 male employed methadone patients, no severe physical disorders	52 weeks: (1) LAAM at 1.3 × methadone dose Mon, Wed and 50% higher Fri dose, or (2) daily methadone. Flexible dosing (minimum needed to prevent withdrawal symptoms), methadone patients were able to get weekend take-aways	Heroin use, retention, preference	Quality score (out of 16) = 6
Johnson 2000[85]	Double-blind, parallel group RCT, methadone vs buprenorphine vs LAAM	220 dependent street heroin users	13 weeks: (1) LAAM tiw and (2) methadone daily low dose (20 mg), (3) high-dose methadone and (4) daily buprenorphine	Heroin use, retention	Quality score = 10; buprenorphine and low-dose methadone groups excluded
Karp-Gelernter 1982[74]	Double-blind, parallel group RCT, 2 × 2 factorial design (methadone vs LAAM, daily vs 3 × per week dosing)	95 male opioid-dependent outpatients, stabilized on methadone	40 weeks, flexible dosing with (1) LAAM or (2) methadone at a dispensing frequency of (1) daily or (2) thrice weekly with 1:1 LAAM:methadone dose ratio initially, 3-day dose 5–10 mg higher than 2-day dose	Heroin use, retention, safety	Quality score = 8; both the two methadone groups and the two LAAM groups were pooled for the analysis

(*Continued*)

Table 5.8 (*Continued*)

Study	*Methods*	*Participants*	*Interventions*	*Outcomes*	*Notes*
Ling 1978[22]	Open label, parallel group RCT	636 male heroin-dependent outpatients, stabilized for at least 1 month on methadone (mean 59.5 mg)	40 weeks flexible dosing with (1) thrice weekly LAAM or (2) daily methadone, up to 100 mg, higher Friday LAAM dose if necessary	Retention, heroin use, symptoms, and side-effects	Quality score = 9
Lehmann 1976[89]	Mixed open/blind parallel group RCT	42 heroin-dependent outpatients in a detoxification program in Norwalk, Connecticut, between 16 and 21 years old	16 weeks of (1) methadone daily in doses sufficient to maintain a comfortable state, or (2) LAAM (10 mg) every third day either open or blinded with placebo	Heroin use, subjective experience of medication, work performance, athletic involvement	Quality score = (unable to be determined); not used in the analysis due to inadequate data
Longshore 2005[34]	Open label, parallel group RCT	315 heroin-dependent outpatients	26 weeks flexible dosing with (1) LAAM (n = 209) or (2) methadone (n = 206)	Heroin use, retention	Subsequent 52 week analysis[22] Quality score = 12

Ritter 2003[78]	Open label, parallel group RCT	99 methadone-maintained outpatients in clinic and community setting	52 weeks flexible dosing with (1) LAAM (with the option of switching to methadone) or (2) methadone	Heroin use, retention	Quality score = 11
Ritter 2001[91]	Open label, parallel group RCT	76 dependent street heroin users, outpatients in clinic and community setting	52 weeks flexible dosing with (1) LAAM (with the option of switching to methadone) or (2) methadone	Heroin use, retention	Quality score = 12
Savage 1976[92]	Double-blind, cross-over design RCT	99 male dependent street heroin users	26 weeks of (1) daily methadone or (2) three times a week LAAM at 1.3 x methadone dose with placebo on intervening days then reverse. Take-aways given under some circumstances	Heroin use, retention	Quality score = 7; first 3 months only used in the meta-analysis

(Continued)

Table 5.8 (*Continued*)

Study	*Methods*	*Participants*	*Interventions*	*Outcomes*	*Notes*
Senay 1974[18]	Double-blind, parallel group RCT	157 male dependent street heroin users	48 weeks flexible dosing: (1) LAAM (mean dose 93.9 mg) 3 x per week with full services; (2) methadone (mean dose 51.7 mg) daily with full services; (3) methadone (mean dose 70.9 mg) daily with no support services	Heroin use, retention, employment, crime	Quality score = 6; comparison between LAAM (full services) and methadone (full services) only. Methadone (minimal services) group excluded
Senay 1977[93]	Open-label, parallel group RCT	193 males aged 21–50 with at least 2 years heroin addiction recruited from the Illinois Drug Abuse Program Central Intake facility, stable on methadone for at least 3 months	14 weeks maintenance treatment. After an initial dose of methadone (1) 6 days a week methadone at a methadone clinic; (2) thrice weekly LAAM at a LAAM clinic. Flexible dosing, 10 mg more LAAM on Fridays, than Mondays and Wednesdays	Retention, heroin use, crime, employment, symptoms and side-effects	Quality score = 6

White 2002[94]	Open label, cross-over design RCT	62 methadone maintained outpatients	13 weeks flexible dosing with (1) daily methadone or (2) alternate daily LAAM then 3 months cross-over then 6 months drug of choice	Heroin use, retention, preference, quality of life	Quality score = 6; first 3 months only used in the meta-analysis
Whysner 1978[73]	Open label RCT	1341 methadone maintained or street heroin dependent users	40 weeks of (1) methadone ($n = 525$) or (2) thrice weekly LAAM ($n = 816$). LAAM flexible dosing commencing at 20 mg, increasing by 10 mg per week or 1.2 x methadone dose	Retention, heroin use	Quality score = 5; multicenter study, largely unpublished. The only data adequate for meta-analysis were published by the VA Drug Dependence Treatment and Research Centre, Philadelphia (Marcovici 1981), which reported on the 130 participants at their site

(Continued)

Table 5.8 (*Continued*)

Study	*Methods*	*Participants*	*Interventions*	*Outcomes*	*Notes*
Zaks 1972[19]	Open label, parallel group RCT	20 male opioid-dependent outpatients, >21 years of age, with >2 year duration of treatment, and >1 treatment failure, all treated with decreasing doses of methadone as an inpatient prior to the study, i.e. drug-free for 1 week	26-week study flexible dosing with (1) thrice weekly LAAM or (2) daily methadone. Initially inpatient, then daily attendance for 1 month, followed by 2–3 × week attendance for 5 months. Methadone doses all 100 mg with 5 take-home doses per week; pickup 2 × per week. LAAM doses 30–80 mg LAAM with no take-aways	Retention, heroin use, cross-tolerance, withdrawal symptoms, side-effects, behavioral change	Quality score = 6

Table 5.9 Methadone/LAAM controlled prospective studies

Study	*Methods*	*Participants*	*Interventions*	*Outcomes*	*Notes*
Grevert 1977[95]	Controlled prospective study	30 LAAM-treated outpatients at an opioid maintenance clinic and 31 methadone-matched controls	13 weeks of (1) LAAM or (2) methadone maintenance	Memory	Quality score = 4; not included in meta-analysis as no comparable outcome measure
Irwin 1976[96]	Controlled prospective study, 3 group, patient selecting parallel design	85 dependent street heroin users and 24 non-addicted volunteers	34 weeks, 3 treatment groups: (1) methadone daily, (2) LAAM daily, and (3) LAAM alt daily	Retention, dosing levels, side-effects	Quality score = 0; daily LAAM used in one group. Not included in meta-analysis due to inadequate data
Resnick 1982[97]	Controlled prospective study	19 dependent street heroin users	8 months of (1) thrice weekly LAAM or (2) daily methadone (one take-away per week), patient selected, with the option of switching medication at any time	Retention	Quality score = 0

Table 5.10 Methadone versus LAAM cross-sectional comparative studies

Study	*Methods*	*Participants*	*Interventions*	*Outcomes*	*Notes*
Casadonte 1996[98]	Opportunistic retrospective comparison of LAAM vs methadone as a result of changes in clinic prescribing practices	94 patients at a clinic in New York, 17 on LAAM (from heroin), 18 on methadone (from heroin) – retrospective control, 19 on LAAM (from methadone), and 40 still on methadone	tiw LAAM vs daily methadone (2 takeaway per week), 6-month follow-up	Preference, cocaine use, side-effects	
Irwin 1976[59]	Cross-sectional study of a matched group of methadone-maintained and LAAM-maintained subjects	20 methadone and 21 LAAM maintenance subjects matched for age, sex, race, and years of opiate use	Methadone (17.9 months mean); LAAM (8 months mean) preceded by methadone (13.9 months mean)	EEG, cognitive performance, biochemistry	
Lenné 2001[99]	Cross-sectional study	10 methadone, 13 LAAM, and 11 buprenorphine patients, and 21 age-matched controls	Alcohol challenge	Driving simulation task	No differences in driving skills across the four groups
Rosenberg 2002[100]	Cross-sectional survey	265 substance misuse service users	All substance misuse services	Availability and acceptability	

100 mg group and the LAAM 80 mg group used similar amounts of heroin during the study, with a trend for less heroin use with LAAM in the final month. Once stabilized on medication, there were fewer morphine-positive urines on LAAM 80 mg than methadone 100 mg at 24 weeks and 40 weeks. The main reason given by patients stopping LAAM was 'medication not holding' and this was thought to be due, in part, to the slow induction schedule and the lack of dose increase for the 3-day dose.

The SAODAP study was an open label RCT comparing LAAM with methadone in 636 methadone patients.[22] To reduce the rate of drop-out due to fixed dosing schedules, flexible methadone and LAAM dosing was used. As an open label study, LAAM patients were able to attend on a three times a week basis, enabling a more realistic assessment of treatment with LAAM compared to methadone. While there were no LAAM take-away doses, the methadone group was able to get take-away doses, in some cases up to 6 days a week, depending on the treating physician and the policy of the clinic. There was a marked difference in retention between the two groups, with 60% of the methadone group completing the study compared with 39% for the LAAM group. Almost one third of the LAAM patients who dropped out of the study gave as their reason that the medication was not holding. This accounted for almost all the differences in retention between the groups. Heroin use in those who were still in the study was similar, although there were more LAAM patients who were abstinent throughout the study.

The authors ascribed some of the poor retention on LAAM to the (a) lack of flexibility in dosing by doctors who were still reluctant to increase LAAM doses for three-day doses; (b) the lack of 'take-aways'; and (c) a perception that LAAM was 'bad' by patients.

The study by Johnson et al is significant in that it is the only study comparing methadone, LAAM, and buprenorphine. It was a double-blind RCT involving 220 heroin users seeking opioid substitution treatment.[85] In addition to the three treatment groups there was a low-dose methadone 'control' group. Participants were randomized equally to the four groups. Treatment was initiated according to a fixed protocol and then adjusted according to pre-established criteria based on clinic attendance and urine results. Mean maximal doses of LAAM (2-day dose), methadone, and buprenorphine (2-day dose) were 100 mg, 90 mg, and 27 mg, respectively. All participants attended 3 days a week and received take-home doses of methadone or placebo on the remaining days.

Retention and heroin use between LAAM, high-dose methadone, and buprenorphine were similar and better than for low-dose (20 mg) methadone. As a four-group study, the sample size was too small to detect small to moderate differences in treatment efficacy and there were no statistically significant differences between high-dose methadone, LAAM, and buprenorphine. These findings were consistent with other studies. Study retention was better with methadone than buprenorphine or LAAM (73% vs 58% vs 53%) and there was a trend for fewer opioid-positive urines with LAAM than methadone or buprenorphine (52% vs 62% vs 62%).

The most recent, and perhaps the final, study comparing LAAM and methadone is a study conducted in California.[34,86,87] It is was an open label study of 315 dependent opioid users randomized in a 2:1 ratio to LAAM or methadone with excellent participant follow-up rates (over 90%). The study was high quality with well-conducted treatment (as indicated by the high retention rate overall) and the use of intention to treat analysis (with high follow-up rates of those not in treatment). The rates of retention in treatment at 6 months did not differ by group (75.5% for the LAAM group and 77% for methadone group), and there was significantly less illicit opioid use (as indicated by positive urine tests) in the LAAM group both during the study (40% vs 60%) and at the 6-month follow-up time point (30.8% vs 60.2%) ($p > 0.01$).

As the only methodologically sound study to date with sufficient sample size to detect clinically significant differences in treatment outcome, the study of Longshore et al[34] validates the findings of the Cochrane meta-analysis that LAAM is more effective than methadone and that the findings of lesser retention with LAAM in earlier studies need to be interpreted with caution.

Meta-analyses

There have been three meta-analyses published comparing methadone and LAAM; one by Glantz et al in 1997,[101] the Cochrane review published in 2002,[33] and a study by Farré et al,[102] also published in 2002. The study by Glantz et al[101] included 12 RCTs, with a total of 1622 participants included in the analysis, although it appears that the outcome of one group of 40 participants[103] was also reported in a separate publication[21] and was counted twice. This meta-analysis found no significant difference in heroin use with LAAM (risk difference 0.01, NS) and greater retention in methadone treatment (risk difference 0.13, $p<0.003$). More LAAM patients discontinued due to side-effects (risk difference 0.04, $p<0.0001$). However, this meta-analysis suffers from a significant methodologic flaw in the handling of urinalysis data,[33] not all relevant studies were included in the review.

The meta-analysis by Farré et al[102] included only double-blind studies that met their quality criteria and, as a result, only included three studies (524 participants), one which used DLAAM (dextro/levo-alpha-acetylmethadol) instead of LAAM.[14] The other two were the multicenter VA Co-operative study,[21] and a third study which was really one site of the VA study, effectively being counted twice.[103] The meta-analysis was dominated by the VA Cooperative study,[21] which was much larger than the other two, and the findings are essentially consistent with the findings of the VA Cooperative study.

Cross-over studies

Cross-over studies can be a powerful way of comparing the effects of medications where there is significant variation between individuals in the response to treatment, because they make within-subject comparisons. There are two cross-over trials comparing methadone and LAAM. The first, conducted in Veterans Administration hospitals in Baltimore in the early 1970s,[92] was a double-blind study treating 99 patients over 6 months, but only between-subject comparisons were made in the analysis. The second study was conducted in South Australia.[94] This was an open label study involving 62 subjects, also over a 6-month period. In the 42 who completed the study, there were significantly fewer days in which heroin was used per month with LAAM than methadone (0.7 vs 2.6 days). There were also fewer hair samples containing evidence of heroin use. Sixty-nine percent of participants stated a preference for LAAM, citing as the main reasons less withdrawal symptoms (39%), fewer side-effects (28.5%), less cravings for heroin (18%), and fewer pick-up days (14%). In this study, LAAM patients also demonstrated more vitality on the SF-36 health outcome survey than methadone patients.

Two non-randomized cross-over studies have also addressed preference for LAAM or methadone. Casadonte[98] treated all new patients with LAAM for a period of time. Of the 35 who had previously been on methadone, 72% of them preferred LAAM, reporting that they did not 'feel' LAAM the way they felt methadone. Deutsch et al[104] examined 44 patients at the completion of a LAAM study and found 'strong preferences' for LAAM on 13 of the 16 treatment characteristics. Eighty percent of patients chose to continue on LAAM at the end of the study.

LAAM instead of methadone take-home doses

One of the proposed benefits of LAAM is a reduction in take-home doses or 'take-aways'. Methadone take-home doses are occasionally associated with fatal overdoses, either for the person to whom they were dispensed, other drug users, or occasionally to young children.[105,106] In addition, when LAAM was being developed, many clinics in North America were not open on Sundays and so they had difficulties dispensing medication to people who had not qualified for methadone take-aways. The two RCTs that have addressed this issue are described in Table 5.11. The first, a pilot study by Jaffe et al,[16] administered a LAAM dose 1.2 times the methadone dose on Fridays with placebos on Saturday and Sunday over a series of three weekends. After the first 3-day LAAM dose, some of the LAAM group complained of mild withdrawal symptoms and the ratio was increased to an average of 1.3 (range 1.2 to 1.5).

The second study[107] compared daily methadone (with take-home doses) to Monday–Thursday methadone and Friday LAAM (initially at the same dose as methadone) in 136 patients over 40 weeks. Although 35% of the LAAM group completed the study, there were more patients who ceased the study in the LAAM group (65% vs 47%), with the majority citing 'medication not holding' as the reason for ceasing. There was also more heroin use and withdrawal symptoms in the LAAM group. It is not clear to what extent these results reflect the difficulties in giving a single 3-day LAAM dose once a week or whether it was just that the doses were inadequate. Most clinics were reluctant to increase LAAM doses despite patients complaining of withdrawal symptoms.[22]

More recently, Valdivia and Raza[109] evaluated the withdrawal symptoms over the 48-hour dosing interval in patients receiving a 2-day LAAM dose on Saturday as an alternative to methadone take-aways. The subjective and objective withdrawal features and cravings before the Saturday dose were

Table 5.11 Studies of LAAM versus methadone take-home doses

Study	*Methods*	*Participants*	*Interventions*	*Outcomes*	*Notes*
Jaffe 1971[15]	RCT, double-blind	10 methadone-maintained patients	1 weekend of (1) methadone on Saturday and a take-home dose for Sunday or (2) LAAM on Saturday (same as methadone dose) and a take-home placebo for Sunday followed by 2 weekends of (1) Friday methadone dose and 2 take-home doses or (2) Friday LAAM dose (1.2 × methadone dose) and placebo take-home doses	Withdrawal symptoms	3-day LAAM dose at 1.2 times the 2-day dose felt to be inadequate and increased up to 1.5 times the 2-day dose
Ling 1980[107]	RCT	136 methadone-maintained patients	40 weeks of (1) methadone (2) methadone (Monday–Thursday) + LAAM (Friday). Methadone take-away doses according to clinic policy for both groups	Retention, withdrawal symptoms, heroin use	Retention better in the methadone group (53% vs 35%), most dropouts due to medication not holding. More heroin use and withdrawal symptoms in the LAAM group
Casadonte 1999[108]	Case series	61 patients seeking opioid detoxification	30-day outpatient opioid reduction using methadone (Monday to Friday) and LAAM (Saturday)		

measured and compared with the withdrawal features before the Monday methadone dose. Sixty participants received methadone Monday to Friday and LAAM Saturday using a methadone:LAAM dose conversion of 1:1.2. The sum of the withdrawal and cravings scores was less in the LAAM group. Valdivia later reported[109] that the practice of giving a Saturday LAAM dose to methadone patients was incorporated into routine practice at the VA clinic he directed in Illinois. In New York, Casadonte[108] was routinely using LAAM instead of a Sunday take-home methadone dose in patients undergoing a 30-day outpatient detoxification. The first 61 patients given LAAM had no problem with LAAM, with 57% transferred to LAAM maintenance when abandoning their detoxification attempt.

LAAM for opiate detoxification

Two studies have addressed this issue (see Table 5.12). The long duration of action of LAAM may offer advantages over shorter-acting agents in the management of heroin withdrawal. Sorensen et al[110] conducted a 4-group, double-blind randomized comparison of methadone with LAAM over 3 or 6 weeks (n=61). Withdrawal severity was similar with LAAM and methadone. Both LAAM groups experienced similar levels of opiate withdrawal when nearing the end of LAAM treatment. A second study was conducted by Lehman[89] in the 1970s, although it was unpublished except in brief summary form. A small number of young heroin users were given low-dose LAAM or methadone to withdraw from heroin in a residential setting. Both approaches were reported as being successful.

LAAM for methadone 'failure'

There are a number of recent case series in the US which demonstrate the effectiveness of LAAM as a second-line agent. Malkerneker[111] converted 20 methadone 'failures' to LAAM and reported a reduction in heroin use from a mean of 18.76 days in the month prior to the transfer, to 10 days in the month following. Opioid withdrawal symptoms between doses were also reduced. Borg et al[112] found that 4 out of 12 patients who had been unable to cease heroin use with methadone were able to with LAAM. Tennant[113] found that 9 out of 10 patients who were unable to stabilize on methadone due to low trough methadone levels were able to stabilize on LAAM without additional drug use.

Table 5.12 Detoxification studies – methadone vs LAAM

Study	*Methods*	*Participants*	*Interventions*	*Outcomes*	*Notes*
Lehmann 1976[89]	Mixed open/blind parallel group RCT	42 dependent heroin users aged between 16 and 21	Residential treatment: (1) methadone daily in doses sufficient to maintain a comfortable state, (2) LAAM (10 mg) every third day, sometimes with placebo in between	Heroin use, subjective experience of medication, work performance	
Sorensen 1982[110]	4-group RCT, blind to drug but not dose regimen	61 male dependent opiate injectors	(1) Methadone 3 weeks commencing at 40 mg; (2) methadone 6 weeks; (3) LAAM 3 weeks commencing at 40 mg; (4) LAAM 6 weeks commencing at 40 mg	Retention, drug use, withdrawal symptoms	No real differences between the groups

Safety of LAAM

Life-threatening cardiac arrhythmias

Ultimately, it has been concerns about the safety of LAAM, not its efficacy, that have removed LAAM from the European and the United States markets. LAAM is one of many medications that have been withdrawn in recent years because of concerns about potential life-threatening arrhythmias due to QT prolongation. Medications that prolong the QT interval increase the amount of time it takes for cardiac cells to repolarize in preparation to receive the signal to contract. Thus cardiac cells will be vulnerable to aberrant electrical pathways initiating muscle contraction, and may result in unsynchronized cardiac muscle contraction. This form of ventricular tachycardia, referred to as *torsades de pointes,* can be fatal.

Initial studies did not detect a significant effect of LAAM on cardiac conduction, although ECGs were conducted only in a minority of studies. Slight QT prolongation was first noticed in 1993, but it was not thought to be of clinical significance.[114] A prolonged QT of 8 milliseconds was again reported in 1998,[115] but was again thought to be clinically insignificant. Reports of cardiac arrhythmias, in particular *torsades de pointes*, led to the issue being re-examined.[30,31]

On 11 April 2001, the manufacturer of LAAM in the US, Roxanne Laboratories, issued a statement confirming that they had received reports of seven cases of known or suspected *torsades de pointes* and three additional cases of symptomatic arrhythmia associated with a prolonged QT interval that had been submitted via ongoing safety surveillance activities. These were the only reports from an estimated 33,000 patients treated with LAAM, with some of these known to have had other risk factors for cardiac disease and arrhythmias including cocaine use.[31]

Subsequent studies have confirmed a small but definite QT prolonging effect of LAAM.[32,116–118] It appears that it is LAAM itself, rather than its active metabolites, which is responsible for the prolongation of the QT interval, raising the possibility of the use of nor-LAAM as an alternative treatment. Although the risks of QT prolongation are small in comparison to the risks of untreated opioid dependence, it appears that pharmaceutical companies are reluctant to promote products with QT prolongation effects.

Other adverse effects

LAAM repeatedly produces unwanted opioid effects including sleepiness, sweating, constipation, reduced sexual function, nausea and vomiting.[83] The evidence for the prevalence of common adverse events comes from the larger randomized trials, the studies by Whysner and Levine,[73] and the labeling assessment study.[27] Non life-threatening adverse effects were common, including difficulty sleeping (55%), constipation (54%), and excessive sweating (43%). These are also common in methadone-maintained patients.

In the VA Cooperative study of 430 patients,[21] there were no LAAM deaths. Eight LAAM patients ceased due to side-effects, one with fatigue and chest pains which were deemed not to be study drug related, others due to difficult ejaculation, swollen joints, nausea, and vomiting. There was no difference in side-effects for patients between treatment with methadone or LAAM.

In the SOADAP study of 636 patients[22] there were two LAAM deaths in the LAAM group, with one due to gunshot wound and the other due to alcohol toxicity, and 11 terminations for side-effects such as constipation, nausea, headache, allergy, sexual problems, speediness, hyperactivity, hallucinations, and patient irritability/anxiety about not taking daily medication. Side-effects of speediness, hyperactivity, and hallucinations have not traditionally been reported with methadone and may represent specific effects of LAAM. There is some evidence from a variety of sources to support a differential effect of LAAM and methadone on mood.[53,59–61,119]

In the study conducted by Whysner and Levine involving more than 3,000 participants[73] a systematic analysis of side-effects was not published. A preliminary paper on 1,267 patients on LAAM indicated that only 2% of patients in this group stopped taking LAAM due to side-effects or adverse reactions. Overall, five deaths were observed in the first week of LAAM treatment.[24]

In the Australian National Evaluation of Pharmacotherapies for Opioid Dependence (NEPOD) project, a meta-analysis of recent Australian studies in which 115 patients were treated with LAAM and over one thousand patients with methadone, buprenorphine, and naltrexone, there was no evidence of significant differences in serious adverse event rates between methadone, LAAM, and buprenorphine, with most of the deaths occurring in people who had ceased treatment.[120]

Other studies have found a slight (2%) decrease in red blood cell hemoglobin.[121,122] Individual studies have found a 1% increase in systolic and diastolic blood pressure,[121] a slight increase in liver transaminases,[122] and a 14% increase in blood sugar with LAAM compared to methadone;[13] these results are of uncertain significance. LAAM and methadone may both raise immunoglobulin levels, the clinical significance of which is also uncertain.[123]

Other studies indicate that LAAM does not appear to have a significant effect on memory[101] or induce human chromosome damage,[124] and is not associated with abnormalities on EEGs.[13]

When taken regularly as prescribed, LAAM does not appear to impact on driving safety,[51] either alone or in combination with alcohol (up to the legal limit).

Deaths

The main cause of death for illicit opioid users is overdose leading to respiratory depression.[125] While LAAM probably reduces this risk significantly, there have been a number of deaths of patients on LAAM. Sedation and fatal overdose can occur with all full μ agonists, particularly in combination with other sedatives such as alcohol and benzodiazepines. As with methadone, the high-risk period for overdoses is during induction to treatment.[126,127] Fatalities during induction from heroin have been reported for a range of treatment protocols including after daily consecutive LAAM dosing (20, 30, 40, and 50 mg), following two doses of 40 mg and 50 mg, and following two doses of 30 mg and 40 mg with 10 mg methadone in between. Deaths following transfer from methadone appear to be due to excessive LAAM dosing, but in all of these cases, other sedative medications or alcohol were also found in the blood.[68,128]

In randomized trials identified in this review of LAAM there were 5 deaths out of 760 patients who commenced LAAM (one death was an overdose during the first week of treatment, the others were violent deaths or due to alcohol-induced liver failure) and one death out of 755 patients who started the trials on methadone. The largely unpublished Whysner study[24] found a mortality rate of 1.3% per annum in a cohort of 3042 patients,[24,129–131] which was similar to contemporary American methadone cohorts of 1.5% to 2% per annum. These mortality rates are consistent with estimates of mortality in other samples of methadone patients and are lower than for heroin users not in treatment.[24,129–131]

Potential for abuse

Safety may also be compromised if a maintenance drug has high potential for abuse, leading to diversion and intravenous use. Initial reports by Fraser and Isbell[7,9] suggested that intravenous LAAM produced no immediate reinforcing effects. This has been contradicted by early research in which subcutaneous LAAM (5–20 mg) was used for acute pain[6] and more recent work by Walsh et al[26] indicating that intravenous LAAM (20 and 40 mg) doses produce acute effects experienced within 5 minutes of administration and last for the same duration as orally administered LAAM. Initial plasma concentrations by intravenous administration of 20 and 40 mg LAAM were respectively 5- and 12-fold higher than the same dose orally. There is no evidence of widespread abuse of LAAM either in clinical trials of opioid dependence or since registration in the US.

Conclusion

LAAM has many characteristics that would seem to make it an ideal opioid substitution treatment. It can be taken every second or third day, and its long duration of action provides a stable opioid effect between doses. For these reasons, there was a considerable research effort in the US to have LAAM made available as an alternative to methadone. LAAM was registered in the US in the absence of a pharmaceutical company to pursue its development. Recent studies and meta-analysis of earlier studies have confirmed the findings of some of the earlier studies indicating less heroin use with LAAM.[34,78,94,132] In addition, most of those who have taken both LAAM and methadone indicate a preference for LAAM. Although earlier studies showed higher rates of dropping out of treatment with LAAM, this appears to have been due to treatment and study design factors and has not been replicated in recent studies.

Despite this evidence of its increased efficacy over methadone, LAAM was only slowly taken up in the US after registration, probably related more to regulatory and funding issues than to the efficacy of LAAM itself.

Since the QT prolongation effects of LAAM became apparent, LAAM has been withdrawn from European markets, and although still registered in the US, production has ceased. LAAM is one of many useful drugs withdrawn in recent years for QT prolongation and an association with *torsades de pointes*. Although there is little doubt that LAAM has the potential to cause life-threatening cardiac arrhythmias, it is unclear just what this risk is in any given individual. Mortality studies certainly do not indicate an obvious risk above that expected in patients on methadone maintenance. On the other hand, if there was reason to believe that a particular patient or group of patients would benefit from LAAM treatment over other available treatments, the small risk of an arrhythmia would be a reasonable one to take.

There have been some recent calls from prominent researchers in the US for LAAM to make a comeback,[133] although with the availability of office-based buprenorphine now in the US, the potential demand for LAAM as an alternative to methadone is uncertain. Meanwhile, opioid agonist treatment is expanding in regions of Eastern Europe and Asia, as the full extent of the injection-driven HIV epidemic has become clear. Perhaps in some of the states in this region, where authorities have been reluctant to approve the take-home use of methadone or buprenorphine, there will once again be a role for LAAM.

References

1. Chen KK. Pharmacology of methadone and related compounds. Annals New York Sci 1948; 51: 83–97.
2. Isbell H, Wickler A, Eisenman AJ, Daingerfield M, Frank E. Liability of addiction to 6-dimethylamino-4-4-diphenyl-3-hepatone in man. Arch Intern Med 1948; 82: 362–92.
3. Pohland A, Marshall FJ, Carney TP. Optically activite compounds related to methadone. J Am Chem Soc 1949; 71: 460–2.
4. Speeter ME, Byrd WM, Cheney LC, Binkley SB. Analgesic carbinols and esters related to amidone (methadone). J Am Chem Soc 1949; 71: 57–60.
5. Eddy NB, Touchberry CF, Lieberman JE, Khazan N. Synthetic analgesics. 1 Methadone isomers and derivatives. J Pharmacol Exp Ther 1950; 98: 121–37.
6. Keats AS, Beecher HK. Analgesic activity and toxic effects of acetylmethadol isomers in man. J Pharmacol Exp Ther 1952; 105: 210–15.
7. Fraser H, Isbell H. Actions and addiction liabilities of alpha-acetylmethadols in man. J Pharmacol Exp Ther 1952; 105(4): 458–65.
8. Billings RE, McMahon RE, Blake DA. l-Acetylmethadol (LAM) treatment of opiate dependence: plasma and urine levels of two pharmacologically active metabolites. Life Sci 1974; 14: 1437.

9. Fraser HF, Nash TL, Vanhorn GD, Isbell H. Use of miotic effect in evaluating analgesic drugs in man. Arch Int Pharmacodyn Ther 1954; 98: 443–51.
10. Isbell H, Fraser HF. Addictive properties of methadone derivatives. J Pharmacol Expl Ther 1954; 13: 369–70.
11. David NA, Semler HJ, Burgner PR. Control of chronic pain by d-l-alpha-acetylmethadol. JAMA 1956; 161: 599–603.
12. Dole V, Nyswander M. A medical treatment for diacetylmorphine (heroin) addiction. JAMA 1965; 193: 80–4.
13. Blachly PH, David NA, Irwin S. L-Alpha-acetylmethadol (LAM): comparison of laboratory findings, electroencephalograms, and Cornell Medical Index of patients stabilized on LAM with those on methadone. 1972 [proceedings]. NIDA Res Monogr, 1976: 57.
14. Jaffe JH, Senay EC, Schuster CR, Renault PR, Smith B, DiMenza S. Methadyl acetate vs methadone. A double-blind study in heroin users. JAMA 1972; 222(4): 437–42.
15. Jaffe JH, Senay EC. Methadone and l-methadyl acetate. Use in management of narcotics addicts. JAMA 1971; 216(8): 1303–5.
16. Jaffe JH, Schuster CR, Smith BB, Blachley PH. Comparison of acetylmethadol and methadone in the treatment of long-term heroin users. A pilot study. JAMA 1970; 211(11): 1834–6.
17. Jaffe JH, Schuster CR, Smith BB, Blachly PH. Comparison of dl-alpha-acetylmethadol and methadone in the treatment of narcotics addicts. Pharmacologist 1969; 11(2): 256.
18. Senay EC, Jaffe JH, DiMenza S, Renault PR. A 48-week study of methadone, methadyl acetate, and minimal services. In: Fisher S, Freedman AM, eds. Opioid Addiction: Origins and Treatment. Washington: V.H. Winston & Sons, 1974.
19. Zaks A, Fink M, Freedman AM. Levomethadyl in maintenance treatment of opiate dependence. JAMA 1972; 220: 811–13.
20. Goldstein A, Judson BA. Three critical issues in the management of methadone programs. In: Bourne PG, ed. Addiction. NY: Academic Press, 1974: 129–48.
21. Ling W, Charuvastra C, Kaim SC, Klett CJ. Methadyl acetate and methadone as maintenance treatments for heroin addicts. A Veterans Administration Cooperative study. Arch Gen Psychiat 1976; 33(6): 709–20.
22. Ling W, Klett CJ, Gillis R. A cooperative clinical study of methadyl acetate. 1. Three-times-a-week regimen. Arch Gen Psychiat 1978; 35: 345–53.
23. Trueblood B, Judson BA, Goldstein A. Acceptability of methadyl acetate (LAAM) as compared with methadone in a treatment program for heroin addicts. Drug Alcohol Depen 1978; 3(2): 125–32.
24. Thomas DB, Whysner JA, Newmann MC. The phase III clinical evaluation of LAAM: I. Comparative epidemiology of mortality in LAAM and methadone. NIDA Res Monogr 1979; 27: 289–95.
25. Whysner JA, Thomas DB, Ling W, Charuvastra C. On the relative efficacy of LAAM and methadone. NIDA Res Monogr 1979; 27: 429–33.
26. Walsh SL, Johnson RE, Cone EJ, Bigelow GE. Intravenous and oral l-alpha-acetylmethadol: pharmacodynamics and pharmacokinetics in humans. J Pharmacol Exp Ther 1998; 285(1): 71–82.

27. Fudala PJ, Vocci F, Montgomery A, Trachtenberg AI. Levomethadyl acetate (LAAM) for the treatment of opioid dependence: a multisite, open-label study of LAAM safety and an evaluation of the product labeling and treatment regulations. J Maint Addict 1997; 1(2): 9–39.
28. Goldstein A, Judson B. Can the community be protected against the hazards of take-home methadone? NIDA Res Monogr 1976(8): 62–3.
29. Kreek MJ, Vocci FJ. History and current status of opioid maintenance treatments: blending conference session. J Subst Abuse Treat 2002; 23(2): 93–105.
30. Schwetz BA. From the Food and Drug Administration. JAMA 2001; 285(21): 2705.
31. Deamer RL, Wilson DR, Clark DS, Prichard JG. Torsades de pointes associated with high dose levomethadyl acetate (ORLAAM). J Addict Dis 2001; 20(4): 7–14.
32. Huber A, Ling W, Fradis J, Charavastra C. Comparison of the effects of methadone and LAAM on the human electrocardiogram. Drug Alcohol Depen 2001; 63(Suppl 1): S70.
33. Clark N, Lintzeris N, Gijsbers A, et al. LAAM maintenance vs methadone maintenance for heroin dependence (Cochrane Review). Cochrane Database Syst Rev 2002; 2.
34. Longshore D, Annon J, Anglin MD, Rawson RA. Levo-alpha-acetylmethadol (LAAM) versus methadone: treatment retention and opiate use. Addiction 2005; 100(8): 1131–9.
35. National Health and Medical Research Council. A Guide to the Development, Implementation and Evaluation of Clinical Practice Guidelines. Canberra: National Health and Medical Research Council, 1998.
36. Huang W, Bemis PA, Slawson MH, Moody DE. Determination of l-alpha-acetylmethadol (LAAM), norLAAM, and dinorLAAM in clinical and in vitro samples using liquid chromatography with electrospray ionization and tandem mass spectrometry. J Pharm Sci 2003; 92(1): 10–20.
37. Neff JA, Moody DE. Differential N-demethylation of l-alpha-acetylmethadol (LAAM) and norLAAM by cytochrome P450s 2B6, 2C18. and 3A4. Biochem Biophys Res Commun 2001; 284(3): 751–6.
38. Oda Y, Kharasch ED. Metabolism of levo-alpha-acetylmethadol (LAAM) by human liver cytochrome P450: involvement of CYP3A4 characterized by atypical kinetics with two binding sites. J Pharmacol Exp Ther 2001; 297(1): 410–22.
39. Oda Y, Kharasch ED. Metabolism of methadone and levo-alpha-acetylmethadol (LAAM) by human intestinal cytochrome P450 3A4 (CYP3A4): potential contribution of intestinal metabolism to presystemic clearance and bioactivation. J Pharmacol Exp Ther 2001; 298(3): 1021–32.
40. Moody DE, Walsh SL, Rollins DE, Neff JA, Huang W. Ketoconazole, a cytochrome P450 3A4 inhibitor, markedly increases concentrations of levo-acetyl-alpha-methadol in opioid-naive individuals. Clin Pharmacol Ther 2004; 76(2): 154–66.
41. BioDevelopment Corporation. Levomethadyl acetate hydrochloride oral solution (ORLAAM) – for the management of opiate dependence – information for physicians. BioDevelopment Corporation, 1994.
42. Henderson GL. Pharmacodynamics of LAAM in man: plasma levels of LAAM and its metabolites following acute and chronic administration in man (fourth

and sixth quarter progress reports). 1974–5 [proceedings]. NIDA Res Monogr 1976; 8: 64–5.
43. Henderson GL, Wilson BK, Lau DH. Plasma l-alpha-acetylmethadol (LAAM) after acute and chronic administration. Clin Pharmacol Ther 1977; 21(1): 16–25.
44. Finkle BS, Jennison TA, Chinn DM, Ling W, Holmes ED. Plasma and urine disposition of 1-alpha-acetylmethadol and its principal metabolites in man. J Anal Toxicol 1982; 6(2): 100–5.
45. The pharmacokinetics of LAAM, norLAAM and dinorLAAM following oral dosage of LAAM. CPDD 1994; 1994. NIDA.
46. Kharasch ED, Whittington D, Hoffer C, et al. Paradoxical role of cytochrome P450 3A in the bioactivation and clinical effects of levo-alpha-acetylmethadol: importance of clinical investigations to validate in vitro drug metabolism studies. Clin Pharmacokinet 2005; 44(7): 731–51.
47. Iribarne C, Picart D, Dreano Y, Berthou F. In vitro interactions between fluoxetine or fluvoxamine and methadone or buprenorphine. Fundam Clin Pharmacol 1998; 12(2): 194–9.
48. McCance-Katz EF, Rainey PM, Smith P, et al. Drug interactions between opioids and antiretroviral medications: interaction between methadone, LAAM, and nelfinavir. Am J Addict 2004; 13(2): 163–80.
49. McCance-Katz EF, Rainey PM, Friedland G, Kosten TR, Jatlow P. Effect of opioid dependence pharmacotherapies on zidovudine disposition. Am J Addict 2001; 10(4): 296–307.
50. McCance-Katz EF, Rainey PM, Smith P, et al. Drug interactions between opioids and antiretroviral medications: interaction between methadone, LAAM, and delavirdine. Am J Addict 2006; 15(1): 23–34.
51. Lenne MG, Dietze P, Rumbold GR, Redman JR, Triggs TJ. The effects of the opioid pharmacotherapies methadone, LAAM and buprenorphine, alone and in combination with alcohol, on simulated driving. Drug Alcohol Depen 2003; 72(3): 271–8.
52. Clark NC, Dietze P, Lenne MG, Redman JR. Effect of opioid substitution therapy on alcohol metabolism. J Subst Abuse Treat 2006; 30(3): 191–6.
53. Sollod RM, Goldstein MG. Rx: 3x/week LAAM: alternative to methadone. Clinical studies: Phase I. NIDA Res Monogr 1976; 8: 39–51.
54. Resnick RB, Orlin L, Geyer G, Schuyten-Resnick E, Kestenbaum RS, Freedman AM. l-Alpha-acetylmethadol (LAAM): prognostic considerations. Am J Psychiat 1976; 133(7): 814–19.
55. Eissenberg T, Stitzer ML, Bigelow GE, Buchhalter AR, Walsh SL. Relative potency of levo-alpha-acetylmethadol and methadone in humans under acute dosing conditions. J Pharmacol Exp Ther 1999; 289(2): 936–45.
56. Brandt MR, Cabansag SR, France CP. Discriminative stimulus effects of l-alpha-acetylmethadol (LAAM), buprenorphine and methadone in morphine-treated rhesus monkeys. J Pharmacol Exp Ther 1997; 282(2): 574–84.
57. Vaupel DB, Jasinski DR. l-alpha-acetylmethadol, l-alpha-acetyl-N-normethadol and l-alpha-acetyl-N,N-dinormethadol: comparisons with morphine and methadone in suppression of the opioid withdrawal syndrome in the dog. J Pharmacol Exp Ther 1997; 283(2): 833–42.

58. Kaiko RF, Inturrisi CE. Disposition of acetylmethadol in relation to pharmacologic action. Clin Pharmacol Ther 1975; 18(1): 96–103.
59. Irwin S, Kinohi RG, Cooler PM, Bottomly DR. Acute time-dose-response effects of cyclazocine, methadone, and methadyl in man. 1975 [proceedings]. NIDA Res Monogr 1976; 8: 70–1.
60. Crowley TJ, Jones RH, Hydinger-Macdonald MJ, Lingle JR, Wagner JE, Egan DJ. Every-other-day acetylmethadol disturbs circadian cycles of human motility. Psychopharmacology (Berl) 1979; 62(2): 151–5.
61. Crowley TJ, Macdonald MJ, Wagner JE, Zerbe G. Acetylmethadol versus methadone: human mood and motility. Psychopharmacology (Berl) 1985; 86(4): 458–63.
62. Marcovici M, O'Brien C, McLellan AT, Kacian J. A clinical controlled study of L-alpha-acetylmethadol in the treatment of narcotic addiction. Am J Psychiat 1981; 138(2): 234–6.
63. Newcombe DA, Bochner F, White JM, Somogyi AA. Evaluation of levo-alpha-acetylmethdol (LAAM) as an alternative treatment for methadone maintenance patients who regularly experience withdrawal: a pharmacokinetic and pharmacodynamic analysis. Drug Alcohol Depen 2004; 76(1): 63–72.
64. Houtsmuller EJ, Walsh SL, Schuh KJ, Johnson RE, Stitzer ML, Bigelow GE. Dose-response analysis of opioid cross-tolerance and withdrawal suppression during LAAM maintenance. J Pharmacol Exp Ther 1998; 285(2): 387–96.
65. Zaks A, Feldman M. Private methadone maintenance. Analysis of a program after one year. JAMA 1972; 222(10): 1279–80.
66. Levine R, Zaks A, Fink M, Freedman AM. Levomethadyl acetate: prolonged duration of opioid effects, including cross-tolerance to heroin. In: Blaine JD, Renault PF, eds. Rx: 3x/week LAAM, Alternative to Methadone. NIDA Research Monograph Series. Rockville, Maryland: National Institute on Drug Abuse, 1976.
67. Tennant F. Alpha-acetylmethadol for treatment of chronic pain patients who abuse opiads. Drug Alcohol Depen 1983; 1983(12): 243–7.
68. Chinn DM, Finkle BS, Crouch DJ, Jennison TA. The biodisposition of l-alpha-acetyl methadol and its principal metabolites: some fatal and nonfatal cases. J Anal Toxicol 1979; 3: 143–9.
69. Ling W, Dorus W, Hargreaves WA, Resnick R, Senay E, Tuason VB. Alternative induction and crossover schedules for methadyl acetate. Arch Gen Psychiat 1984; 41(2): 193–9.
70. Jones HE, Strain EC, Bigelow GE, et al. Induction with levomethadyl acetate: safety and efficacy. Arch Gen Psychiat 1998; 55(8): 729–36.
71. Judson BA, Goldstein A. Levo-alpha-acetylmethadol (LAAM) in the treatment of heroin addicts. I. Dosage schedule for induction and stabilization. Drug Alcohol Depen 1979; 4(6): 461–6.
72. Tennant FS Jr, Rawson RA, Pumphrey E, Seecof R. Clinical experiences with 959 opioid-dependent patients treated with levo-alpha-acetylmethadol (LAAM). J Subst Abuse Treat 1986; 3(3): 195–202.
73. Whysner JA, Levine GL. Phase III clinical study of LAAM: report of current status and analysis of early terminations. NIDA Res Monogr 1978; 19: 277–90.

74. Karp-Gelernter E, Savage C, McCabe OL. Evaluation of clinic attendance schedules for LAAM and methadone: a controlled study. Int J Addict 1982; 17(5): 805–13.
75. Effective maintenance treatment of opioid dependence with twice weekly LAAM dosing. Proceedings from the 59th Annual Scientific Meeting of the College on Problems of Drug Dependence, Inc.; 1997. NIDA.
76. Casadonte P, O'Donnell E, Rotrosen JP. Effective maintenance treatment of opioid dependence with twice weekly LAAM dosing. Proceedings from the 59th Annual Scientific Meeting of the College on Problems of Drug Dependence, Inc. 1997.
77. Segal R, Everson A, Sellers EM, Thakur R. Failure of acetylmethadol in treatment of narcotic addicts due to nonpharmocological factors. CMA Journal 1976; 115: 1014–16.
78. Ritter AJ, Lintzeris N, Clark N, Kutin JJ, Bammer G, Panjari M. A randomized trial comparing levo-alpha acetylmethadol with methadone maintenance for patients in primary care settings in Australia. Addiction 2003; 98(11): 1605–13.
79. Eissenberg T, Bigelow GE, Strain EC, et al. Dose-related efficacy of levomethadyl acetate for treatment of opioid dependence. A randomized clinical trial. JAMA 1997; 277(24): 1945–51.
80. Effective medical treatment of heroin addiction. NIH consensus development conference. Program and abstracts. National Institutes of Health, 1997.
81. Oliveto AH, Farren C, Kosten TR. Effect of LAAM dose on opiate use in opioid-dependent patients. A pilot study. Am J Addict 1998; 7(4): 272–82.
82. Valdivia JF, Khattak S. Effects of LAAM and methadone utilization in an opiate agonist treatment program. Mt Sinai J Med 2000; 67(5–6): 398–403.
83. Judson BA, Goldstein A, Inturrisi CE. Methadyl acetate (LAAM) in the treatment of heroin addicts. II. Double-blind comparison of gradual and abrupt detoxification. Arch Gen Psychiat 1983; 40(8): 834–40.
84. Kinlock TW, Battjes RJ, Schwartz RP. A novel opioid maintenance program for prisoners: report of post-release outcomes. Am J Drug Alcohol Ab 2005; 31(3): 433–54.
85. Johnson RE, Chutuape MA, Strain EC, Walsh SL, Stitzer ML, Bigelow GE. A comparison of levomethadyl acetate, buprenorphine, and methadone for opioid dependence. N Engl J Med 2000; 343(18): 1290–7.
86. LAAM and methadone maintenance treatment: retention, drug use and HIV risk behaviors. Problems of Drug Dependence, 2000: Proceedings from the 62nd Annual Scientific Meeting of the College on Problems of Drug Dependence, Inc. 2001. NIDA.
87. Annon J, Longshore D, Rawson R, Anglin MD. LAAM and methadone maintenance treatment: retention, drug use and HIV risk behaviors. Problems of Drug Dependence, 2000: Proceedings from the 62nd Annual Scientific Meeting of the College on Problems of Drug Dependence, Inc. 2001; 181.
88. Freedman RR, Czertko G. A comparison of thrice weekly LAAM and daily methadone in employed heroin addicts. Drug Alcohol Depend 1981; 8: 215–22.
89. Lehmann WX. The use of 1-alpha-acetyl-methadol (LAAM) as compared to methadone in the maintenance and detoxification of young heroin addicts. 1973 [proceedings]. NIDA Res Monogr 1976(8): 82–3.

90. Anglin MD, Conner BT, Annon J, Longshore D. Levo-alpha-acetylmethadol (LAAM) versus methadone maintenance: 1-year treatment retention, outcomes and status. Addiction 2007; 102(9): 1432–42.
91. Ritter A, Lintzeris N, Clark N, Kutin J, Bammer G. A randomised trial of buprenorphine maintenance in primary care office-based settings: clinical guidelines, training programs and efficacy. Drug Alcohol Depen 2001; 63(Suppl 1): S131.
92. Savage C, Karp EG, Curran SF, Hanlon TE, McCabe OL. Methadone/LAAM maintenance: a comparison study. Compr Psychiat 1976; 17(3): 415–24.
93. Senay EC, Dorus W, Renault PF. Methadyl acetate and methadone. An open comparison. JAMA 1977; 237: 138–42.
94. White JM, Danz C, Kneebone J, La Vincente SF, Newcombe DA, Ali RL. Relationship between LAAM-methadone preference and treatment outcomes. Drug Alcohol Depen 2002; 66(3): 295–301.
95. Grevert P, Masover B, Goldstein A. Failure of methadone and levomethadyl acetate (levo-alpha-acetylmethadol, LAAM) maintenance to affect memory. Arch Gen Psychiat 1977; 34(7): 849–53.
96. Irwin S, Blachly PH, Marks J, Carlson E, Loewen J, Reade N. The behavioral, cognitive and physiologic effects of long-term methadone and methadyl treatment. 1973 [proceedings]. NIDA Res Monogr 1976; 8: 66–7.
97. Resnick RB, Washton AM, Garwood J, Perzel J. LAAM instead of take-home methadone. NIDA Res Monogr 1982; 41: 473–5.
98. Casadonte P, Butler P, Rostrosen J, et al. Integration of LAAM into an opiate substitution treatment program. CPDD 1996: NIDA, 1996: 144.
99. Lenné M, Lintzeris N, Breen C, et al. Withdrawal from methadone maintenance treatment: prognosis and participant perspectives. Aust NZ J Public Health 2001; 2: 121–5.
100. Rosenberg H, Melville J, McLean PC. Acceptability and availability of pharmacological interventions for substance misuse by British NHS treatment services. Addiction 2002; 97: 59–65.
101. Glanz M, Klawansky S, McAullife W, Chalmers T. Methadone vs. l-alpha-acetylmethadol (LAAM) in the treatment of opiate addiction. A meta-analysis of the randomized, controlled trials. Am J Addict 1997; 6(4): 339–49.
102. Farré M, Mas A, Torrens M, Moreno V, Cami J. Retention rate and illicit opioid use during methadone maintenance interventions: a meta-analysis. Drug Alcohol Depen 2002; 65(3): 283–90.
103. Panell J, Charuvastra VC, Ouren J. Methadyl acetate versus methadone: the experience of one hospital. Med J Aust 1977; 2(5): 150–2.
104. Deutsch SI, Huber A, Rawson RA, et al. Opiate treatment options: patients prefer LAAM. CPDD 1997: NIDA, 1998: 315.
105. Spadari M, Arditti J, Affaton MF, David JM, Valli M. [Accidental narcotic and buprenorphine poisoning in children notified at the Marseille Poison Center between 1993 and 1999]. Therapie 2000; 55(6): 705–8.
106. Robinson BJ, Kwiterovich P, Lietman P, Vavich J. The hazard of narcotics in the home: accidental ingestion by infants and young children. J Pediatr 1971; 79(4): 688–90.

107. Ling W, Klett JC, Gillis RD. A cooperative clinical study of methadyl acetate. II. Friday-only regimen. Arch Gen Psychiat 1980; 37(8): 908–11.
108. LAAM and methadone maintenance treatment: retention, drug use and HIV risk behaviors. Problems of Drug Dependence, 1999: Proceedings from the 61st Annual Scientific Meeting of the College on Problems of Drug Dependence, Inc. 1999. NIDA.
109. Valdivia J, Raza S. Utilization of LAAM in the Management of Methadone Take-Home Doses. Problems of Drug Dependence, 1999: Proceedings from the 61st Annual Scientific Meeting of the College on Problems of Drug Dependence, Inc.: NIDA, 2000.
110. Sorensen JL, Hargreaves WA, Weinberg JA. Withdrawal from heroin in three or six weeks: comparison of LAAM versus methadone. NIDA Res Monogr 1982; 41: 230–1.
111. Abstinence and occurrence of withdrawal symptoms in methadone failure patients converted to LAAM. CPDD 1996; 1996. NIDA.
112. Borg L, Ho A, Wells A, Joseph H, Appel P, Moody D, et al. The use of levo-alpha-acetylmethadol (LAAM) in methadone patients who have not achieved heroin abstinence. J Addict Dis 2002; 21(3): 13–22.
113. Tennant F Jr. LAAM maintenance for opioid addicts who cannot maintain with methadone. CPDD: NIDA, 1987: 294.
114. Kampman K, Bartzokis G, Lange R, Nuite Belleville A, Nademanee K, Beckson M, et al. LAAM and methadone maintenance treatment: retention, drug use and HIV risk behaviors. Problems of Drug Dependence, 1993: Proceedings from the 55th Annual Scientific Meeting of the College on Problems of Drug Dependence, Inc.: NIDA, 1994: 381.
115. Kut J, Valdivia J, Parikh B. LAAM and EKG changes. CPDD. Scottsdale, 1998: 76.
116. Kang J, Chen XL, Wang H, Rampe D. Interactions of the narcotic l-alpha-acetylmethadol with human cardiac K+ channels. Eur J Pharmacol 2003; 458(1–2): 25–9.
117. Katchman AN, McGroary KA, Kilborn MJ, et al. Influence of opioid agonists on cardiac human ether-a-go-go-related gene K(+) currents. J Pharmacol Exp Ther 2002; 303(2): 688–94.
118. Wedam EF, Bigelow GE, Johnson RE, Nuzzo PA, Haigney MC. QT-interval effects of methadone, levomethadyl, and buprenorphine in a randomized trial. Arch Intern Med 2007; 167(22): 2469–75.
119. Karp-Gelernter E, Wurmser L, Savage C. Therapeutic effects of methadone and 1-alpha-acetylmethadol. Am J Psychiat 1976; 133: 955–7.
120. Digiusto E, Shakeshaft A, Ritter A, O'Brien S, Mattick RP. Serious adverse events in the Australian National Evaluation of Pharmacotherapies for Opioid Dependence (NEPOD). Addiction 2004; 99(4): 450–60.
121. Blaine JD, Renault PR, Thomas DB, Whysner JA. Clinical status of methadyl acetate (LAAM). Ann NY Acad Sci 1981; 362: 101–15.
122. Wilson BK, Spannagel V, Thomson CP. The use of l-alpha-acetylmethadol in treatment of heroin addiction: an open study. Int J Addict 1976; 11(6): 1091–100.

123. Matsuyama SS, Charuvastra VC, Ouren J, Schwartz J, Jarvik L. Immunoglobulin levels in heroin addicts after treatment with methadone and methadyl acetate. Drug Alcohol Depen 1980; 6(5): 345–8.
124. Matsuyama SS, Charuvastra VC, Jarvik LF, Fu TK, Sanders K, Yen FS. Chromosomes in patients receiving methadone and methadyl acetate. Arch Gen Psychiat 1978; 35(8): 989–91.
125. Goldstein A, Herrera J. Heroin addicts and methadone treatment in Albuquerque: a 22-year follow-up. Drug Alcohol Depend 1995; 40(2): 139–50.
126. Caplehorn JRM. Deaths in the first two weeks of maintenance treatment in NSW in 1994: identifying cases of iatrogenic methadone toxicity. Drug Alcohol Rev 1998; 17: 9–17.
127. Drummer OH, Syrjanen M, Opeskin K, Cordner S. Deaths of heroin addicts starting on a methadone maintenance programme [letter] [see comments]. Lancet 1990; 335(8681): 108.
128. Schecter A, Kauders F. Patient deaths in a narcotic antagonist (naltrexone) and l-alpha-acetylmethadol program. Am J Drug Alcohol Ab 1975; 2(3–4): 443–9.
129. Gronbladh L, Ohlund LS, Gunne LM. Mortality in heroin addiction: impact of methadone treatment. Acta Psychiatr Scand 1990; 82(3): 223–7.
130. Concool B, Smith H, Stimmel B. Mortality rates of persons entering methadone maintenance: a seven-year study. Am J Drug Alcohol Ab 1979; 6(3): 345–53.
131. Zanis DA, Woody GE. One-year mortality rates following methadone treatment discharge. Drug Alcohol Depend 1998; 52(3): 257–60.
132. Clark N, Ritter A, Lintzeris N, Kutin J, Bammer G. Office-based LAAM maintenance for opioid dependence: a randomised comparison with methadone. Drug Alcohol Depen 2001; 63(Suppl 1): S28.
133. Jaffe JH. Can LAAM, like Lazarus, come back from the dead? Addiction 2007; 102(9): 1342–3.

chapter 6

The place of buprenorphine in the management of opioid dependence

Richard P. Mattick, Courtney Breen, and Amy Gibson

Introduction

Buprenorphine is a partial agonist at μ opioid receptors and has been used extensively in pain management. Its use in the management of opioid dependence has occurred in the last decade although its potential has been recognized from the late 1970s.[1] Buprenorphine provides several advantages in the management of opioid dependence. The medication has a good margin of safety,[2] and its partial agonist effect reduces buprenorphine's ability to cause the fatal respiratory depression which is associated with ingestion of full agonist opioids.[3] This margin of safety allows multiples of the daily dose to be dispensed less than daily.[4–8] This has provided an advantage over methadone, which cannot be safely administered in multiples of the daily dose due to fatal overdose risk.

The elimination of buprenorphine in humans comprises a relatively short distribution half-life of 3 to 5 hours[9] and a long terminal elimination half-life of 32 hours or more.[10] The medication binds very tightly to receptor sites, causing a very slow release from opioid receptors, and this property produces the kinetics that are important in bringing about the long duration of action.[11] This strong binding to opioid receptor sites has also been observed in studies of pure opioid antagonists which show that it is quite difficult to displace buprenorphine from opioid receptors once it is bound.[12,13]

The tightness of binding of buprenorphine to, and slow dissociation from, opioid receptor sites has been one explanation for the low level of withdrawal symptoms associated with abrupt cessation of chronic dosing with buprenorphine compared with other opioids such as morphine.[11] Others have considered whether the partial agonist effect of buprenorphine may reduce the extent of significant physical dependence (or neuroadaptation) and that this may be the mechanism whereby less severe withdrawal symptoms occur.[1] Although the withdrawal syndrome from buprenorphine may be less severe than from full agonists,[14,15] research into the nature and severity of withdrawal from buprenorphine maintenance remains limited.

The relative ease of cessation gives buprenorphine a role in allowing individuals to be either (a) stabilized on buprenorphine and to be maintained on it; or (b) to withdraw from it without the severity of withdrawing directly from heroin or methadone. Randomized research has shown that the buprenorphine is as effective in managing withdrawal as clonidine (see Chapter 3). If an individual continues taking buprenorphine, they may easily transfer to methadone[16] if that appears to be a more appropriate treatment. This flexibility of stabilization and detoxification, or stabilization and maintenance, either on buprenorphine or subsequently on methadone, offers an advantage given the ambivalence concerning methadone maintenance treatment sometimes expressed in the community. In summary, the less than daily dosing, the safety profile, and the relative ease of withdrawal from buprenorphine provide a number of interesting advantages over full agonist therapies (such as methadone) for the management of opioid dependence.

Buprenorphine products

There are two buprenorphine products approved for use in the treatment of opioid dependence: the mono product, a sublingual tablet containing buprenorphine hydrochloride, and the combination product, a sublingual tablet containing buprenorphine hydrochloride and naloxone hydrochloride in a ratio of 4:1.

Buprenorphine compared to methadone or placebo

Reviews of the studies comparing methadone and buprenorphine in the management of opioid dependence have been published elsewhere.[17–19] As methadone is an effective treatment, it is an appropriate comparison treatment for buprenorphine. The first section reviews early clinical trials of the mono product using an ethanol-based sublingual solution, which has a slightly higher bioavailability than the marketed sublingual tablet formulation.[20,21] The following section reviews trials using the mono product tablet preparation. Trials comparing buprenorphine to placebo and evidence from trials of the combination product are also reported.

Clinical trials comparing buprenorphine solution with methadone

The first randomized double-blind trial comparing buprenorphine with methadone was conducted by Bickel and colleagues.[22] The participants were stabilized on relatively low doses of either buprenorphine (2 mg) or methadone (30 mg) for 3 weeks followed by a reduction over 4 weeks. There were no differences between treatment groups with respect to retention, symptom report, or reduction of illicit opioid use, although the outcomes for both groups were poor. Buprenorphine was less effective than methadone in its ability to attenuate the physiologic and subjective effects of a hydromorphone challenge. The short duration and low doses in the trial limited interpretation of the results.

In a 6-month randomized double-blind trial using higher doses of buprenorphine, Johnson and colleagues[23] allocated participants to three treatment groups: 8 mg buprenorphine, 20 mg methadone, or 60 mg methadone. The 20 mg methadone group showed significantly poorer retention than the other groups, while there was no difference in retention between the buprenorphine and the methadone 60 mg groups. Buprenorphine treatment yielded significantly more morphine-free urine results than either 20 mg or 60 mg of methadone. The authors concluded that 8 mg buprenorphine was at least as effective as 60 mg methadone per day, and that both were superior to 20 mg methadone in reducing illicit opioid use and maintaining patients in treatment.

Subsequently, Kosten and his colleagues reached less clear conclusions when they compared two relatively low doses of sublingual buprenorphine (2 mg or 6 mg) with methadone maintenance (35 mg or 65 mg).[24] There was less illicit opioid use in the 6 mg buprenorphine group than in the 2 mg buprenorphine group, as demonstrated by urinalysis and patient self-report. Continued opioid withdrawal symptoms in the 2 mg buprenorphine group suggested that on average, this is not an adequate maintenance dose. Participants in methadone treatment had better retention, more opioid-free urine samples, and better 3-week abstinence results than those in buprenorphine treatment. The authors and others[25] were critical of the low buprenorphine doses used in the study, especially considering the suggestion of a dose–response relationship for buprenorphine. The fixed (rather than flexible) dose regimen also provided little information about the relative dose equivalence of buprenorphine and methadone.

Clearer conclusions were reached by Strain and colleagues, who used higher doses of buprenorphine in their 26-week study of buprenorphine and methadone dose-equivalence. They used a flexible dose regimen after initial stabilization on 8 mg buprenorphine or 50 mg methadone.[26] Patients could increase or decrease their dose up to a maximum 90 mg methadone or 16 mg buprenorphine. The mean doses achieved were 8.9 mg buprenorphine and 54 mg methadone. There were no differences between buprenorphine and methadone in: the number of dose increases requested, participants completing the induction/maintenance phase, treatment retention, the number of opioid-positive urine samples, and compliance with medication and counseling. These data suggested that an 8 mg dose of buprenorphine was similar to a moderate dose of methadone.

Importantly, in a literature where replication is limited, Strain and colleagues repeated the same study design in a group of patients who were using both opioids and cocaine.[27] This time, average daily doses were 11.2 mg of buprenorphine and 66 mg of methadone, with half the patients receiving the maximum dose possible (90 mg methadone or 16 mg buprenorphine). Again, both methadone and buprenorphine were equally effective in reducing illicit opioid use, in treatment retention, and in compliance with the attendance and counseling. Both groups showed significant decreases in cocaine-positive urines.

In another fixed dose study, Ling and colleagues reached less clear conclusions when they compared 30 mg methadone, 80 mg methadone, and 8 mg buprenorphine doses in opioid-dependent individuals.[28] The 80 mg methadone dose was found to be superior to both 30 mg methadone and 8 mg buprenorphine in retaining patients in treatment, reducing illicit opioid use, and decreasing craving for opioids. The 30 mg methadone and 8 mg buprenorphine doses were largely equivalent, and there were no differences in the occurrence of adverse events. Ling and colleagues noted that 8 mg buprenorphine was not an optimal dosage, and that higher doses would probably provide a better outcome. They also noted the discrepancy between their results and those of earlier research,[23] and pointed out the need to use effective and flexible rather than pre-determined doses of buprenorphine.

Schottenfeld and colleagues used fixed doses to compare buprenorphine (12 or 4 mg) and methadone (65 or 20 mg) in a 6-month, double-blind clinical trial.[29] They reported no significant differences in retention rates or cocaine use between treatment groups. Rates of opioid-positive toxicology tests were lowest for the 65 mg of methadone group followed by the 12 mg buprenorphine group, 20 mg methadone group, and 4 mg buprenorphine group.

Oliveto and colleagues also recruited opioid-dependent cocaine users in their 13-week study, and allocated them to desipramine hydrochloride (a tricyclic antidepressant) or placebo in addition to 12 mg buprenorphine or 65 mg methadone.[30] There were no significant differences in retention between the four treatment groups. Analysis showed that opioid abstinence was obtained more quickly with methadone treatment and cocaine abstinence obtained more quickly with buprenorphine treatment. Opioid abstinence was obtained more quickly in patients with high plasma desipramine levels regardless of opioid medication type. Buprenorphine was not considered more effective than methadone in reducing opioid use, and the authors agreed that more flexible dosing levels would assist in optimizing abstinence. Again, the problem of fixed doses was a limitation.

Flexible dosing was used in a study comparing thrice-weekly buprenorphine (16 to 32 mg on Mondays and Wednesdays, 24 to 48 mg on Fridays), thrice-weekly levomethadyl acetate (75 to 115 mg), high-dose daily methadone (60 to 100 mg), and low-dose (20 mg) daily methadone maintenance treatment.[31] The retention in study treatment was significantly higher for those receiving LAAM, buprenorphine, or high-dose methadone in comparison to low-dose methadone. LAAM, buprenorphine, and high-dose methadone all significantly reduced illicit opioid use in comparison to low-dose methadone. The different treatments all had similar side-effects and no toxic interactions with illicit drug use. Buprenorphine and high-dose methadone participants showed a trend towards higher rates of continuous abstinence than participants in low-dose methadone treatment. Thrice-weekly buprenorphine dosing showed approximately equivalent abstinence compared with daily methadone treatment and equivalent study retention to thrice-weekly LAAM, suggesting similar effects from the medications. This study largely replicated the earlier flexible-dose study results.

Like Strain and colleagues previously,[27] Montoya et al recruited a sample of opioid- and cocaine-dependent participants in their randomized, double-blind study of four different buprenorphine dosing regimens.[32] Participants were allocated to 2 mg daily, 8 mg daily, 16 mg daily, or 16 mg on alternate days for 13 weeks. Participants in the 8 mg or 16 mg daily buprenorphine groups showed significant reductions in urine morphine and benzoyleconine levels during the 10-week maintenance period and the 16 mg group showed reductions in both opiate and cocaine use. There were no reductions in opiate use in participants receiving the lowest (2 mg) dose of buprenorphine. No significant group differences were found in treatment retention or adverse events. Nearly half of the participants experienced adverse events, and there was a trend towards higher adverse events in the 16 mg alternate-day dosing group, which may be attributed to withdrawal symptoms as opposed to toxic adverse events.

In another randomized, double-blind, double-dummy study of participants with concomitant cocaine and opioid dependence, Schottenfeld and colleagues allocated participants to daily buprenorphine or methadone.[33] Participants receiving methadone treatment were retained in treatment significantly longer over the 6-month study, and had longer continuous periods of drug-free urine tests in comparison to buprenorphine patients.

Overall, the results of these studies are contradictory; this apparent contradiction is due to the differing designs, especially the dosing approach (flexible to reflect clinical practice or fixed and unchanging in response to patient needs). However, the results suggested that buprenorphine at moderate doses could have clinical utility. Where flexible doses were administered the issues of inadequate dosing were less marked, and the results of the two medications were more similar and consistent.

Clinical trials comparing buprenorphine tablet with methadone

All the studies reviewed in the previous section used the buprenorphine sublingual solution, while the current mono-buprenorphine product marketed for general clinical use is a sublingual tablet. A number of controlled studies have compared this formulation of buprenorphine with methadone.

A small Austrian study of buprenorphine tablet versus methadone employed a maximum dose of 8 mg buprenorphine and an 80 mg dose limit for methadone.[34,35] Retention in the buprenorphine group (38%) was significantly less than in the methadone group (71%). This difference was attributed to the maximum dose of the buprenorphine tablet being set too low.[35] Buprenorphine participants had significantly lower levels of opioid use than methadone participants.

Methadone retention was also reported as superior in a 6-week study by Petitjean and colleagues who used a flexible dosing regimen in their study of buprenorphine versus methadone maintenance.[36] Mean doses were 10.5 mg for buprenorphine and 69.8 mg for methadone. Retention rate was significantly better in the methadone group (90%) compared to the buprenorphine group (56%), possibly due to inadequate induction doses of buprenorphine. Survival analysis confirmed the significant difference in retention, and almost all of the buprenorphine patients who dropped out did so within the first 10 days, two thirds of them reporting withdrawal symptoms. Both treatment groups had similar illicit opioid and cocaine use, measured through urine samples.

A 6-month, fixed-dose Italian double-blind study[36] compared 8 mg buprenorphine with 60 mg methadone and reported a non-significant trend in favor of methadone for retaining participants in treatment. Again, many of the drop-outs from the buprenorphine group occurred during the induction phase, which was relatively slow compared with other studies, and took over a week to reach a maximum daily dose of 8 mg buprenorphine. No significant differences were found between groups in heroin use. No significant differences between groups were noticed in the reporting of adverse events. The non-significant trend to lower retention in the buprenorphine group might be explained by insufficient buprenorphine dosage or too slow an induction period, however the relevance of the result was limited by low recruitment to the study (n=72).

Restricted doses of buprenorphine and methadone were used to comply with national guidelines in two Iranian studies by Ahmadi and colleagues. The first study compared 50 mg naltrexone, 50 mg methadone, and 5 mg buprenorphine over 6 months.[37] Retention in methadone was found to be significantly better than both buprenorphine and naltrexone groups, and retention in buprenorphine was better than in the naltrexone group. No significant side-effects were reported for any of the medications.

The second Iranian study compared buprenorphine (1, 3, or 8 mg) with methadone (30 mg) in a double-blind, randomized trial over a period of 18 weeks.[38] Retention at 18 weeks in the 8 mg buprenorphine group (68%) was significantly better than the 1 mg (29%) and 3 mg (46%) groups, and retention in methadone (61%) was significantly better than the 1 mg buprenorphine group. The authors suggested that better results may have been possible with higher medication doses or more psychosocial treatment.

A non-randomized, flexible dose study comparing buprenorphine (mean dose 9.2 mg) and methadone (mean dose 81.5 mg) found no differences in treatment retention between the two groups at 12 weeks.[39] Methadone patients, however, did have significantly higher treatment retention in week 4, and buprenorphine patients had significantly lower rates of opioid-positive urines at week 12.

The largest comparison of buprenorphine versus methadone maintenance so far was a randomized, double-blind, double-dummy study conducted in three Australian methadone clinics.[40] The formulations of medications, flexibility in dose levels, and criteria for study discontinuation (non-attendance after 5 to 7 days) reflected clinical practice. The first 6 weeks of the 13-week study duration consisted of daily dosing for all participants, then buprenorphine participants were transferred to alternate-day dosing for the remainder of the study. Methadone treatment was significantly superior to buprenorphine in terms of retention. It was suggested that low doses during the buprenorphine induction phase could have led to earlier drop-out. No differences in illicit drug use were found between methadone and buprenorphine treatment groups,

85% of buprenorphine participants transferred to alternate-day dosing were maintained on this dosing schedule, and both methadone and buprenorphine maintenance were considered effective in treating opioid dependence.

Another Australian study by Lintzeris and colleagues compared buprenorphine versus methadone under naturalistic conditions in a randomized, controlled, open-label trial including treatment by general practitioners and community pharmacies.[41] Treatment protocols followed the established national guidelines: methadone patients had supervised dosing at pharmacies with one weekly take-away for stable patients; buprenorphine patients had daily supervised dosing at induction, but were permitted to change to alternate-daily or thrice-weekly dosing when stable. At 12 months, there were no significant differences in treatment retention for either treatment group.

A study by Neri and colleagues compared methadone and buprenorphine in a 12-month randomized double-blind trial.[42] Participants receiving methadone could receive a maximum of 100 mg and the majority of participants were on this dose. Buprenorphine tablets were dispensed at a mean dose of 10 mg/day for the first 3 weeks, a mean of 20 mg every second day for the next 2 weeks, and a mean of 30 mg every third day for the remainder of the study period. Retention in both treatment groups was high and not significantly different. Significantly more urine tests in methadone participants were positive for opiates than in buprenorphine participants. Fewer side-effects were also reported in buprenorphine participants. The authors concluded buprenorphine was a valid alternative to methadone treatment in opioid-dependent participants.

In Norway, Kristensen and colleagues[43] conducted a randomized study comparing fixed 16 mg buprenorphine to flexible methadone (mean 106 mg, range 80–160 mg). Retention in treatment after 180 days was better in the methadone group (85%) compared to the buprenorphine group (36%). The buprenorphine group had more opiate-positive urines (24% to 20%) and showed greater self-reported risk behavior and psychologic distress. The buprenorphine group rated better on physical health. The authors concluded that high-dose methadone should be the treatment of choice, but in cases where methadone is not tolerated buprenorphine may be an appropriate alternative. The appropriateness of comparing a fixed buprenorphine dose with a flexible methadone dose is debatable.

A recent German study[44] used flexible doses to compare methadone and buprenorphine. Mean doses at 6 months were 10.7 mg for the buprenorphine group and 49.1 mg for the methadone group. There was no difference in retention in the buprenorphine group (48%) compared to the methadone group (55%). Participants were allowed to transfer medications if they wanted and 8 patients from the buprenorphine group and 3 from the methadone group transferred medication. If these patients are excluded from the analysis, the retention remains the same between groups (54%). There was no significant difference between groups in terms of drug use.

Overall results from these studies show that methadone is superior to buprenorphine in retaining patients in treatment. Studies frequently showed equivalence between methadone and buprenorphine in terms of suppressing opioid use. Once again, it is acknowledged in many of the studies that adequate and flexible dose regimens and appropriate dose inductions may influence treatment outcome.

Placebo controlled studies

Johnson and colleagues were the first to compare buprenorphine treatment with a placebo control condition, rather than with methadone.[45] Participants were randomly assigned placebo ($n=60$), buprenorphine 2 mg ($n=60$), or buprenorphine 8 mg ($n=30$). The sublingual solution formulation was used. Analyses showed that buprenorphine participants spent a greater time on initial dose, requested fewer dose changes, used less illicit opioids, and rated dose adequacy higher than those on placebo, but that the two active medication groups did not differ from each other. This result is somewhat surprising given other results suggestive of a dose–response relationship for buprenorphine, but the failure to detect differences between the two buprenorphine dose levels may have been due to the short study period.

The second major placebo controlled trial was reported by Fudala and colleagues.[46] Patients were randomly assigned to receive 16 mg of buprenorphine, 16 mg of buprenorphine combined with 4 mg naloxone, or placebo medication.[46] The double-blind phase of the trial ran over a 4-week period. The number of urines negative for opiates were similar in the two active treatment conditions, but significantly lower in the placebo group. As a result, the double-blind component of the trial was terminated early.

These authors then continued with an open-label phase wherein they examined the combination buprenorphine/naloxone therapy for adverse events. A total of 461 participants participated in this study. They found few and mild treatment-related adverse events, most commonly headache and symptoms of withdrawal, but little evidence of any significant changes in liver function or hematology tests. These authors concluded that buprenorphine alone and in combination with naloxone are safe interventions to administer on an outpatient basis to opiate-dependent individuals.

In Norway, Krook and colleagues randomized opioid-dependent participants to either 16 mg daily buprenorphine or placebo on a waiting list for medication-assisted rehabilitation.[47] Buprenorphine participants performed better than those receiving placebo on retention in treatment, reported opioid use, reported other drug use, and in well-being. No serious adverse events were reported in either treatment group.

A Swedish study by Kakko and colleagues randomized 40 opiate-dependent individuals who were ineligible for methadone maintenance treatment to either buprenorphine maintenance (fixed dose of 16 mg) or to 6 days of buprenorphine treatment followed by placebo maintenance treatment.[48] Retention in treatment was significantly better in the buprenorphine group compared to the placebo group: all 20 patients receiving placebo dropped out of treatment within the first 2 months of the study, after urine analysis results showed drug use. In contrast, 1-year retention in the buprenorphine group was 75% and a mean of 75% of the urine analysis results was negative for all substances tested. Four participants died during the treatment period, all in the placebo group. Despite such high (20%) mortality in the controls, these participants did not fulfill Swedish criteria for entry into methadone programs, and buprenorphine was not yet available to patients outside of research studies due to regulatory problems.

Schottenfeld and colleagues conducted a double-dummy, double-blind, fixed-dose study of buprenorphine, naltrexone, and placebo in Malaysia.[49] Patients were randomly allocated to receive 8 mg buprenorphine (or matching placebo) and 50 mg naltrexone (matching placebo) for the first week and 16 mg buprenorphine (or placebo) and 100 mg tablets of naltrexone (or placebo) every Monday and Wednesday, and 24 mg of buprenorphine (or placebo) and 150 mg naltrexone (or placebo) on Fridays. Retention was significantly better for buprenorphine than both naltrexone and placebo. Buprenorphine was also significantly better than naltrexone and placebo in days to first heroin use, days to heroin relapse, and consecutive days of heroin abstinence. The authors concluded that buprenorphine maintenance treatment is superior to naltrexone and placebo in retaining patients in treatment, sustaining abstinence, delaying the resumption of heroin use, and relapse.

An early study to assess the safety and efficacy of an 8 mg dose of buprenorphine[50] used 1 mg buprenorphine as placebo compared to 4 mg, 8 mg, and 16 mg in a 16-week study. The 1 mg group had significantly poorer retention (40%) compared to the 8 mg group (52%) and the 16 mg group (61%). The placebo group had significantly more positive urines than those receiving 8 mg. There was no increase in frequency of adverse events with increased dose.

All the studies comparing buprenorphine to placebo have shown buprenorphine to be superior to placebo.

Relevance and generalizability of the trial results

The results of the major trials of buprenorphine compared to methadone or placebo treatment suggest that buprenorphine is an effective maintenance agent, with the caveat that adequate doses of buprenorphine are used and the induction period is rapid enough to relieve withdrawal symptoms. Buprenorphine is superior to placebo in terms of retaining patients in treatment and suppressing illicit opioid use. Overall the results show methadone to be superior to buprenorphine in terms of retaining patients in treatment and suppressing illicit opioid use.

The generalizability of these results must consider the buprenorphine formulation used. There is evidence that the bioavailability of the ethanol-based solution (predominantly used in early North American studies) is greater than the bioavailability of the marketed buprenorphine tablet formulation.[20] Results from a small (n=24) subject comparative study showed that the bioavailability of buprenorphine from the sublingual tablet was 70% of that from the sublingual solution.[21]

The participants in the majority of trials have remarkably similar demographics. Approximately two thirds are male, they are generally in their early 30s, with a history of opioid use of a number of years (typically between 5 and 7 years), and they tend to be unemployed and use other drugs. It is important to recognize that opioid dependence is a chronic relapsing disorder and the most important clinical feature is dependence on opioid drugs. Differences across countries in study populations become less important than the fact that the individual is opioid dependent. The studies have been conducted in many countries with similar results. There is no reason to believe there should be any difference in efficacy or safety between international settings.

The experience in France is relevant here. Until the beginning of the 1990s, very little pharmacotherapy for opioid dependence was available until there was recognition of the public health problems of opiate dependence and the potential for infectious disease (such as HIV) spreading in injecting drug users. Once pharmacotherapy was introduced by the French Government, the number of patients in buprenorphine treatment expanded rapidly to approximately 74,300, with another 9,600 in methadone treatment in 2001.[51] It is now estimated that more than half of the estimated 180,000 problem heroin users in France are being treated by about 20% of all physicians in France.[52] While methadone is provided by registered clinics, all registered medical doctors are allowed to prescribe buprenorphine without any special education or licensing. Buprenorphine prescriptions are filled at pharmacies for the patients to take the medication away. The medication is generally considered to be quite safe, although there have been deaths associated with buprenorphine use, particularly in cases where patients appear to have taken buprenorphine in combination with benzodiazepines[53,54] or other opioids.[55] Buprenorphine misuse and diversion occur with reports suggesting that the intravenous diversion of buprenorphine may occur in up to 20% of buprenorphine patients in France.[52] However, overall buprenorphine maintenance treatment in France has been associated with consistent public health, social, individual, and economic benefits.[52] Contextual factors contribute to the uptake of buprenorphine treatment in France, including: the role of buprenorphine's safety compared to methadone, the involvement of general practitioners compared to registered specialists, and the importance of the office-based setting compared to the center-based, allowing for greater patient access to treatment and the French health system, which has universal medical coverage.[52]

Buprenorphine safety

Pharmacology of buprenorphine

Buprenorphine is an opioid derived from an alkaloid of morphine that acts as a partial agonist at the μ opioid receptor and an antagonist at the κ opioid receptor.[56] These qualities mean that it has sufficient opioid activity to act as a maintenance treatment and it is also used successfully to help relieve the symptoms of opioid withdrawal.

Slow to dissociate from receptors, buprenorphine produces a long-acting response so that dosing regimens between daily and thrice-weekly administration are possible. Once bound to the μ receptor, buprenorphine acts as a competitive inhibitor, producing a partial blockade of the actions of other opioids at that receptor. Strong binding of buprenorphine to receptors also means that it should take larger amounts of naloxone (an opioid antagonist) to successfully reverse the actions of buprenorphine. While this is supported in laboratory studies, clinical experience in Helsinki suggests that normal doses of naloxone were effective in managing 11 patients with buprenorphine overdoses.[57]

In both tablet and solution form, buprenorphine is given sublingually to avoid high first-pass metabolism through the gastrointestinal tract. The commercial preparation of buprenorphine is in tablet form and has a lower bioavailability than the solution, as demonstrated by the 8 mg buprenorphine tablet producing significantly lower mean plasma concentrations than that of the 8 mg buprenorphine liquid.[58]

Buprenorphine has a ceiling effect in high doses, and beyond therapeutic levels of approximately 12 to 16 mg per day,[59] very little additional physiologic effect occurs. While methadone, a full opioid agonist, is capable of causing fatal respiratory depression in high doses, the ceiling effect of buprenorphine limits the extent of respiratory depression possible. For this reason, buprenorphine is considered to possess markedly greater safety in overdose than methadone, and is well tolerated in users who have detoxified from opioid use.[2] Buprenorphine's safety margin also makes double dosing on alternate days a possible mode of treatment delivery in opioid-dependent patients.

Buprenorphine and benzodiazepines

Various drug interactions have important effects on the safety of buprenorphine. In particular, there have been a number of deaths recorded where patients have been found to have both benzodiazepines and buprenorphine found on toxicologic examination. Of 34 deaths in Paris where buprenorphine was detected, one benzodiazepine was also detected in 16 cases, two benzodiazepines were detected in four cases, and three and four benzodiazepines were both detected in one case each.[60]

It is likely that buprenorphine has a lower rate of death than a full agonist mixed with high-dose benzodiazepines. Australian research has shown clearly that most of the deaths attributable to full agonist opioids such as heroin and methadone involve alcohol and benzodiazepines.[61] It is, however, important to recognize that whilst buprenorphine alone is a relatively safe medication, when administered in combination with benzodiazepines or alcohol the safety margin may be decreased.

A small case series looking at the deaths of six known heroin abusers in two regions of France found buprenorphine and benzodiazepines detected in the blood samples of all bodies.[54] Buprenorphine was found at higher than therapeutic levels in three bodies, and all benzodiazepines detected were in the therapeutic range. In a slightly larger case series of 20 French fatalities involving high-dose buprenorphine, all levels of buprenorphine detected in the blood were within or slightly over the therapeutic range.[53] All but one of the cases had concomitant psychotropic drugs detected (mostly benzodiazepines), but whether other drugs such as opioids were detected was not discussed.

It is clear from clinical practice that normal therapeutic doses of benzodiazepines and buprenorphine have been safely co-administered.

Lintzeris and colleagues examined co-administration of buprenorphine or methadone with single doses of diazepam within the therapeutic range and found minimal impairment in respiratory or other physiologic measures but significant effects in performance effects, with psychomotor changes being greater for methadone-maintained patients.[62] These findings suggest that, although acute benzodiazepine use at therapeutic doses seem safe for both methadone- and buprenorphine-maintained patients, they should be aware of the psychomotor changes and warned against driving or operating machinery. Lintzeris and colleagues also examined diazepam co-administration with methadone and buprenorphine under high doses and found high-dose diazepam significantly influenced response to methadone and buprenorphine, impacting on sedation, attention, and psychomotor skills. The authors suggest caution when prescribing high doses of benzodiazepines to this population.[63]

Other drug interactions

Levo-acetylmethadol (LAAM) was withdrawn as a treatment for opioid patients in 2003 due to QT prolongation and methadone has also been shown to prolong the QT interval.[64,65] One randomized controlled trial that was conducted to compare LAAM, methadone, and buprenorphine found that patients receiving buprenorphine had significantly less QT prolongation than the other medications.[66]

HIV-positive patients often have conditions that place them at risk for QT prolongation. As opioid addiction and HIV co-occur, and patients may be on antiretroviral medication, this is an important issue for treatment. An investigation of five antiretroviral medications (efavirenz, nelfinavir, delavirdine, ritonavir, and lopinavir/ritonavir) in combination with buprenorphine naloxone found QT interval increases with buprenorphine naloxone in combination with either delavirdine or ritonavir, but not with the other antiretrovirals or buprenorphine naloxone alone.[67]

There is evidence to suggest that atanzanavir and antazanavir/ritonavir co-administered with buprenorphine may result in an increase in buprenorphine and metabolite concentration and require decreased doses of buprenorphine.[68] Patients may need increased monitoring for opioid excess and doses may need adjustment.[69]

Mortality data

It has been recognized for a number of years that methadone (either alone or combined with benzodiazepines or alcohol) is associated with fatal overdose.[70–73] Buprenorphine appears to have a greater safety profile than methadone, with deaths due to buprenorphine being rare.

French data form the majority of information about mortality associated with buprenorphine due to the longer history and widespread use of buprenorphine in France.[51]

Auriacombe and colleagues used overdose deaths, average estimated daily doses of methadone and buprenorphine in clinical practice, and quantity of medications sold in France to examine overdose deaths attributed to buprenorphine and methadone from 1994 to 1998.[74] An estimated 1.4 times more buprenorphine-related deaths than methadone-related deaths occurred, while there were 14 times more buprenorphine than methadone patients and greater restrictions for methadone patients. Buprenorphine is prescribed for up to a month at a time by general practitioners with prescriptions filled at community pharmacies, whereas methadone is only available from specialist clinics, usually under supervised dosing. The yearly death rate for methadone was estimated to be at least three times greater than for buprenorphine, and the authors consider buprenorphine to be a safe alternative to methadone treatment, even under the relatively easy French access conditions.[74] A later report mentions that opiate overdose deaths in France have decreased by 79% since buprenorphine was introduced in 1995.[51]

These reports are acknowledged to contain several possible sources of inaccuracy. Not all deaths are necessarily captured using these methods, and since treatment duration may not necessarily be the same, the incidence of deaths may vary. Different treatment types may also attract patient demographics with different risks of mortality. Despite this, the authors estimate that biases are likely to be equally likely in methadone- and buprenorphine-related death data.

A retrospective data review conducted by Gueye and colleagues considered trends in number, mortality, and nature of severe opioid poisonings between 1995 and 1999 in north-eastern Paris and surrounding suburbs.[75] Data reviewed were obtained from a toxicologic intensive care unit (TICU), a pre-hospital emergency service, and coronial data. Coronial data do not include information on all deaths and only began testing for the presence of buprenorphine in 1998, so trend analysis was not possible. The number of people receiving buprenorphine treatment in the region was estimated from drug company sales figures.

From 1995 to 1999, the detection of buprenorphine in opioid poisons patients in the TICU increased from an average of two to eight occurrences per year, coinciding with a decrease in opioid poisoning mortality from 12 to 0% in the TICU and from 9 to 0% in the pre-hospital emergency service. Buprenorphine was detected in 19 of the 80 TICU poisonings cases and 10 of these had another opiate or opioid detected in addition to buprenorphine, and one (non-fatal) case of poisoning where buprenorphine was the only opioid detected. All cases of opioid deaths recorded had other drugs detected, and 9 of 13 deaths where buprenorphine was detected also had another opioid detected. Benzodiazepines were the most common non-opioid drug to be detected in the poisoning cases.[75]

From 1996 to 1999 there was a 2.7-fold increase in buprenorphine detection in the TICU data and a 2.6-fold increase in buprenorphine sales, supporting the hypothesis of the relative safety of high-dose buprenorphine treatment, in agreement with Auriacombe and colleagues.[74] When considering the lower availability of methadone in the region, methadone was detected in a greater proportion of poisonings than buprenorphine. The authors concluded that high-dose buprenorphine availability has not been associated with an inordinate number of severe poisonings or deaths.[75]

A retrospective study has considered forensic cases where buprenorphine or methadone was detected between 1997 and 2002 in Paris.[60] Data reviewed included pre-mortem, autopsy, police data, hospital data, and toxicologic analyses. It should be noted that not all fatal opioid deaths in Paris are referred to the coroner for toxicology, and limited data were available on the therapeutic and toxic ranges of buprenorphine. Some difficulty was noted in determining the role of substitution drugs in the death process.

In 5 years of deaths there were 34 cases where buprenorphine was detected and 35 cases where methadone was detected (of which 9 cases had both drugs). Of these fatalities, buprenorphine and methadone were judged to be directly implicated in 4 and 3 deaths respectively, and had a strongly plausible participation in the lethal process in 8 and 11 additional deaths. In the 4 fatalities in which buprenorphine was implicated, 3 also had methadone and two to four other drugs detected; while the remaining fatality also had cocaine and alcohol detected. Buprenorphine was uniformly detected with other drugs (median number of other drugs detected was 4.5), and all but one methadone case was detected with other drugs (median number of other drugs detected was 5). The authors also comment on the similar numbers of deaths where buprenorphine and methadone were detected despite the greater availability of buprenorphine in the country.[60]

In the 13 fatalities involving buprenorphine recorded at the Institute of Legal Medicine of Strasbourg between August 2000 and October 2001, mean values of buprenorphine detected in the post-mortem specimens were within the therapeutic range.[76] Another small report discussed 11 serious overdoses in Helsinki where buprenorphine was involved between 1996 and 2002.[57] Plasma concentrations of buprenorphine were not measured and most information on drugs used was from self-report. Most cases of overdoses had concomitant use of other central nervous system depressants, alcohol, or intravenous use of buprenorphine. Seven fatal overdoses in the UK where buprenorphine was the only drug detected at toxicology have been reported.[55] Four deaths occurred by accident, two were suicides and one was undetermined causes.[55]

In a comparative review of Australian coronial records from 2000 to 2003 one death attributed to buprenorphine was identified compared to 282 to methadone and 32 to oral naltrexone.[77] The buprenorphine mortality rate was 0.02 per 1,000 episodes compared to the French estimate of 0.24 per 1,000 patients.[74] The authors note that as only a single death was detected caution should be used when comparing rates. Significant differences in buprenorphine mortality to methadone and naltrexone were not tested.

Severe adverse events

Serious adverse events (SAEs) have been defined as any untoward medical occurrence that results in death or persistent or significant disability/incapacity; is life-threatening; requires in-patient hospitalization or prolongation of existing hospitalization; or is a congenital anomaly or birth defect.[78] In a longitudinal study using data from 12 clinical trials and 1244 participants, Digiusto and colleagues reported on the incidence of SAEs during and after trial treatment.[78] These trials formed part of the Australian National Evaluation of Pharmacotherapies for Opioid Dependence (NEPOD) studies and investigated naltrexone, LAAM, methadone, and buprenorphine interventions. Five heroin overdoses occurred in the buprenorphine groups, all of which occurred during treatment. Similar numbers of SAEs occurred in the methadone and buprenorphine treatment groups.

In another study of 8 mg buprenorphine solution, low-dose methadone, and high-dose methadone for a duration of 1 year, no severe adverse effects attributable to buprenorphine occurred.[28]

Adverse events

A number of studies have examined adverse events experienced by participants. In one US study, opioid-dependent participants ($n=225$) were randomized to either 8 mg daily buprenorphine solution, 30 mg daily methadone, or 80 mg daily methadone in a double-blind manner for 52 weeks.[28] Although the authors did not believe the 8 mg buprenorphine dose was optimal, adverse events were about equally represented in all three groups, except for low-dose methadone patients experiencing significantly more nausea that either of the other two groups.

A study of 1, 4, 8, or 16 mg daily doses by Ling and colleagues[79] was primarily designed to consider differences in outcomes between 1 and 8 mg daily dosing groups. No increase in adverse event frequency was noted in the 8 mg group in comparison to the 1 mg group, and adverse events were those commonly seen in opioid-treated patients. Thirty-one percent of all buprenorphine patients experienced headaches, but there were no differences between the study groups.

In a small, 6-week, double-blinded, randomized study of flexible dosing of buprenorphine tablets versus methadone maintenance, Petitjean and colleagues reported that the frequency of most adverse events was not different between treatment groups, although methadone recipients reported significantly more sedation than buprenorphine recipients.[36] Thirty-three percent of those receiving buprenorphine reported headaches, but this was not significantly different from the 23% of the methadone group experiencing headaches,[36] and similar to the rate of headaches reported previously.[79]

The issue of buprenorphine and liver function needs to be better studied as some indications of hepatic toxicity suggest caution.

Dose levels

Ling and colleagues compared different fixed daily doses (1, 4, 8, or 16 mg) of buprenorphine solution in this large randomized, double-blind trial involving daily dosing and weekly counseling.[79] Retention in treatment was significantly better in the 16 mg group (61%) and the 8 mg group (52%) than the 1 mg group (40%). Log-rank tests also confirmed that time to drop-out was significantly less in the 1 mg group than either the 8 mg or 16 mg groups. Illicit opioid use, opioid craving, and global ratings were all significantly better in the 8 mg dose than the 1 mg dose, however the study was not designed to detect significant differences between the 8 mg and 16 mg doses.

An Iranian research group led by Ahmadi and colleagues has also investigated lower dose levels of buprenorphine by randomizing patients to double-blind daily administration of 1, 3, or 8 mg of buprenorphine tablets for 1 year.[80] There was a significant dose-dependent effect on retention in treatment. Twelve-month treatment retention was 27% for the 1 mg group, 60% for the 3 mg group, and 78% for the 8 mg group. It should be noted that the maximum daily dose permitted in Iran at the time of this study was 8 mg.

Frequency of dosing

A number of randomized controlled studies have demonstrated the apparent safety and efficacy of alternate-day and less frequent buprenorphine dosing. A small (n=13), randomized, double-blind, daily versus alternate-daily buprenorphine cross-over study was conducted by Amass and colleagues. The majority of measured effects did not differ significantly between alternate and daily dosing, participants rarely detected dose increases, and no adverse reactions to the dosing procedures were detected.[5] A larger study (n=99) randomly assigned participants in a double-blind manner to daily 8 mg or alternate-daily 8 mg buprenorphine solution over 11 weeks after a 4-week lead-in period.[6] Despite doses of buprenorphine not being doubled for the alternate-day dosing group, no significant differences were noted between groups on retention, opiate-positive urine, clinical attendance, dose adequacy, withdrawal symptoms, or cocaine-positive urines.

Consistent results came from a small (n=18) cross-over randomized study that compared open daily dosing, blind daily dosing, blind alternate-day dosing, and open alternate-day dosing.[81] Alternate-day dosing used double the daily dose on Mondays, Wednesdays, and Fridays, and a single dose on Sundays. Maintenance doses were determined in the first week and cross-overs began on the 14th day. Participants were paid for clinic attendance and opioid abstinence so drug use and retention outcomes were influenced by this. Acceptability and safety were similar in alternate and daily dosing, and alternate-day dosing was preferred in the 7 participants receiving two cycles of treatment. No adverse reactions were noted in doubling the dose for alternate-day dosing, although ratings of withdrawal, feeling 'sick', and sedation were slightly lower in daily rather than alternate dosing.

Bickel and colleagues compared buprenorphine solution daily, second, or third daily to see if triple the maintenance dose could be administered without complications.[82] This was a small sample ($n=16$) double-blind, placebo-controlled cross-over study running for 3 weeks after a 2-week induction period onto buprenorphine. No significant differences on measures of agonist effects, adverse reactions, or excessive opioid intoxication between the doses were noted. The results suggest that tripling the dose is safe and only results in minimal withdrawal complaints.

Schottenfeld and colleagues considered opiate-dependent patients randomly allocated to daily or thrice-weekly dosing at fixed double-blind doses of 34 mg/70 kg (Fridays and Sundays) and 44 mg/70 kg (Tuesdays) after a 3-day induction onto buprenorphine.[83] Thrice weekly dosing was comparable in efficacy, retention, and drug use to daily dosing. No adverse medication effects were reported and the medication was well tolerated. Some increased cocaine use occurred, but this was not different between the treatment groups. Substantial decreases in illicit opioid use occurred in both treatment groups.

In a randomized double-blind study of participants receiving either thrice-weekly (16 mg Monday, Wednesday and 24 mg Fridays) or daily (8 mg) buprenorphine for 12 weeks, no significant differences were found in treatment retention.[84] However, there were significantly more opioid-positive tests in the thrice-weekly dosing participants (58.5%) than in the daily dosing participants (46.6%). Only eight participants reported adverse effects including constipation, nausea, and asthenia, and adverse effects did not differ significantly between treatment groups. The authors mentioned insufficient buprenorphine doses and fixed dosing levels as possible limitations of the study, and advise daily buprenorphine dosing at least at the start of maintenance treatment.

A 24-week clinical study using buprenorphine solution at doses of 4, 8, 10, or 12 mg randomized participants to daily, 3, or 2 days per week.[85]

Participants presenting three times a week received double doses on Monday and Wednesday and a triple dose on Friday. Participants presenting twice a week received quadruple their dose on Monday and triple their dose on Fridays. The authors noted that all dosing regimens had comparable efficacy in terms of treatment retention, opioid abstinence, and reductions in HIV risk behavior.

A study comparing three dosing regimens – daily the maintenance dose every 24 hours, triple the maintenance dose every 72 hours, and quintuple the maintenance dose every 120 hours – found that opioid withdrawal symptoms increased significantly during the every fifth day dosing regimen, suggesting that the maximum duration of action of buprenorphine is less than 5 days.[86] Another study[87] comparing quintuple and sextuple the maintenance dose every 5 days also found significant withdrawal after 96 hours, indicating dosing every 5 days is not recommended.

In summary, the trials suggest alternate-day dosing is possible with many patients. However, experience in real clinical practice may suggest that not all patients cope with this form of dosing. It is important to have treatment flexibility and to not simply endorse mandatory alternate-day dispensing for all clients. Up to one third of patients will likely prefer daily dispensing of this medication, despite the increased need for clinic attendance.

Buprenorphine/naloxone combination product

The abuse potential of buprenorphine has been acknowledged since its introduction.[88] There have been reports of buprenorphine diversion and injection from many countries,[89–93] with reports of significant associated infection. In response to this misuse, a combination tablet was developed which includes buprenorphine and naloxone in a 4:1 ratio. The combined buprenorphine/naloxone product is specifically designed to reduce the extent of misuse of the medication by injection, and to reduce diversion of it to illicit drug users outside treatment. The 4:1 ratio preserves the therapeutic effects of buprenorphine and minimizes the opiate antagonist effects of naloxone when taken sublingually, but if injected it precipitates withdrawal.[94]

The safety, efficacy, and dosing capabilities of the buprenorphine/ naloxone sublingual tablet is reportedly the same as the buprenorphine tablet.[7] However, comparison studies of mono buprenorphine and the combination buprenorphine/naloxone products are limited. The only direct comparison randomized controlled trial was the 4-week study by Fudala and colleagues, which concluded 16 mg buprenorphine and 16 mg of the buprenorphine/naloxone combination therapy were superior to placebo and similar in terms of efficacy and safety.[46]

An Iranian study[95] compared the combination product to placebo by randomly assigning 35 patients to either 1 mg, 2 mg, or 4 mg sublingual buprenorphine/naloxone for 17 weeks. The retention in the 4 mg group (62.9%) was significantly better than the 1 mg group.

Following involvement in a clinical trial of buprenorphine/naloxone and counseling[96] participants were followed up for 2 to 5 years.[97] Comparable to results of clinic-based methadone treatment, 38% of patients were retained in treatment at 2 years. No serious adverse events related to buprenorphine/naloxone occurred.

A retrospective study in Finland that involved switching 64 patients from buprenorphine to the combination product[98] found that the majority (91%) switched to the same dose of buprenorphine/naloxone. One patient discontinued buprenorphine/naloxone due to adverse events during the transfer, and 5 discontinued during the 4-month follow-up. Over a quarter reported adverse events within the 4-month follow-up period and over half of the patients requested dose reductions. The authors suggest that the adverse events could be related to higher buprenorphine serum levels. At 4 months 26 patients (40%) remained in buprenorphine/naloxone treatment. They concluded that when patients are transferred from high-dose buprenorphine (>22 mg) to the combination product dose adjustments may be required.

There have been reports that the use of the combination product may require higher doses than the monotherapy at low doses,[99] although the available studies suggest equal potency.[100]

A Swedish randomized study examined a stepped care into treatment using buprenorphine/naloxone compared to conventional methadone maintenance.[101] It was a flexible-dose study with a double-blind induction phase followed by a maintenance phase where patients could request a dose increase every 2 weeks. Patients already receiving 32 mg of buprenorphine were switched to methadone. At 180 days, of the 48 patients allocated to buprenorphine naloxone 17 remained on buprenorphine/naloxone (35%)

with 20 (41%) switching to methadone maintenance. In the methadone group 38 were retained in treatment (79%). The mean buprenorphine/naloxone dose was 29.6 mg and the mean methadone dose was 111 mg for those who switched from buprenorphine/naloxone and 110 mg for those in the methadone group. The proportion of drug-free urines increased over time for both groups. The authors concluded that the outcomes for stepped treatment and methadone maintenance treatment were similar. They noted that the retention outcomes were high and suggested that the flexible dosing and comparatively high doses may have contributed to the results.

There have been reports of misuse of the combination product. Alho and colleagues[102] surveyed an untreated population through a needle exchange program to examine the abuse of buprenorphine and the buprenorphine/naloxone combination product in Finland. Almost three-quarters of the sample reported that buprenorphine was their most frequently injected drug. About two-thirds of the sample of 176 had tried injecting buprenorphine/naloxone and of those who tried it, two-thirds repeated injection with some reporting regular injection. Respondents were asked to compare the experience of injecting the combination product with injecting buprenorphine. Of the 107 respondents, 80% reported the injection of the buprenorphine combination product as a 'bad' experience and 20% reported it as similar to their experience with injecting buprenorphine. The street price for buprenorphine was reportedly higher than the combination product, indicating a higher value among users. Although the authors conclude that results should be considered tentatively due to the response rate and study design, the study provides evidence that misuse of the combination product occurs.

An Australian study randomly allocated participants to observed or unobserved administration of buprenorphine/naloxone. All participants had weekly clinical interviews but the unobserved group were given weekly take-home medication. The study found that retention and heroin use were not significantly different. Treatment with close clinical monitoring but no observed dosing was significantly cheaper and therefore more cost-effective.[103] A follow-up from this study found that there was a high drop-out rate for unstable participants to attend for observed dosing. There was a greater tendency for participants who had been initially allocated to unobserved dosing but were then required to attend for observed dosing due to instability to drop out.[104] The authors conclude that it may be better to initiate treatment with observation and then select unobserved treatment for those responding well. Restricting access to unobserved dosing may limit diversion.

Comparison studies are limited and therefore it is unknown to what extent the combination product limits diversion while maintaining retention. It is advised in individuals or situations in which diversion is an issue, consideration should be given to increasing supervision, adjusting doses or switching treatment.[105]

Conclusions

Role of buprenorphine

Buprenorphine has the potential to take on a major role in the management of opioid dependence. Buprenorphine is a medication with unique features that make it a useful addition to the current approaches to managing opioid dependence. The place of buprenorphine is as a 'gateway' intervention, given the evidence that it is able to be used as an effective withdrawal medication, or that it can be used for maintenance therapy. Buprenorphine has demonstrated effectiveness in retaining patients in treatment and suppressing illicit opioid use. It appears that the partial agonist buprenorphine is not as effective as methadone maintenance treatment in retaining patients in treatment but is similar to methadone in terms of reducing illicit opioid use.

Safety profile

Buprenorphine also appears to possess markedly greater safety in overdose among opioid-exposed individuals than methadone, since it produces relatively limited respiratory depression, and is extremely well tolerated by non-dependent humans who have had some experience with opioids in the past.[2] The safety margin means that it has the potential for alternate-day dosing (i.e., double dosing on alternate days). Utilization of an alternate-day dosing regimen may provide a significant advantage over methadone as a maintenance medication in terms of patient convenience, risk of diversion of take-home doses, and possibly in terms of the economic costs of treatment delivery.

Likely doses

It appears that the appropriate daily doses of this medication will be between 12 mg and 16 mg of buprenorphine. A higher (double) dose seems likely to be required for alternate-day dosing. The maximum daily dose is likely to be no more than 24 mg per day for the great majority of patients. At these doses, there is no evidence of adverse events and, as noted earlier, the medication appears to be markedly safer than full agonists, with a lower risk of overdose death. Nonetheless, there are drug interactions relevant to the use of buprenorphine in the management of patients with opioid dependence. In particular, there have been deaths recorded where patients have been found to have high levels of benzodiazepines and to have buprenorphine found on toxicology examination.

Reducing diversion and misuse

Related to the safety issue is the possible misuse of buprenorphine. In some countries there have been reports of widespread injecting of buprenorphine. In response, a buprenorphine/naloxone combination has been developed. The combined buprenorphine/naloxone product is specifically designed to reduce the misuse of the medication by injection, and to reduce diversion of it to illicit drug users outside treatment. Injection of dissolved buprenorphine/naloxone tablets will result in an acute withdrawal state (by the action of the antagonist naloxone), and this potential should discourage inappropriate self-administration by injection. Comparison studies are limited and therefore it is unknown to what extent the combination product limits diversion while maintaining retention.

Summary

While methadone maintenance is a widely used medication for the management of opioid dependence, there is a large pool of untreated individuals. There is reasonable information to suggest that many of these individuals do not wish to enter methadone treatment because of their negative perceptions of it and particularly because of their belief that they may become dependent on it. Buprenorphine has the potential to bring many of these patients into treatment and to provide them with some assurance that the level of dependence that they will develop on buprenorphine will not be as great as that on full agonists such as methadone. Given the prevalence of opioid dependence, the limitations of methadone (even though it is an efficacious treatment), and the evidence that buprenorphine exerts positive effects on opioid users, it seems that buprenorphine is a useful maintenance agent. It may have a place in some countries, depending on attitudes to full agonists such as methadone, and depending on cost factors. It is an important addition to the range of pharmacotherapeutic responses to the opioid-dependent population.

References

1. Jasinski DR, Pevnick JS, Griffith JD. Human pharmacology and abuse potential of the analgesic buprenorphine. Arch Gen Psychiat 1978; 35: 501–16.
2. Walsh S, Preston K, Stitzer M, Cone E, Bigelow G. Clinical pharmacology of buprenorphine: ceiling effect at high doses. Clin Pharm Th 1994; 55(5): 569–80.
3. Umbricht A, Huestis MA, Cone EJ, Preston KL. Effects of high dose intraveneous buprenorphine in experienced opioid abusers. J Clin Psychop 2004; 24(8): 479–87.
4. Amass L, Kamien JB, Mikulich SK. Thrice-weekly supervised dosing with the combination buprenorphine-naloxone tablet is preferred to daily supervised dosing by opioid dependent humans. Drug Alcohol Depen 2001; 61: 173–81.
5. Amass L, Bickel WK, Higgins ST, Badger GJ. Alternate-day dosing during buprenorphine treatment of opioid dependence. Life Sci 1994; 54: 1215–28.
6. Johnson RE, Eissenberg T, Stitzer ML, Strain EC, Liebson IA, Bigelow GE. Buprenorphine treatment of opioid dependence: clinical trial of daily versus alternate-day dosing. Drug Alcohol Depen 1995; 40: 27–35.
7. Amass L, Kamien JB, Mikulich SK. Efficacy of daily and alternate daily dosing regimes with the combination buprenorphine-naloxone tablet. Drug Alcohol Depen 2000; 58: 143–52.
8. Petry NM, Bickel WK, Badger GJ. A comparison of four buprenorphine dosing regimens using open-dosing procedures: is twice-weekly dosing possible? Addiction 2000; 95(7): 1069–77.
9. Jaffe JH, Martin WR. Opioid analgesics and antagonists. In: Gilman AG, Rall TW, Nies AS, Taylor P, eds. The Pharmacological Basis of Therapeutics. 8th ed. New York: Pergamon Press; 1990: 485–521.
10. Kuhlman JJ, Levine B, Johnson RE, Fudala PJ, Cone EJ. Relationship of plasma buprenorphine and norbuprenorphine to withdrawal symptoms during dose induction, maintenance and withdrawal from sublingual buprenorphine. Addiction 1998; 93(4): 549–59.
11. Lewis JW. Buprenorphine. Drug Alcohol Depen 1985; 14: 363–72.
12. Kreek MJ. Long-term pharmacotherapy for opiate (primarily heroin) addiction: opioid antagonists and partial agonists. In: Schuster CR, Kuhar MJ, eds.

Pharmacological Aspects of Drug Dependence: Toward an Integrated Neurobehavioural Approach. Berlin: Springer; 1996: 563–98.

13. Lehmann KA, Reichling U, Wirtz R. Influence of naloxone on the post-operative analgesic and respiratory effects of buprenorphine. Eur J Clin Pharmacol 1988; 34: 343–52.
14. San L, Cami J, Fernandez T, Olle JM, Peri JM, Torrens M. Assessment and management of opioid withdrawal symptoms in buprenorphine-dependent subjects. Br J Addict 1992; 87: 55–62.
15. Mello NK, Mendelson JE. Buprenorphine suppresses heroin use by heroin addicts. Life Sci 1980; 207(4431): 657–9.
16. Breen C, Harris S, Hawken L, et al. Cessation of methadone maintenance treatment using buprenorphine: transfer from methadone to buprenorphine and subsequent buprenorphine reductions. Drug Alcohol Depen 2003; 71(1): 49–55.
17. Mattick RP, Oliphant D, Hall W, Ward J. The effectiveness of other opioid replacement therapies: buprenorphine, LAAM, heroin and injectable methadone. In: Ward J, Mattick RP, Hall W, eds. Methadone Maintenance Treatment and Other Opioid Replacement Therapies. London: Harwood Press; 1998.
18. Mattick RP, Kimber J, Breen C, Davoli M. Buprenorphine maintenance versus placebo or methadone maintenance for opioid dependence. The Cochrane Database of Systematic Reviews 2008; Issue 2.
19. Connock M, Juarez-Garcia A, Jowett S, et al. Methadone and buprenorphine for the management of opioid dependence: a systematic review and economic evaluation. Health Technol Assess 2007; 11(9).
20. Mendelson J, Upton R, Jones RT, Jacob P, eds. Buprenorphine pharmacokinetics: bioequivalence of an 8mg sublingual tablet formulation. Problems of drug dependence, 1995: Proceedings of the 55th annual scientific meeting of the College on problems of drug dependence, Inc; 1995; Phoenix, AZ. National Instiutute on Drug Abuse.
21. Ling W. Pharmacokinetics and bioavailability of liquid vs tablet buprenorphine. Los Angeles: West Los Angeles Veterans Affairs Medical Centre; 1998. Contract No.: Document Number.
22. Bickel WK, Stitzer ML, Bigelow GE, Liebson IA, Jasinski DR, Johnson RE. A clinical trial of buprenorphine: Comparison with methadone in the detoxification of heroin addicts. Clin Pharmacol Ther 1988; 43: 72–8.
23. Johnson RE, Jaffe JH, Fudala PJ. A controlled trial of buprenorphine treatment for opioid dependence. JAMA 1992; 267(20): 2750–5.
24. Kosten TR, Schottenfeld R, Ziedonis D, Falcioni J. Buprenorphine versus methadone maintenance for opioid dependence. J Nerv Ment Dis 1993; 181(6): 358–64.
25. Newman RG. Comparing buprenorphine and methadone maintenance. J Nerv Ment Dis 1994; 182: 245–6.
26. Strain EC, Stitzer ML, Liebson IA, Bigelow GE. Comparison of buprenorphine and methadone in the treatment of opioid dependence. Am J Psychiat 1994; 151(7): 1025–30.

27. Strain EC, Stitzer ML, Liebson IA, Bigelow GE. Buprenorphine versus methadone in the treatment of opioid-dependent cocaine users. Psychopharmacol (Berl) 1994; 116: 401–6.
28. Ling W, Wesson DR, Charuvastra C, Klett CJ. A controlled trial comparing buprenorphine and methadone maintenance in opioid dependence. Arch Gen Psychiat 1996; 53: 401–7.
29. Schottenfeld RS, Pakes JR, Oliveto A, Ziedonis D, Kosten TR. Buprenorphine vs methadone maintenance treatment for concurrent opioid dependence and cocaine abuse. Arch Gen Psychiat 1997; 54: 713–20.
30. Oliveto AH, Feingold A, Schottenfeld R, Jatlow P, Kosten TR. Desipramine in opioid-dependent cocaine abusers maintained on buprenorphine vs methadone. Arch Gen Psychiat 1999; 56(9): 812–20.
31. Johnson RE, Chutuape MA, Strain EC, Walsh SL, Stitzer ML, Bigelow GE. A comparison of levomethadyl acetate, buprenorphine, and methadone for opioid dependence. N Engl J Med 2000; 343: 1290–7.
32. Montoya ID, Gorelick DA, Preston KL, et al. Randomized trial of buprenorphine for treatment of concurrent opiate and cocaine dependence. Clin Pharmacol Ther 2004; 75: 34–48.
33. Schottenfeld RS, Chawarski MC, Pakes JR, Pantalon MV, Carroll KM, Kosten TR. Methadone versus buprenorphine with contingency management or performance feedback for cocaine and opioid dependency. Am J Psychiat 2005; 162(2): 340–9.
34. Eder H, Fischer G, Gombas W, Jagsch R, Stuhlinger G, Kasper S. Comparison of buprenorphine and methadone in opiate addicts. Eur Addict Res 1998; 4(Suppl 1): 3–7.
35. Fischer G, Gombas W, Eder H, et al. Buprenorphine versus methadone maintenance for the treatment of opioid dependence. Addiction 1999; 94(9): 1337–47.
36. Petitjean S, Stohler R, Deglon JJ, et al. Double-blind randomized trial of buprenorphine and methadone in opiate dependence. Drug Alcohol Depen 2001; 62: 97–104.
37. Ahmadi J, Ahmadi K, Ohaeri J. Controlled, randomized trial in maintenance treatment of intravenous buprenorphine dependence with naltrexone, methadone or buprenorphine: A novel study. Eur J Clin Invest 2003; 33: 824–9.
38. Ahmadi J. Methadone vs buprenorphine maintenance for the treatment of heroin-dependent outpatients. J Subst Abuse Treat 2003; 24: 217–20.
39. Gerra G, Borella F, Zaimovic A, et al. Buprenorphine versus methadone for opioid dependence: predictor variables for treatment outcome. Drug Alcohol Depen 2004; 75: 37–45.
40. Mattick RP, Ali R, White J, O'Brien S, Wolk S, Danz C. Buprenorphine versus methadone maintenance therapy: a randomized double-blind trial with 405 opioid-dependent patients. Addiction 2003; 98: 441–52.
41. Lintzeris N, Ritter A, Panjari M, Clark N, Kutin J, Bammer G. Implementing buprenorphine treatment in community settings in Australia: experiences from the buprenorphine implementation trial. Am J Addic 2004; 13: S29–S41.

42. Neri S, Bruno CM, Pulvirenti D, et al. Randomized clinical trial to compare the effects of methadone and buprenorphine on the immune system in drug abusers. Psychopsychology 2005; 179: 700–4.
43. Kristensen O, Espergen O, Asland R, Jakobsen E, Lie O, Seiler S. Buprenorphine and methadone to opiate addicts – a randomised trial. Tidsskr Nor Laegeforen 2005; 125(2): 148–51.
44. Soyka M, Zingg C, Koller G, Kuefner H. Retention rate and substance use in methadone and buprenorphine maintenance therapy and predictors of outcome: results from a randomized study. Interl J Neuropsychop 2008; 11: 641–53.
45. Johnson RE, Eissenberg T, Stitzer ML, Strain EC, Leibson IA, Bigelow GE. A placebo controlled clinical trial of buprenorphine as a treatment for opioid dependence. Drug Alcohol Depen 1995; 40: 17–25.
46. Fudala PJ, Bridge TP, Herbert S, et al. Office-based treatment of opiate addiction with a sublingual-tablet formulation of buprenorphine and naloxone. N Engl J Med 2003; 349: 949–58.
47. Krook AL, Brors O, Dahlberg J, et al. A placebo-controlled study of high dose buprenorphine in opiate dependents waiting for medication-assisted rehabilitation in Oslo, Norway. Addiction 2002; 97: 533–42.
48. Kakko J, Svanborg D, Kreek MJ, Hellig M. 1-year retention and social function after buprenorphine-assisted relapse prevention treatment for heroin dependence in Sweden: a randomised, placebo controlled trial. Lancet 2003; 361: 662–8.
49. Schottenfeld RS, Charwarski MC, Mazlan M. Maintenance treatment with buprenorphine and naltrexone for heroin dependence in Malaysia: a randomised, double-blind, placebo-controlled trial. The Lancet 2008; 371: 2192–200.
50. Ling W, Charuvastra C, Collins JF, et al. Buprenorphine maintenance treatment of opiate dependence: a multicenter, randomized clinical trial. Addiction 1998; 93(4): 475–86.
51. Auriacombe M, Fatseas M, Dubernet J, Daulouede JP, Tignol J. French field experience with buprenorphine. Am J Addict 2004; 13(Suppl 1): S17–S28.
52. Fatseas M, Auriacombe M. Why buprenorphine is so successful in treating opiate addiction in France. Current Psychiatry Reports 2007; 9(5): 358–64.
53. Tracqui A, Kintz P, Ludes B. Buprenorphine-related deaths among drug addicts in France: A report on 20 fatalities. J Anal Toxicol 1998; 22(6): 430–4.
54. Reynaud M, Petit G, Potard D, Courty P. Six deaths linked to concomitant use of buprenorphine and benzodiazepines. Addiction 1998; 93(9): 1385–92.
55. Schifano F, Corkery J, Gilvarry E, Deluca P, Oyefeso A, Ghodse AH. Buprenorphine mortality, seizures and prescription data in the UK, 1980–2002. Human Psychopharmacology: Clin Exp 2005; 20: 343–8.
56. Robinson SE. Buprenorphine: an analgesic with an expanding role in the treatment of opioid addiction. CNS Drug Rev 2002; 8(4): 377–90.
57. Boyd J, Randell T, Luurila H, Kuisma M. Serious overdoses involving buprenorphine in Helsinki. Acta Anaesth Scand 2003; 47: 1031–3.

58. Schuh KJ, Johanson CE. Pharmacokinetic comparison of the buprenorphine sublingual liquid and tablet. Drug Alcohol Depen 1999; 56(1): 55–60.
59. Lintzeris N, Clark N, Winstock A, et al. National Clinical Guidelines and Procedures for the use of Buprenorphine in the Treatment of Heroin Dependence. In: Intergovernmental Committee on Drugs (IGCD) sub-committee methadone and other treatments, editor. Canberra: Australian Government Department of Health and Ageing; 2006.
60. Pirnay S, Borron SW, Giudicelli CP, Tourneau J, Baud FJ, Ricordel I. A critical review of the causes of death among post-mortem toxicological investigations: analysis of 34 buprenorphine-associated and 35 methadone-associated deaths. Addiction 2004; 99(8): 978–88.
61. Darke S, Ross J, Zador D, Sunjic S. Heroin-related deaths in New South Wales, Australia, 1992–1996. Drug Alcohol Depen 2000; 60: 141–50.
62. Lintzeris N, Mitchell T, Bond A, Nestor L, Strang J. Interactions on mixing diazepam with methadone or buprenorphine in maintenance patients. J Clin Psychopharmacol 2006; 26(3): 274–83.
63. Lintzeris N, Mitchell TB, Bond AJ, Nestor L, Strang J. Pharmacodynamics of diazepam co-administered with methadone or buprenorphine under high dose conditions in opioid dependent patients. Drug Alcohol Depen 2007; 91: 187–94.
64. Krantz MJ, Lewkowiez L, Hays H, Woodroffe M, Robertson AD, Mehler PS. Torades de pointes associated with very high dose methadone. Ann Med Intern 2002; 137: 501–4.
65. Maremmani I, Pacini M, Cesaroni C, Lovrecic M, Perugi G, Tagliamonte A. QTc interval prolongation in patients on long-term methadone maintenance therapy. Eur Addict Res 2005; 11: 44–9.
66. Wedam EF, Bigelow GE, Johnson RE, Nuzzo PA, Haigney MCP. QT-interval effects of methadone, levomethadyl, and buprenorphine in a randomized trial. Arch Intern Med 2007; 167(22): 2469–74.
67. Baker JR, Best AM, Pade PA, McCance-Katz EF. Effect of buprenorphine and antiretroviral agents on the QT interval in opioid-dependent patients. Drug Alcohol Subst Ab 2006; 40: 392–6.
68. McCance-Katz EF, Moody DE, Morse GD, et al. Interaction between buprenorphine and atazanavir or atazanavir/ritonavir. Drug Alcohol Depen 2007; 91: 269–78.
69. Bruce RD, McCance-Katz EF, Kharasch ED, Moody D, Morse GD. Pharmacokinetic interactions between buprenorphine and antiretroviral medications. Clin Infect Dis 2006; 43(Suppl 4): S216–23.
70. Drummer OH, Syrjanen M, Opeskin K, Cordner S. Deaths of heroin addicts starting on a methadone maintenance programme. Lancet 1990; 335: 108.
71. Gardner R. Methadone misuse and death by overdosage. Br J Addict 1970; 65: 113–18.
72. State Coroner of Victoria. Records of Investigation into Deaths: Case Nos. 623/89, 3273/89, 4439/88. Melbourne: State Coroner's Office; 1990.
73. Wu CH, Henry JA. Deaths of heroin addicts starting on methadone maintenance. Lancet 1990; 335: 424.

74. Auriacombe M, Franques P, Tignol J. Deaths attributable to methadone vs buprenorphine in France. JAMA 2001; 285(1): 45.
75. Gueye PN, Megarbane B, Borron SW, et al. Trends in opiate and opioid poisonings in addicts in north-east Paris and suburbs, 1995–99. Addiction 2002; 97(10): 1295–304.
76. Kintz P. A new series of 13 buprenorphine-related deaths. Clin Biochem 2002; 35(7): 513–16.
77. Gibson A, Degenhardt L. Mortality related to pharmacotherapies for opioid dependence: a comparative analysis of coronial records. Drug Alcohol Rev 2007; 26: 405–10.
78. Digiusto E, Shakeshaft A, Ritter A, O'Brien S, Mattick RP, the-NEPOD-Research-Group. Serious adverse events in the Australian National Evaluation of Pharmacotherapies for Opioid Dependence (NEPOD). Addiction 2004; 99: 450–60.
79. Ling W, Charuvastra C, Collins JF, et al. Buprenorphine maintenance treatment of opiate dependence: a multicenter, randomized clinical trial. Addiction 1998; 93(4): 475–86.
80. Ahmadi J, Babaee-Beigi M, Alishahi M, Maany I, Hidari T. Twelve-month maintenance treatment of opium-dependent patients. J Subst Abuse Treat 2004; 26: 61–4.
81. Amass L, Bickel WK, Crean JP, Blake J, Higgins ST. Alternate-day buprenorphine dosing is preferred to daily dosing by opioid-dependent humans. Psychopharmacol (Berl) 1998; 136: 217–25.
82. Bickel WK, Amass L, Crean JP, Badger GJ. Buprenorphine dosing every 1, 2, or 3 days in opioid-dependent patients. Psychopharmacol (Berl) 1999; 146: 111–18.
83. Schottenfeld RS, Pakes J, O'Connor P, Chawarski M, Oliveto A, Kosten TR. Thrice-weekly versus daily buprenorphine maintenance. Biol Psychiat 2000; 47: 1072–9.
84. Perez de los Cobos J, Martin S, Etcheberrigaray A, et al. A controlled trial of daily versus thrice-weekly buprenorphine administration for the treatment of opioid dependence. Drug Alcohol Depen 2000; 59: 223–33.
85. Marsch LA, Bickel WK, Badger GJ, Jacobs EA. Buprenorphine treatment for opioid dependence: the relative efficacy of daily, twice and thrice weekly dosing. Drug Alcohol Depen 2005; 77: 195–204.
86. Petry NM, Bickel WK, Badger GJ. Examining the limits of buprenorphine interdosing interval: daily, every third day and every fifth day dosing regimes. Addiction 2001; 96(6): 823–34.
87. Gross A, Jacobs EA, Petry NM, Badger GJ, Bickel WK. Limits to buprenorphine dosing: a comparison between quintuple and sextuple the maintenance dose every five days. Drug Alcohol Depen 2001; 64: 111–16.
88. Strang J. Abuse of buprenorphine. Lancet 1985; 28(8457): 725.
89. Robinson GM, Dukes PD, Robinson BJ, Cooke RR, Mahoney GN. The misuse of buprenorphine and buprenorphine-naloxone combination in Wellington, New Zealand. Drug Alcohol Depen 1993; 33: 81–6.
90. Obadia Y, Perrin V, Feroni I, Vlahov D, Moatti JP. Injecting misuse of buprenorphine among French drug users. Addiction 2001; 96: 267–72.

91. Jenkinson RA, Clark NC, Fry CL, Dobbin M. Buprenorphine diversion and injection in Melbourne, Australia: an emerging problem? Addiction. 2005; 100(2): 197–205.
92. O'Connor JJ, Maloney E, Travers R, Campbell A. Buprenorphine abuse among opiate addicts. Br J Addict 1988; 83: 1085–7.
93. Singh RA, Mattoo SK, Malhotra A, Varma VK. Cases of buprenorphine abuse in India. Acta Psychiatrica Scandinavia 1992; 86: 46–8.
94. Mendelson J, Jones T. Clinical and pharmacological evaluation of buprenorphine and naloxone combinations: why the 4:1 ratio for treatment? Drug Alcohol Depen 2003; 70: S29–S37.
95. Ahmadi J. Buprenorphine maintenance treatment of heroin dependence: the first experience from Iran. J Subst Abuse Treat 2002; 22: 157–9.
96. Fiellin DA, Pantalon MV, Chawarski MC, et al. Counseling plus buprenorphine-naloxone maintenance therapy for opioid dependence. New Engl J Med 2006; 355(4): 365–7.
97. Fiellin DA, Moore BA, Sullivan LE, et al. Long-term treatment with buprenorphine/naloxone in primary care: results at 2–5 years. Am J Addict 2008; 17: 116–20.
98. Simojoki K, Vorma H, Alho H. A retrospective evaluation of patients switched from buprenorphine (Subutex) to the buprenorphine/naloxone combination (Suboxone). Substance Abuse Treatment, Prevention, and Policy 2008; 3(16).
99. Bell J, Byron G, Gibson A, Morris A. A pilot study of buprenorphine-naloxone combination tablet (Suboxone) in treatment for opioid dependence. Drug Alcohol Rev 2004; 23: 311–18.
100. Johnson RE, McCagh JC. Buprenorphine and naloxone for heroin dependence. Current Psychiatry Reports 2000; 2(6): 519–26.
101. Kakko J, Gronbladh L, Dybrandt Svanborg K, et al. A stepped care strategy using buprenorphine and methadone versus conventional methadone maintenance in heroin dependence: a randomized controlled trial. Am J Psychiat 2007; 164(5): 797–803.
102. Alho H, Sinclair D, Vuori E, Holopainen A. Abuse liability of buprenorohine-naloxone tablets in untreated IV drug users. Drug Alcohol Depen 2007; 88: 75–8.
103. Bell J, Shanahan M, Mutch C, et al. A randomized trial of effectiveness and cost-effectiveness of observed versus unobserved administration of buprenorphine-naloxone for heroin dependence [see comment]. Addiction 2007; 102(12): 1899–907.
104. Bell JR, Ryan A, Mutch C, Batey R, Rea F. Optimising the benefits of unobserved dose administration for stable opioid maintenance patients: follow-up of a randomised trial. Drug Alcohol Depen 2008; 96(1–2): 183–6.
105. Carrieri MP, Amass L, Lucas GM, Vlahov D, Wodak A, Woody GE. Buprenorphine use: the international experience. Clin Infect Dis 2006; 43: S197–215.

chapter 7

Treating heroin dependence with diamorphine (pharmaceutical heroin)

Gabriele Bammer

Introduction

Treating dependence with the drug of dependence may seem like an odd notion, but has, in fact, been practiced for some dependencies since the early 1900s. Most documentation of these initial practices comes from the United States of America and the United Kingdom.[1,2] Diamorphine (pharmaceutical heroin) prescribing became illegal in the US after 1919[1] and fell out of favor in the UK in the late 1960s.[3] The advent of HIV/AIDS in the 1980s provided a stimulus for re-examining diamorphine prescription.[4,5] This was in response to recognition that unsafe injecting practices placed illicit drug users at heightened risk of contracting HIV/AIDS, and also that getting users into treatment markedly reduced unsafe practices. Interest in diamorphine prescribing has also come from those who have advocated innovation in drug treatment and policy. While other short-acting opioids, such as morphine, codeine, and fentanyl, and other injectables, such as injectable methadone, have also been suggested as possible treatments and used in some countries, the focus of this review will be on diamorphine, as considerable evidence on this treatment option has been amassed in recent years.

This chapter draws predominantly on the relatively recent Swiss and Dutch clinical trials of diamorphine, and to a lesser extent on assessment of the long-standing British experience, which allows registered specialist prescribing of diamorphine as a standard practice (this is extensively reviewed elsewhere).[2,6] It does not draw on the more recent clinical trials from Germany, Spain, and Canada. An early Cochrane review[7,8] found that there were few eligible studies and that non-comparability meant that definitive conclusions could not be arrived at; however, this should be remedied when the results of further trials are added.

This review begins by examining the context of diamorphine prescribing, including the legal constraints; the social and treatment environment; and the way treatment is provided. It then moves on to examining the evidence for the effectiveness and cost-effectiveness of diamorphine prescribing. The third section examines risks associated with diamorphine prescription.

The context of diamorphine prescribing

The prescription of diamorphine is more constrained than is the case for other pharmacotherapies and this affects its use in clinical trials and in practice. A brief review of the legal limitations is therefore presented. From the early 1900s to the 1960s, treatment options for heroin dependence, especially pharmacotherapies, were very limited. That is no longer the case, so that the wider availability of other treatments influences who is likely to be suitable for diamorphine treatment. This is also briefly discussed. Finally, the potential risk of diversion of diamorphine to the illegal market is great and must be considered in the provision of clinical services. This has to be counter-balanced by the treatment aim of effectively reintegrating treatment clients into society. The way these conflicting objectives have been dealt with in the UK, Switzerland, and the Netherlands is discussed, along with what has been learnt from those experiences about dosing and routes of administration.

Legal constraints

Two international treaties significantly circumscribe the conditions under which diamorphine can be prescribed:

- the Single Convention on Narcotic Drugs, 1961, as amended by the 1972 protocol; and

- the United Nations Convention Against Illicit Traffic in Narcotic Drugs and Psychotropic Substances, 1988.[9]

The most significant aspect of these Conventions is that they 'limit exclusively to medical and scientific purposes the production, manufacture, export, import, distribution of, trade in, use and possession of drugs' (Article 4 of the Single Convention).[9] In addition, the Single Convention requires countries to report to the International Narcotics Control Board on the quantities of narcotic drugs required and actually used.[9]

Significant pressures are placed on countries to abide by both the spirit and letter of these conventions. The UK was the only country which permitted doctors, albeit a small number, to continue to prescribe diamorphine after the 1961 Convention was introduced. The more recent clinical trials in Switzerland and the Netherlands have had both medical and scientific rationales in keeping with the Conventions.

Social and treatment milieu

The social and treatment milieu in which diamorphine prescription takes place affects both its acceptability and its outcomes. Given that there are now a number of pharmacotherapies (methadone, buprenorphine, naltrexone, and, to a lesser extent, levo-alpha-acetylmethadol [LAAM]) and other treatment approaches for heroin dependence, it is generally agreed that diamorphine prescription is a treatment of last resort. There is some evidence to support this stance:

- In both the Swiss and the Dutch trials, the demand for diamorphine treatment was not as high as anticipated, with some available treatment places remaining vacant. In the Dutch trials only 549 of the 750 available trial places were filled.[10] It is not clear if users were put off by the restrictions associated with being in a research study, by diamorphine as treatment, or by treatment per se.
- Results from the UK suggest that a high proportion (36%) of those attracted to treatment with injectables may prefer methadone to diamorphine.[11] Injectable methadone has been available for many years in the UK and familiarity with the pharmacotherapy may be important. In Switzerland, where injectable methadone was introduced at the same

time as diamorphine, its acceptability was low.[12] This was also the case for injectable morphine.

- In the Geneva arm of the Swiss trials, oral methadone maintenance was found to be more attractive than diamorphine for many of those clients who were put on a 6-month waiting list before having access to diamorphine treatment. During that time they received oral methadone and at the end of the waiting time, only 38% (9 people) took up the diamorphine option.[13] It is noteworthy that, prior to the expansion of all treatment options which occurred at the time of the diamorphine trial, methadone maintenance was not widely available in Geneva. This suggests that the demand for diamorphine prescription can be reduced if a sound array of other options is in place.

While not conclusive, all of these results support the current approach to diamorphine prescription, which is that other effective and less expensive treatment options should be widely available and offered first.

As well as this generally agreed criterion for client suitability and treatment milieu, diamorphine is also largely seen as an adjunct both to other pharmacotherapies and to non-pharmacologic options, rather than a replacement for them. This, in turn, influences how clinical trials are conducted. Nowadays, it makes little therapeutic sense to assess diamorphine in standard phase 3 clinical trials, where the new treatment (diamorphine) is evaluated against the current gold standard (in this case oral methadone). In clinical practice, diamorphine would not replace a long-acting therapy like methadone, but might be used in conjunction with it. The most common alternative design for a 'phase 3' randomized controlled trial is therefore to examine methadone plus diamorphine versus methadone alone. This was the design used in the Dutch trials. Some would also argue that ancillary treatments like counseling and occupational therapy should be provided, given that they are known to be helpful. Assessment of diamorphine therefore has to balance scientific rigor against clinical realities. A scientifically rigorous trial aims to minimize the number of confounders so that both the comparison and its interpretation are straightforward. However, this often has limited real-world applicability. A trial that mimics ideal clinical conditions generally does not allow the separate contributions of different pharmacotherapies and adjunct treatments to be easily assessed. This was the case with most of the Swiss trials.

Having said this, it is worth pointing out that there has been one trial which can be viewed as a phase 3 trial, namely the 1970s trial undertaken by Hartnoll and colleagues[14] in the UK. Although oral methadone was already available then, the trial can be seen as comparing the best available treatment at that time, injectable diamorphine, with the new treatment, oral methadone, not the other way round. The authors also point out that it was a trial of a confrontational versus a non-confrontational approach. All participants came into treatment requesting injectable diamorphine. Some were given the treatment modality they requested (non-confrontational), whereas others were given oral methadone (confrontational). In the event, the results were equivocal. Those receiving a prescription for diamorphine tended to stay in treatment but continued to inject and use illicit drugs, although in smaller amounts than before entering treatment. Those receiving oral methadone went to one extreme or the other: either they became abstinent or nearly so, or they continued to be heavily involved in drug use (using more than the diamorphine group) and dropped out of treatment. The point being made here is that the context in which a trial occurs influences the kind of scientific design that is possible and also the results that are achieved.

The diamorphine treatment service

As outlined above, the manner in which diamorphine prescribing takes place is governed by two countervailing concerns. On the one hand, service provision aims to ensure that the prescribed diamorphine is effective as treatment, and not simply as another source of mood-altering substance, and at the same time entry of prescribed diamorphine onto the illegal market is prevented. On the other hand, service providers aim to normalize treatment for illicit drug use, so that users not only have a range of treatment options, but that they are accessible and attractive.

The 1960s experience in the UK showed that unrestricted and poorly regulated prescribing and dispensing by medical practitioners and pharmacists could contribute to the entry of diamorphine to the illegal market and lead to disenchantment among service providers about their therapeutic role.[3] This also showed that, even if only a small number of prescribers behave inappropriately, it can create an environment and expectations that bring the whole system into disrepute. One way of overcoming this is through careful regulation and monitoring. Another is to prescribe and dispense through clinics, where the pharmacotherapies are also administered.

A major, and under-recognized, contribution of the Swiss trials was that they demonstrated a workable clinic-based system for prescribing, dispensing, and administration. This system has been able to maximize the effectiveness of diamorphine as treatment and virtually eliminate any contribution to the illegal drug market, but at a cost of reducing normalization of treatment. This system of service provision has largely been used in the Dutch, German, Spanish, and Canadian trials.

In general, this system has restricted opening hours, usually for 2 to 3 hours, two or three times per day. Patients are carefully supervised to prevent drugs being brought into or taken out of the clinic. Strenuous accounting and monitoring procedures prevent staff diversion and enhanced security limits the possibility of break-ins and robbery. Cleanliness and safe practices are emphasized. Doses are carefully regulated. Take-away diamorphine is not available, but oral methadone is provided to prevent withdrawal overnight. Medical treatment and psychosocial therapies are available to help reintegrate users into society.

Examination of the detail of service provision, in the Swiss and Dutch trials in particular, has provided insights into:

- workable routes of diamorphine administration, and
- appropriate doses of diamorphine, depending on the route of administration and the adjunct pharmacotherapies used.

Routes of diamorphine administration

Most diamorphine administration in the Swiss trials was by injection. Diamorphine cigarettes were developed, but were found to be relatively ineffective, with 90% of the diamorphine being destroyed by the burning process.[12] Given that illegal heroin is mostly administered by injection in Switzerland, this was not a major problem, although it did severely restrict the ability to move trial participants to a safer route of administration.

However, inhalation ('chasing the dragon'), rather than injection, was the most common route of self-administration in the Netherlands, being practiced by 75–90% of heroin users by the late 1990s.[15] An effective method of producing inhalable diamorphine therefore had to be devised.[16]

The Swiss also undertook pilot studies of immediate- and slow-release diamorphine tablets,[17] diamorphine capsules, diamorphine suppositories, a liquid inhalation aerosol, and a powder inhalation aerosol. Limited information about these can be found in the book by Uchtenhagen and colleagues.[12] There were also Dutch studies on various preparations.[18]

Appropriate doses of diamorphine

An important service provision challenge was to determine the doses of diamorphine which should be prescribed, depending on whether the drug was administered by injection or inhalation, and depending on treatment with adjunct pharmacotherapies. In the Swiss trials, participants had the option of using diamorphine as the only pharmacotherapy, whereas in the Dutch trials diamorphine was always prescribed in conjunction with oral methadone.

Both the Swiss and the Dutch trials showed that the doses prescribed could be successfully stabilized. In the Swiss trials, the average dose of injectable diamorphine was 474 mg (SD=206 mg; median: 460 mg, 25th percentile: 340 mg, 75th percentile: 600 mg).[19] As methadone was prescribed on an as-needs basis, this varied from participant to participant. On average, participants received methadone on 30% of trial days; the average dose was 53 mg (SD=44 mg; median: 40 mg, 25th percentile: 30 mg, 75th percentile: 75 mg). In the Dutch trials, where diamorphine was coprescribed with methadone, the average daily diamorphine dose among treatment completers was 549 mg (SD=193 mg) in the injecting trial and 547 mg (SD=174 mg) in the inhaling trial. These diamorphine doses were supplemented with an average dose of 60 mg (SD=17 mg) of oral methadone and 57 mg (SD=18 mg) of oral methadone in the experimental groups of the respective trials and 71 mg (SD=24 mg) and 67 mg (SD=23 mg) in the control groups. Put another way, in the Dutch trials, participants who completed treatment visited the clinics 2.1 times per day and used 260 mg of diamorphine per visit with an average dose 548 mg of diamorphine per day.[20]

Comparison of the prescribed doses in the Swiss and Dutch trials suggests that making oral methadone available on request (as in Switzerland), rather than mandatory (as in the Netherlands), reduces the dose of diamorphine needed to produce stabilization. Even more noteworthy is comparison of the doses prescribed in the Swiss and Dutch trials with those prescribed in the UK, which are considerably lower. Metrebian and colleagues[21] surveyed prescribers and found that the median minimum daily dose was 90 mg (range 5 mg to 500 mg) and the median maximum daily dose was 350 mg (range 60 mg to 1500 mg). As Carnwath and Merrill[22] point out, much more work on appropriate doses and on dose equivalence, especially between diamorphine and methadone, is needed.

Effectiveness and cost-effectivenesss

There are three broad classes of outcomes that are of interest. First is retention in treatment, which is a prerequisite for treatment to be effective. Second is a reduction in or cessation of illicit drug use. Third is reduction in harmful behaviors and other negative consequences associated with illicit drug use, particularly criminal behavior, exposure to HIV/AIDS and other blood-borne infections, other health problems, and social dislocation. The importance of these three classes of outcomes is not usually differentiated in evaluations of diamorphine and other treatments, although more emphasis is placed on the distinction by commentators, policy makers, and the broader community, who often have a particular interest in the achievement of abstinence.

This section begins with a brief overview of the Swiss and Dutch trial designs and a synopsis of the conclusions about effectiveness and cost-effectiveness. It then examines in more detail (a) retention in treatment, (b) effects on illicit drug use and abstinence, (c) effects on health, (d) effects on criminal behavior (other than illicit drug use), (e) effects on social functioning, and (f) cost-effectiveness.

Overview of the Swiss and Dutch trial designs

In the Swiss trials, injectable diamorphine was provided in the context of substantial mandatory psychosocial and medical treatment, with oral methadone available as needed to provide additional stabilization. In this context, diamorphine prescription is more accurately described as 'diamorphine-assisted treatment'. In the Dutch context, injectable or inhalable diamorphine was provided as an adjunct to oral methadone maintenance, with standard psychosocial treatment also available, and is more accurately described as 'coprescribed diamorphine'. For convenience, the short-hand 'diamorphine prescription' will continue to be used, except when a specific trial is being referred to.

The Swiss trials involved two double-blind studies, three randomized studies, and 11 studies where treatment was allocated based on previous prescriber experience and patient preference, and where a before–after analysis of the cohort was used. One trial was conducted in a penal institution.[12] There are a number of analyses that have been conducted and published at various times. The primary results presented here are based on Rehm et al,[23] who conducted analyses using the largest number of participants. The retention in treatment data are based on the provision of injectable diamorphine-assisted treatment to 1,969 participants (in 2,166 admissions) who were seen between January 1994 and December 2000 at 21 centers in 19 cities. The results on treatment effectiveness are based on before–after analysis of outcomes for 237 patients who began treatment in the 15 months after January 1994 and who stayed in treatment for at least 18 months. Eligibility criteria for the Swiss trials were a minimum age of 20 years, heroin dependency of at least 2 years, and repeated failure in previous treatments.[12]

In the Netherlands an open-label randomized controlled multicenter study was conducted in six cities from 1998 to 2002. There were separate trials examining the effectiveness of injectable diamorphine (n=174) and inhalable diamorphine (n=375). The experimental condition consisted of 12 months of treatment with oral methadone plus coprescribed diamorphine and these participants were compared with methadone-only controls. (There was also a group who received 6 months of treatment with oral methadone plus inhalable diamorphine, but their results are not reported here.) The controls were prescribed methadone for 12 months and at the end of that time were offered 6 months of oral methadone plus coprescribed diamorphine. Diamorphine prescription was discontinued for at least 2 months at the end of the experimental treatment period.[10,20]

The main outcome variable was prespecified and was a composite, as follows. To be classified as a 'responder', trial participants had to show at least 40% improvement in at least one of three domains – physical, mental or social – compared with baseline and also not show a decrement of 40%

or more in any of the other areas. Further, use of cocaine or amphetamines could not increase by 20% or more. An 'intention to treat' analysis was performed; in the injectable trial 7 out of 76 participants did not start diamorphine treatment, in the inhalable trial 6 out of 117 did not start diamorphine treatment. The corresponding figures for methadone treatment were 0/98 and 1/139.[10] The Dutch results presented here are therefore conservative.

To be eligible, participants had to be at least 25 years old and to meet diagnostic criteria for heroin dependence for at least the past 5 years. They had to have regularly attended a methadone maintenance program for the previous 6 months and to have taken 50 mg (inhaling trial) or 60 mg (injecting trial) methadone daily for an uninterrupted period of at least 4 weeks in the previous 5 years. Those eligible for the trials used illicit heroin daily or nearly every day, had poor physical or mental health or social functioning, and had not voluntarily abstained from heroin use for longer than 2 months in the previous year. Women participants could not be pregnant or breastfeeding.[20]

Synopsis of conclusions about effectiveness and cost-effectiveness

In brief, the Swiss results showed that:

- More than 70% of patients remained in treatment for more than a year. More than 60% of those who left diamorphine treatment moved to another form of treatment.
- Consumption of illicit substances, especially illegal heroin, decreased. There was also a significant reduction in cocaine consumption.
- There were marked improvements in both physical and mental health for those who stayed in treatment for 18 months or longer.
- Reduction in criminality was especially marked, regardless of whether self-report or police report measures were used.
- Although not all parameters changed, there were improvements in a range of indicators of social integration.
- There was a considerable reduction in costs for medical care and, in particular, law enforcement; cost–benefit analysis showed that the benefits per day amounted to almost twice the daily treatment costs.

In summary, the Dutch trials showed that:

- On the composite response score, 12 months of coprescribed diamorphine plus methadone treatment was significantly more effective than methadone-only treatment for both the injectable and inhalable trials. The difference in the injectable trial was 24% and in the inhalable trial it was 23%. Fifty-six percent of those receiving coprescribed diamorphine were responders in the injectable trial and the corresponding figure for the inhalable trial was 50%.[20]
- Discontinuation of the coprescribed diamorphine after 12 months resulted in a rapid deterioration in 82% of the participants who had responded to the treatment. Perhaps more noteworthy is that 16% continued to do well.
- While program costs for diamorphine coprescription were considerably higher, they were associated with significantly reduced law enforcement costs, as well as costs of damage to victims. Cost–utility analysis showed that diamorphine coprescription also led to a greater increase in quality-adjusted life years than was the case for those receiving methadone alone.

Effects on treatment retention

Retention in treatment is a prerequisite for effectiveness and is a particularly important outcome when the target group is receiving diamorphine as a last resort, because other treatments had not been successful. There is controversy, however, about the length of treatment which is necessary, which is heightened when the treatment in question is diamorphine. There is much less controversy about long-term naltrexone treatment, for example.

In the Swiss cohort study 86% of participants remained in treatment for at least 3 months, 70% for at least a year, 50% for at least 2.5 years, and 34% for 5 years or longer.[23] The most common reason for leaving treatment at any time point was to transfer to methadone treatment (37%). Transfer to abstinence-based treatment was the next most common reason for leaving (22%) and became more common the longer participants stayed in diamorphine treatment, with 9% of those leaving in the first 4 months moving to abstinence-based treatment, increasing to 29% of those leaving diamorphine treatment after 3 or more years. Lack of compliance was the third most common reason for discharge (15%), but was only really significant early in treatment, accounting for 30% of those leaving in the first 4 months and 15% of those leaving in the next 8 months.

In the Dutch trials, retention at 12 months for those who were coprescribed diamorphine was 72% in the injecting trial and 68% in the inhaling trial,[20] which is comparable to the results of the Swiss trials. It was, however, lower than retention found in the methadone-only control groups: 85% and 87% in the injecting and inhaling trials, respectively. Given that the control groups would be eligible to receive diamorphine prescription after 12 months, the higher retention rate might be expected.

In the Dutch trials diamorphine treatment was terminated at the end of 12 months. In the following 2 months 82% of the treatment responders deteriorated substantially, regressing back to pretrial scores.[20] Perhaps more interesting and surprising is that 16% maintained their improvements after diamorphine was discontinued.[10]

Effects on illicit drug use and abstinence

For the 237 people who persisted with diamorphine-assisted treatment for at least 18 months in the Swiss trials, their use of illicit drugs is shown in Table 7.1. It can be seen that significant reductions occurred for both heroin and cocaine ($p<0.0001$). Although not illegal, benzodiazepine use also decreased from 19% at baseline to 12% at 6 months, 15% at 12 months, and 9% at 18 months. An indirect measure, whether or not participants visited the illegal drug scene in the last month, also corroborates this reduction in drug use.[23]

Little information is available on the achievement of abstinence from both prescribed diamorphine and illegal heroin. As outlined above, 22% of those who left diamophine treatment moved to abstinence-based treatment and 37% to methadone treatment.[23] It is worth noting that, overall, relatively little is known about how best to promote abstinence and that no available treatments have a strong proven track record.

The Dutch trial results were primarily based on the composite score (see above) and only few results on individual variables were reported. No data seem to have been reported on illegal heroin use or on abstinence, but reductions in cocaine and amphetamine use have been described.

After 12 months, the number of days on which cocaine was used among those receiving injectable diamorphine coprescription in the Dutch trials

Table 7.1 Effects of diamorphine-assisted treatment on the percentage using illegal drugs in the Swiss trials[23]

Illicit drug	*Baseline (%)*	*After 6 months (%)*	*After 12 months (%)*	*After 18 months (%)*
Illegal heroin	82	9	4	6
Cocaine	29	7	4	5
Did not visit the illegal drug scene in the last month	14	46	52	59

was 12.8, compared with 15.4 in the control group and 15.5 at baseline. The control group score of 15.4 was also a drop from 18.0 days at baseline. For amphetamine use, the corresponding figures were 0.4 days, 0.6 days, and 0.9 days. Baseline amphetamine use for the control group was 1.2 days.[10] After 12 months, days on which cocaine was used among those receiving inhalable diamorphine coprescription in the Dutch trials was 11.9, compared with 16.5 in the control group and 15.2 at baseline. The control group showed a small increase from 15.2 days at baseline. For amphetamine use, the corresponding figures were 0.4 days, 0.1 days, and 0.1 days. Baseline for the control group was 0.1 days.[10]

The reductions in stimulant use seen in both the Swiss and Dutch trials are noteworthy, because many assumed that other illicit drug use would increase if diamorphine was available on prescription.

Effects on health

Of the 237 people who persisted with diamorphine-assisted treatment for at least 18 months in the Swiss trials, health effects are shown in Table 7.2. It can be seen that marked reductions occurred in severe somatic and mental health problems and in the percentage who were underweight; these were all significant at the $p<0.0001$ level.[23]

Rehm and colleagues[23] also reported a significant reduction in skin infections, anxiety states, delusional disorders, and the need for somatic and mental health treatment. Figures illustrating these reductions on a

Table 7.2 Effects of diamorphine-assisted treatment on the percentage with health problems in the Swiss trials[23]

Health problem	*Baseline (%)*	*After 6 months (%)*	*After 12 months (%)*	*After 18 months (%)*
Severe somatic problems	22	12	13	13
Severe mental problems	37	20	17	19
Bodymass index less than 20 (i.e. underweight)	35	20	21	24

smaller group of participants are shown in the book by Uchtenhagen and colleagues.[12]

In the Dutch trials, the physical health score for those receiving injectable diamorphine coprescription after 12 months was 8.6, compared with 10.5 in the control group and 12.1 at baseline. The control group also showed a drop from a score of 11.1 at baseline. For mental health, the corresponding scores were 55.1, 62.1, and 76.3. The baseline score for the control group was 72.7.[10]

After 12 months, the physical health score for those receiving inhalable diamorphine coprescription in the Dutch trials was 9.3, compared with 11.3 in the control group and 10.6 at baseline. The control group also showed a small drop from a score of 11.6 at baseline. For mental health, the corresponding scores were 50.1, 66.7, and 68.4. The baseline score for the control group was 70.7.[10] The reduction in scores in the Dutch trials indicated that health improved, and again this was in line with the results from the Swiss trials.

Effects on criminal behavior (other than illicit drug use)

Of the 237 people who persisted with diamorphine-assisted treatment for at least 18 months in the Swiss trials, illegal income dropped

Table 7.3 Effects of diamorphine-assisted treatment on criminal behavior (number of offences) in the Swiss trials (n=253[25])

Offence	*Before (previous 4 weeks)*	*Before (previous 4 weeks)*	*After 6 months' treatment (previous 4 weeks)*	*After 6 months' treatment (previous 4 weeks)*
	Self-report	*Police record*	*Self-report*	*Police record*
Shoplifting	8.3	6.7	3.2	4.0
Theft and serious property offences	7.1	5.5	1.2	1.2
Trafficking cannabis	4.3	0.4	1.2	0.8
Trafficking hard drugs	13.8	6.3	2.4	2.4
Total offences (listed in this table)	26.1	17.0	6.3	7.9

from 69% of total income at admission to 17% at 6 months, 14% at 12 months and 11% at 18 months.[23] Extensive information on reduction in criminal behavior has been reported (see also Ribeaud[24]), with just one example shown in Table 7.3.[25] This example is significant because it shows that police records confirmed self-reported reduction in criminal behavior.

In the Dutch trials, days on which illegal activities were undertaken among those receiving injectable diamorphine coprescription after 12 months was 2.9, compared with 8.7 in the control group and 12.9 at baseline. The control group also showed a drop from 11.5 days at baseline.[10] After 12 months, days on which illegal activities were undertaken among those receiving inhalable diamorphine coprescription in the Dutch trials was 3.6, compared with 7.8 in the control group and 11.4 at baseline. The control group also showed a drop from 11.2 days at baseline.[10]

Effects on social functioning

For the 237 people who persisted with diamorphine-assisted treatment for at least 18 months in the Swiss trials, the effects on social functioning are shown in Table 7.4. Statistically significant reductions were seen in the percentage who lived in unstable housing situations, who were homeless, and who were unemployed. There was a slight (but significant) increase in the percentage who received a disability pension, a slight (but significant) reduction in those receiving welfare payments, and a slight increase in the percentage who had no debt.[23]

In the Dutch trials, days on which there was no personal contact with non-drug users among those receiving injectable diamorphine coprescription after 12 months was 14.0, compared with 12.7 in the control group and 17.9 days at baseline. The control group also showed a drop from 16.3 days at baseline.[10] After 12 months, days on which there was no personal contact with non-drug users among those receiving inhalable diamorphine coprescription in the Dutch trials was 11.8,

Table 7.4 Effects of diamorphine-assisted treatment on social functioning in the Swiss trials[23]

Social functioning measure	*Baseline (%)*	*After 6 months (%)*	*After 12 months (%)*	*After 18 months (%)*
Unstable housing situation	43	31	24	21
Homeless	18	8	1	1
Unemployed	73	48	44	45
Receiving disability pension	22	22	25	27
Receiving welfare payments	63	60	61	54
No debt	26	26	27	33

compared with 12.2 in the control group and 14.2 at baseline. The control group also showed a small drop from 13.7 days at baseline.[10]

Cost-effectiveness

The results of the cost–benefit analysis undertaken for the Swiss trials are reported in Gutzwiller and Steffen.[26] Considerably more effort was put into determining costs[27] than benefits,[28] thus the results are likely to be conservative.[29] There has also been some criticism of how the calculations were undertaken,[29,30] but there is general agreement that the benefits outweighed the costs. The total benefit was calculated at CHF (Swiss francs) 95.50 per participant per day, compared with the cost of CHF 51.17 per person per day. Reduced crime contributed most to the benefits (75.5%), followed by improved health (17.9%), improved employment (4.1%), and improved housing (2.5%).[28]

The Dutch undertook a cost–utility analysis.[31] The total program costs over 1 year averaged €16,222 higher per patient for those receiving diamorphine plus methadone compared with those receiving methadone alone. However, there were significantly reduced law enforcement costs (average €4,129) and costs of damage to victims (average €25,374) in the former group. Thus the total cost of treatment with diamorphine plus methadone was on average €12,793 less than for methadone alone. Coprescription of diamorphine was also calculated to increase quality-adjusted life years (QALYs) by an additional 0.058 per patient per year. The increased QALYs after 1 year in the diamorphine plus methadone group were 0.788 and in the methadone group they were 0.730.

Risks

Feasibility research undertaken in Australia in the 1990s was unique in its detailed consideration of the potential risks associated with diamorphine prescribing and of how these risks might be minimized and evaluated.[32,33] Because of the lack of solid empirical evidence, this assessment largely rested on expert opinion – sought primarily from police, providers of treatment and other services, users and ex-users, and particularly from opponents of diamorphine prescribing. The Swiss and Dutch trials begin to provide an empirical base for reassessing those risks.[34] Unless another reference is cited, the findings presented below were first presented in reference 34. A brief summary of the risks, with relevant results from the Swiss and Dutch trials, follows.

Diamorphine prescribing would not achieve positive outcomes

Trial results have been overwhelmingly positive, as indicated earlier.

Diamorphine prescribing was unworkable if it was to occur through a clinic-based system which required user attendance for each administration

As described above, the opposite has occurred, with the Swiss devising a clinic-based system, which has now been widely emulated in other countries.

Diamorphine prescribing could lead to more permissive attitudes towards illicit drug use

Prescription of heroin and permissiveness towards illegal drug use are not inextricably linked, with permissiveness resulting from complex interacting factors, over which a trial can exert relatively little influence. The Swiss and Dutch were very careful to present and discuss their trials in a way which did not support drug use, but neither country undertook general population surveys on changes in attitudes towards illicit drug use during the trials, so that the available evidence is largely circumstantial. Nevertheless, there were no indications of increased permissiveness.

Diamorphine prescribing could attract dependent users from around the country and/or from neighboring countries, in a 'honeypot effect'

In both the Swiss and Dutch trials careful attention was paid to residency criteria and this seems to have prevented an influx of users from other areas or other countries.

Diamorphine prescribing could reduce motivation to completely cease all heroin use and could institutionalize and further marginalize trial participants

As outlined above, there is no information about the impact on abstinence. However, in the Swiss trials, 22% of those who left treatment transferred to abstinence-based treatments.[23] In the Dutch trials 16% of the participants who benefited from the diamorphine treatment ('responders') continued to do well in terms of health, social functioning, and reduced criminal activities when diamorphine coprescription was terminated as planned after 12 months. While this percentage may seem low, this is a surprising finding. The Dutch trials focused on those otherwise unlikely to become abstinent, by restricting trial eligibility to those who had been heroin dependent for at least 5 years and excluding anyone who had been voluntarily abstinent for 2 or more months in the preceding year.

In addition, measures of social functioning in the core trial evaluation of both the Swiss and Dutch trials showed that diamorphine prescription led to social integration rather than institutionalization and further marginalization, through increased contacts outside the drug scene, improved living conditions, and reductions in illegal activities. Further, participants tended to visit the clinic less often than they were eligible to. Rather than three visits per day, Swiss trial participants tended to visit 2.6 times per day[19] and Dutch participants 2.1 times per day.[10]

The evidence for the demotivating effects of diamorphine treatment is therefore not strong.

Diamorphine prescribing could undermine other treatments by encouraging people to drop out in order to qualify for diamorphine. Further, it could have opportunity costs through being funded at the expense of other treatments and it could be unaffordable in the long term

The effect on treatment drop-out of restricting diamorphine prescription to those for whom other treatments have been unsuccessful warrants further investigation. Although the factors influencing the effects of diamorphine prescription on national drug treatment policy are complex and outside the control of those providing diamorphine treatment, the Swiss experience shows that introducing diamorphine prescription can occur in, and even help stimulate, a context of overall improvement in the treatment system.

Diamorphine prescription is expensive. The results from the Swiss trials suggest that the benefits of diamorphine prescription considerably outweigh the costs, but further cost–benefit and cost-effectiveness analysis is needed. This includes assessment of the cost-effectiveness of other forms of treatments for the same patient group.

Diamorphine prescription could make law enforcement more difficult by blurring the differentiation between lawful and unlawful heroin use or by allowing justification of crimes committed under the influence of diamorphine prescription

While these issues were not part of the specific evaluation of either the Swiss or Dutch trials, there were no indications in either country that such blurring or justification occurred. In both trials diamorphine prescription led to marked reductions in criminal behavior, as measured by both self-report and police records (see above). This overwhelmed any other potential effects on law enforcement.

Prescribed diamorphine could be diverted onto the illegal market

As outlined earlier, a number of measures were taken to prevent diversion in both the Swiss and Dutch trials. In Switzerland, no diversion of injectable diamorphine was reported in more than 7 years of diamorphine-assisted prescription. In the Dutch trials, a total of 50 attempts by participants to take small amounts (in all cases smaller than the participant's daily dose) of prescription diamorphine out of the unit were intercepted. These attempts should be seen in context, namely that approximately 140,000 diamorphine doses were dispensed to more than 300 participants over a period of 3 years. In both the Swiss and Dutch trials the penalty for attempted diversion by participants could be exclusion from diamorphine treatment. The Dutch also reported that no aberrations were found in the diamorphine accounting process; thus there were no indications that staff diverted diamorphine. It can be concluded that effective procedures to prevent diamorphine diversion can be enacted.

Prescribed diamorphine could compromise road safety by recipients driving under the influence of heroin

Further research is needed to assess the impact of diamorphine on driving and other motor and perceptual skills, as there may be a significant risk here. In the Netherlands, a controlled clinical side-study investigated the bioavailability and pharmacodynamic effects of inhaled heroin.[16] A 50 mg dose (one-fifth of the average treatment dose) produced a decline in reaction times comparable to that of 0.7 g/kg alcohol. The decline was identifiable 25 minutes following the start of heroin inhalation, reached its maximum after 25–60 minutes, and then returned to normal in the following hours. This strongly suggests that heroin prescription is likely to affect driving skills. It is possible that this risk could be effectively managed by individual titration of diamorphine doses, but this needs further investigation.

Both the Swiss and the Dutch trials took steps to ameliorate this risk. Swiss trial participants were required to relinquish their drivers' licenses, while Dutch participants were warned about likely hazards. Both countries monitored accidents as part of the trial data collection. In Switzerland, from 1997 to 2002, there were 3 reports of accidents with motorized vehicles, all with motorbikes, and none with cars. There may have been an increase in bicycle accidents, but there are no clear comparison data. In the Dutch trials only one serious adverse event of possible relevance occurred during the 12-month experimental study period, where a patient was found wandering in traffic in a confused state.

Diamorphine prescription could increase 'public nuisance' through participants congregating outside clinics or by leading to violence between those who were and were not successful in obtaining a treatment place

These risks were not specifically assessed in the Swiss trials, but some track was kept of problems. There was no evidence to suggest any significant public nuisance. If there had been, it is unlikely that the referendum to continue diamorphine-assisted treatment would have been successful.[12] The likelihood of violence between those who were and those who were not successful in receiving a treatment place was minimal, as treatment places were generally not limited.

In the Netherlands, adverse events in the area of public order and controllability were monitored. There were 48 events outside the clinics, including use of illicit drugs, sleeping or urinating on the street near the clinic, selling drugs, (attempted) burglary, arguing, and begging. Only four were rated as severe.[10] In addition, there were 191 events within the treatment units, mostly of verbal aggression towards the treatment staff.

Unfortunately there seems to be little comparative information about public nuisance associated with other forms of drug treatment and with other facilities. Nevertheless, it seems that public nuisance associated with diamorphine prescription is low and manageable.

Diamorphine prescription could cause problems for babies born to women recipients

Further research on the effects of diamorphine on fetal and subsequent development is warranted, but current evidence provides no indications of substantial risk. There were 12 pregnancies in the Swiss diamorphine-assisted treatment trials between 1994 and 1996.[35] Four of the women were transferred to treatment with oral morphine, one gave up diamorphine treatment 4 months before the birth of the baby and the remaining women were continued on diamorphine treatment. The women were generally in poor health: all had hepatitis B, all but one had hepatitis C, two were HIV positive, and the majority had mental health problems (depression, eating disorders, and personality disorders). There were eight live births, three terminations, and one spontaneous abortion during diamorphine withdrawal in the third month of pregnancy. The abortion may be explained by opioid-induced contractions of the uterus. There were no other complications during the course of pregnancy or at birth. The children had no malformations. All children were underweight and in the smallest 10th percentile of birth weights, which is likely to have resulted from the poor health of the mothers, rather than the diamorphine treatment. There were no reports of sudden infant death syndrome (SIDS).

In the Dutch trials, pregnancy or breastfeeding were among the exclusion criteria at study entry. Women trial participants were tested for pregnancy every month, with the intention of referring any who tested positive to a general practitioner or gynecologist for further prenatal care. No such referrals were necessary.

Finally, not covered in the paper by Bammer and colleagues,[34] there has been discussion about an ethical risk, namely whether people dependent on heroin are competent to give informed consent to participation in a trial of diamorphine prescription.[36] This is unresolved and possibly unresolvable.

Conclusions

As these results illustrate, many of the speculations about the likely effects, especially potential negative effects, of diamorphine prescribing have been found to have no substance. Indeed, the results to date suggest that there may be a place for diamorphine in the treatment armamentarium. Certainly the results are positive enough to warrant further research, especially into the most effective doses, combination with other therapies, and cost-effectiveness. As diamorphine becomes more widely accepted, there is likely to be pressure to find cheaper ways to provide the treatment, which may lead to moves to relax the tight controls, which have minimized the risks. However, given the high level of controversy surrounding diamorphine prescription, it is unlikely that any significant degree of laxness will be allowed.

References

1. Musto DF. The American Disease. Origins of Narcotic Control, 3rd edn. New York: Oxford University Press, 1999.
2. Strang J, Gossop M, eds. Heroin Addiction and Drug Policy: the British System. Oxford: Oxford University Press, 1994.
3. Spear B. The early years of the 'British System' in practice. In: Strang J, Gossop M, eds. Heroin Addiction and Drug Policy: the British System, 3–28. Oxford: Oxford University Press, 1994.
4. van den Brink W, Hendriks VM, van Ree JM. Medical co-prescription of heroin to chronic, treatment-resistant methadone patients in the Netherlands. J Drug Issues 1999; 29: 587–608.
5. Zeltner T. Vorwort: Projekte des Bundesamtes für Gesundheitswesen (BAG) zur ärztlich kontrollierten Abgabe von Betäubungsmitteln. [Foreword: Project of the Federal Office of Public Health for a Medical Prescription of Narcotics]. In: Rihs-Middel M, Lotti H, Stamm R, Clerc J, eds. Ärztliche Verschreibung von Betäubungsmitteln. Wissenschaftliche Grundlagen und praktische Erfahrungen. [The medical prescription of narcotics. Scientific foundations and practical experiences]. Bern: Verlag Hans Huber, 1996.
6. Stimson GV, Metrebian N. Prescribing heroin. What's the evidence? Joseph Rowntree Foundation: York, 2003. www.jrf.org.uk/bookshop/eBooks/1859350836.pdf. Accessed 29 July 2008.
7. Ferri M, Davoli M, Perucci CA. Heroin maintenance for chronic heroin dependents (Cochrane Review). In: The Cochrane Library, Issue 1. John Wiley & Sons: Chichester, UK, 2004.
8. Ferri M, Davoli M, Perucci CA. Heroin maintenance treatment for chronic heroin-dependent individuals: a Cochrane systematic review of effectiveness. J Subst Abuse Treat 2006; 30: 63–72.
9. Norberry J. Legal issues. In: Feasibility research into the controlled availability of opioids. Volume 2 Background Papers, 87–115. National Centre for Epidemiology and Population Health: Canberra, 1991. http://nceph.anu.edu.au/Publications/Opioids/stage1vol2a.pdf. Accessed 29 July 2008.
10. CCBH: Central Committee on the Treatment of Heroin Addicts. Medical co-prescription of heroin: two randomized controlled trials. Central Committee on the Treatment of Heroin Addicts: Utrecht, 2002. www.ccbh.nl/ENG/index.htm Accessed 29 July 2008.
11. Metrebian N, Shanahan W, Stimson GV, et al. Prescribing drug of choice to opiate dependent drug users: a comparison of clients receiving heroin with those receiving injectable methadone at a West London drug clinic. Drug Alcohol Rev 2001; 20: 267–76.
12. Uchtenhagen A, Dobler-Mikola A, Steffen T, Gutzwiller F, Blättler R, Pfeifer S. Prescription of narcotics for heroin addicts. Main results of the Swiss national cohort study. Karger Verlag: Basel, 1999.
13. Perneger TV, Giner F, del Rio M, Mino A. Randomised trial of heroin maintenance programme for addicts who fail in conventional drug treatments. Brit Med J 1998; 317: 13–18.

14. Hartnoll R, Mitcheson M, Battersby A, et al. Evaluation of heroin maintenance in controlled trials. Arch Gen Psychiat 1980; 37: 877–83.
15. Nationale Drug Monitor (NDM). Jaarbericht NDM 2002 [Annual report NDM 2002]. Bureau NDM Utrecht, 2002.
16. Hendriks VM, van den Brink W, Blanken P, et al. Heroin self-administration by means of 'chasing the dragon': Pharmacodynamics and bioavailability of inhaled heroin. Eur Neuropsychopharm 2001; 11: 241–52.
17. Frick U, Rehm J, Kovacic S, et al. A prospective cohort study on orally administered heroin substitution for severely addicted opioid users. Addiction 2006; 101: 1631–9.
18. Information on studies of various preparations of diamorphine undertaken by the Dutch can be found at www.ccbh.nl/ENG/index.htm. Accessed 29 July 2008.
19. Gschwend P, Rehm J, Blättler R, et al. Dosage regimes in the prescription of heroin and other narcotics to chronic opioid addicts in Switzerland – Swiss National Cohort Study. Eur Addict Res 2004; 10: 41–8. Cited in 34.
20. van den Brink W, Hendriks VM, Blanken P, et al. Medical prescription of heroin to treatment resistant heroin addicts: two randomised controlled trials. Brit Med J 2003; 327: 310–12.
21. Metrebian N, Carnwath T, Stimson GV, Storz T. Survey of doctors prescribing diamorphine (heroin) to opiate-dependent drug users in the United Kingdom. Addiction 2002; 97: 1155–61.
22. Carnwath T, Merrill J. Dose equivalents in opioid substitution treatment. Int J Drug Policy 2002; 13: 445–7.
23. Rehm J, Gschwend P, Steffen T, et al. Feasibility, safety, and efficacy of injectable heroin prescription for refractory opioid addicts: a follow-up study. Lancet 2001; 358: 1417–20.
24. Ribeaud, D. Long-term impacts of the Swiss heroin prescription trials on crime of treated heroin users. J Drug Issues 2004; 34: 163–94.
25. Killias M, Aebi M, Ribeaud D. Effects of heroin prescription on police contacts among drug-addicts. Eur J Criminal Policy Res 1998; 6: 433–8.
26. Gutzwiller F, Steffen T, eds. Cost-Benefit Analysis of Heroin Maintenance Treatment, Karger: Basel, 2000.
27. Rossier-Affolter, R. Cost analysis on the medical prescription of narcotics. In: Gutzwiller F, Steffen T, eds. Cost-Benefit Analysis of Heroin Maintenance Treatment, 9–35. Karger: Basel, 2000.
28. Frei A, Greiner R-A, Mehnert, A, Dinkel, R. Socioeconomic evaluation of heroin maintenance treatment. In: Gutzwiller F, Steffen T, eds. Cost-Benefit Analysis of Heroin Maintenance Treatment, 37–128. Karger: Basel, 2000.
29. Jeanrenaud, C. Commentary. In: Gutzwiller F, Steffen T, eds. Cost-Benefit Analysis of Heroin Maintenance Treatment, 1–7. Karger: Basel, 2000.
30. Cook PJ. Book review of Gutzwiller F, Steffen T, eds. Cost-Benefit Analysis of Heroin Maintenance Treatment, Karger: Basel, 2000. Addiction 2001; 96: 1071–2.
31. Dijkgraaf MGW, van der Zanden BP, de Borgie CAJM, et al. Cost utility analysis of co-prescribed heroin compared with methadone maintenance

treatment in heroin addicts in two randomised trials. Brit Med J 2005; 330: 1297–302.

32. Bammer G. Provision of diamorphine (heroin) by prescription for drug dependency: issues and recommendations. CNS Drugs 1999; 11: 253–62.
33. Bammer G, Dobler-Mikola A, Fleming PM, et al. The heroin prescribing debate – integrating science and politics. Science 1999; 284: 1277–8.
34. Bammer G, Brink W van den, Gschwend P, et al., What can the Swiss and Dutch trials tell us about the potential risks associated with heroin prescribing? Drug Alcohol Rev 2003; 22: 363–71.
35. Geistlich S. Schwangerschaftsverlauf und Entzugssymptome Neugeborener in der diversifizierten Opiatabgabe. [Course of pregnancy and withdrawal symptoms in newborns in prescription of opioids.] Zürich: Institut für Suchtforschung, Bericht Nr. 51, 1997. Cited in 34.
36. Charland LC. Cynthia's dilemma: consenting to heroin prescription. Am J Bioethics 2002; 2: 37–47 and a range of commentaries.

chapter 8

Naltrexone maintenance treatment

Amy Gibson and Alison Ritter

Introduction

Naltrexone was first registered in the US in 1984[1] and today is available in many countries as a treatment for both heroin and alcohol dependence. This chapter reviews the safety, efficacy, and effectiveness of naltrexone as a maintenance treatment for opioid dependence. The safety and efficacy of naltrexone as a withdrawal intervention for heroin detoxification was discussed in Chapter 3.

Naltrexone hydrochloride is an orally well-absorbed opioid antagonist with no agonist properties.[2] It binds competitively to the μ opiate receptor to attenuate or completely block the effect of exogenous opioids at that receptor.[3] Peak plasma concentrations of naltrexone in blood plasma are reached within 1 to 2 hours after an oral dose and the duration of action approaches about 24 hours. Its metabolite, 6-beta-naltrexol, is a weaker antagonist with a longer half-life, and some antagonist action remains after approximately 48 hours[2] or even up to 72 hours.[4] Despite both compounds having relatively short half-lives, the duration of naltrexone blockade is much longer. An oral dose of 50 mg naltrexone has been shown to produce 80% inhibition of opioid binding for 72 hours.[5] Naltrexone has few actions besides its opioid-blocking properties.[6] If given to an opioid-dependent subject, naltrexone will precipitate prolonged symptoms of withdrawal.[2]

Discontinuation of naltrexone treatment produces very few symptoms, and the drug has very little or no potential for abuse.[2]

Early studies tested the use of heroin and hydromorphone under experimental conditions whilst participants were taking naltrexone.[7–11] Results consistently support naltrexone as an effective blockade against both the objective and subjective effects of heroin and hydromorphone.

At its recommended maintenance dose of 50 mg per day,[6] naltrexone is well tolerated with few side-effects.[12] The most common side-effects reported are nausea, diarrhea, vomiting, headaches, skin rashes, decreased mental acuity, dysphoria, depression, and loss of energy, with most of these symptoms occurring early in treatment.[13–20] There is no evidence that naltrexone causes or exacerbates clinically significant liver disease.[21] Whilst other rarer reactions such as mania and psychosis may occur,[22] naltrexone is considered to be a safe drug.[23]

One of the reported side-effects of naltrexone is dysphoria.[24,25] Research supports positive associations,[26] as well as non-significant associations[27] between naltrexone and dysphoria, with the most common finding being that the symptoms of depression abate over the course of naltrexone treatment.[28–31] Rea and colleagues found no significant differences in depression scores in patients randomized to 50, 0.5, or 0.05 mg per day naltrexone, or between those retained in versus those who had ceased naltrexone treatment.[32] A randomized study reported that those subjects transferring from methadone to naltrexone treatment did not exhibit any worsening of symptoms, and subjects compliant with naltrexone treatment showed less depressive symptoms than non-compliant subjects.[33] A review has concluded that there is limited evidence to support an association between naltrexone and dysphoria or depression.[34]

The pharmacologic explanation for naltrexone's effectiveness in preventing opiate use is that it blocks the effects of exogenous opioids. Conditioning plays a large role in the initiation and continuation of drug use, with the euphoric effects of opiates acting as strong positive reinforcement for further use. Research has demonstrated that the prolonged use of naltrexone enables the extinction of this conditioned response. If the opiate-dependent individual is exposed to drug-related cues without the positive reinforcement of euphoria, over time drug-seeking behavior and craving is extinguished.[23,35,36]

The first section of this chapter reports on the acceptability of naltrexone as a treatment. This is followed by a review of outcomes of naltrexone maintenance treatment, including retention in treatment, abstinence from heroin, and psychosocial outcomes.

The focus then turns to the combination of naltrexone maintenance with psychosocial treatments, and serious adverse events. The use of sustained-release formulations of naltrexone is then summarized before the chapter concludes with future directions of naltrexone maintenance research and clinical practice.

Acceptability of naltrexone treatment

There is widespread registration of naltrexone as a treatment option for heroin dependence; however this does not ensure treatment uptake. This is demonstrated in a survey of American clinicians: about 44% of private clinics in the US have naltrexone maintenance available as a treatment, but only 11% of clients are actually treated with naltrexone.[37] Thirty-nine percent of the responding clinicians in this survey believe that the availability of naltrexone treatment could be increased.[37] This figure is small compared to the 82% of respondents who stated that more 12-step programs were required.[37]

Organizational factors may play a role in the uptake of naltrexone treatment. One study found that older centers, with administrative leaders with longer tenure, those with a high percentage of managed care clients, and those centers with a high percentage of repeat presentations all had higher levels of naltrexone prescribing.[38] Barriers to the introduction and prescribing of naltrexone have been cited by American medical staff as lack of knowledge about naltrexone and perceived cost issues.[39]

Even if availability were substantially improved, the evidence suggests that the majority of opioid users remain sceptical towards naltrexone treatment.[40] A number of treatment studies have demonstrated the poor client acceptance of naltrexone. A review of naltrexone maintenance[24] calculated the average commencement rate of opiate-dependent clients across five studies.[7,41–44] Twenty-seven percent of those who expressed interest in naltrexone treatment were inducted onto naltrexone. Later studies support this low induction rate. Rothenberg and colleagues demonstrated that 78% of interested clients were eligible for treatment, but only just over half of those deemed eligible completed detoxification and commenced the naltrexone program.[45] Rawson and colleagues reported that 35% of clients who met study criteria and were interested in entering the treatment were successfully inducted onto naltrexone.[31] Likewise, Tucker and colleagues reported a 31% uptake rate from screening to successful induction onto naltrexone.[46] In a study of prisoners, Shearer and colleagues found that only 14% of those assigned to naltrexone treatment actually commenced it.[47] Similar induction rates were noted in an American study; 15% of those originally screened for participation completed inpatient detoxification and entered behavioral naltrexone therapy.[48]

Higher induction rates have been reported from two Russian studies, with Krupitsky and colleagues reporting the proportion of clients commencing treatment after initial screening at 64% and 67%, respectively.[49,50] These acceptance rates have been attributed to the fact that most heroin-dependent individuals in Russia are young, live with their parents, and are usually brought to treatment by family members who remain involved in their treatment and supervise their dosing.[50]

While there are examples of high rates of acceptance and induction onto naltrexone treatment such as those from Russia, the majority of research suggests that, despite high initial interest, only the minority of clients will eventually be inducted onto treatment. Naltrexone induction rates are much lower than agonist treatment induction rates. When heroin-dependent subjects were given a choice of naltrexone, methadone, and buprenorphine maintenance treatments following detoxification treatment with buprenorphine, only 5% chose naltrexone, whereas 60% chose methadone and buprenorphine treatment.[51–53]

Outcomes from naltrexone maintenance treatment

In their Cochrane Review, Kirchmayer and colleagues evaluated the efficacy of naltrexone maintenance treatment in preventing relapse after detoxification in opioid-dependent individuals.[3] While 11 studies met criteria for inclusion, the methodologic quality of the studies was generally poor and the study designs and outcomes measured were too heterogeneous for the authors to conclude whether naltrexone treatment is effective as a maintenance therapy.[3]

Retention in naltrexone maintenance

Retention in treatment is a key variable in understanding the efficacy of naltrexone treatment. Studies with high retention in naltrexone show better results than control groups for opioid-positive urines, psychiatric symptoms, craving, and levels of opioid abuse after cessation of treatment.[54]

Naltrexone treatment has been characterized by early attrition with many clients leaving treatment within the first 2 weeks,[55] and it has been stated that the largest obstacle to maintaining abstinence is retaining patients in the first few weeks of treatment.[45] A review reported an average attrition rate of 39% for the first 2 weeks of treatment,[24] while some later studies have reported lower attrition rates. Tucker and colleagues reported an attrition rate at the end of the second week of treatment of 22%,[56] and in an effectiveness study of 981 consecutive admissions, Bartu and colleagues reported an attrition rate of 21% in the first two weeks.[57]

Given the high early attrition from treatment, low overall retention rates are not surprising. Average retention periods varied between one and a half and eight months.[15,16,27,41,58–60] The average retention period calculated across these studies was 3 months,[24] a figure that remains reasonably consistent with later studies. Rothenberg and colleagues reported 55% of their naltrexone maintenance sample completed 1 month; 40% completed 8 weeks, with 19% of participants remaining in treatment at 6 months.[45] Bartu and colleagues reported an average retention rate of 9 weeks, with 25% of clients achieving 3 months of treatment.[57]

Studies of highly motivated participants generally demonstrate the highest retention and completion rates, for example naltrexone treatment as a component of a prisoner work-release program resulted in a 75% retention rate.[61] Similarly, 61% of clients who were business executives and 74% of those who were physicians remained in naltrexone treatment for 6 months.[62] An Italian study showing a high degree of family participation and cooperation in patient treatment reported 80% retention at 6 months.[63] In contrast, the work by Shearer and colleagues with Australian prisoners did not demonstrate superior retention in prison populations, with only a 7% retention rate at 6 months and a mean retention of 59 days.[47] The absence of incentives and coercion when compared to other studies of prison populations was suggested as a major influence on their results.

An average retention of 3 months for regular opioid-dependent treatment seekers, with higher rates for highly motivated or otherwise coerced populations, is a relatively brief period of treatment for a chronic relapsing condition such as heroin dependence. It is important, then, to consider how retention in naltrexone treatment compares with placebo.

Non-significant differences in retention between naltrexone and placebo groups were found in three studies, two tending towards longer retention in naltrexone treatment,[55,64] and the other showing that placebo-treated participants had longer retention and attendance at more scheduled visits.[26] These studies tend to point towards non-superior retention in naltrexone treatment compared to placebo. In contrast, significant differences in retention and relapse were found between naltrexone and placebo groups in highly motivated participants in Russia.[49] At 6 months, 44% of the naltrexone participants remained in treatment relapse-free compared to only 16% of the placebo participants.[49] A significant difference in retention between naltrexone and placebo groups was confirmed in later work by the same research group examining the role of fluoxetine in improving naltrexone treatment outcomes.[50] Thus, there may be evidence for superior retention in naltrexone treatment compared to placebo.

A more critical comparison for retention rates is between naltrexone treatment and other maintenance treatments for heroin dependence. The evidence so far shows that retention in naltrexone is consistently shorter than in agonist maintenance treatments.[53] Studies comparing retention in naltrexone and methadone treatment found that clients treated with methadone remained in treatment longer than those treated with naltrexone.[47,65–67] A study of Australian prisoners found that the longest retention occurred with the methadone group, followed by the buprenorphine group, and finally the naltrexone maintenance group.[47] While the sample size was small by the end of the study, this result has been supported by other research groups. Ahmadi and Ahmadi investigated retention in a 24-week treatment study for 204 illicit buprenorphine-dependent clients who were randomized to methadone, buprenorphine, or naltrexone maintenance treatment.[67] The study found that clients treated with methadone remained in treatment longer than those treated with naltrexone and retention was significantly better for the buprenorphine group than the naltrexone group.[67]

It is not surprising that naltrexone has shorter treatment retention than agonist treatments. As naltrexone has no agonist properties, it produces no euphoria, tolerance, or dependence. Therefore, no positive or negative reinforcements are offered, and clients may stop treatment at any stage without immediate physiologic consequences. This is in contrast to methadone, which produces agonist effects and which has significant withdrawal symptoms if discontinued suddenly.[55,65,68]

A key challenge for naltrexone treatment appears to be improving retention. When retention is improved, relapse to heroin use is less likely.[16,18,54,59,62,69] Endeavors to improve retention have included the use of psychosocial treatments[20,35] and reinforcement protocols. For example, a study of a voucher-based incentive program demonstrated improved retention for those in the intervention group, with 50% of clients retained in treatment for 3 months compared to 25% of clients in the non-voucher group.[70] The combined use of naltrexone with psychosocial interventions is summarized later. Other ways to improve retention are through alternate medication delivery systems, such as sustained-release naltrexone formulations.[40] These have been in development for some time and are described in full later in the chapter.

Opioid abstinence

Opioid abstinence and relapse to opioid use are commonly reported outcome measures, although large variations exist between studies in how these outcomes are defined[71] and whether abstinence is measured during or after treatment.

Naltrexone substantially improves opioid abstinence rates while subjects remain in treatment. In a review of studies reporting urine test results while subjects were retained in treatment, an average of only 6% of urine tests were positive for opioids.[24]

As with treatment retention, the highest rates of post-treatment abstinence were found in the highly motivated participant groups. A group of naltrexone-treated parolees and probationers only recorded 8% opioid-positive urines after 6 months.[55] All 14 physicians who completed a naltrexone treatment program were still abstinent from opiates (determined by urine drug screens) at 12-month follow-up, and 64% of business executives were still abstinent at 12 and 18 months post-naltrexone treatment.[62] A group of highly motivated clients receiving supportive therapy were followed up 12 months after completion of ultra rapid detoxification under anesthesia and commencement of naltrexone maintenance treatment.[72] Sixty-eight percent of the clients were abstinent at 12 months with 24% having relapsed and 8% lost to follow-up.[72]

Opioid abstinence in naltrexone maintenance treatment has been compared to abstinence in placebo treatment, with mixed results. Several studies found significantly higher abstinence rates amongst their naltrexone participants compared to the placebo groups.[44,73] Again, more highly motivated groups feature in the positive results. A group of naltrexone-treated parolees and probationers only recorded 8% opioid-positive urines after 6 months, significantly lower than the 30% opioid-positive urines in those receiving placebo treatment.[55] In a group of Russian participants with high levels of family support, only 30% (n=8) of the naltrexone participants had relapsed, significantly fewer than the 72% (n=18) of the placebo group participants who had relapsed to opioid use.[49] There have also been reports of no significant difference in abstinence rates between naltrexone and placebo treatments.[26,64]

Studies comparing abstinence outcomes between naltrexone and methadone maintenance treatment have reported differing results: two studies found significantly higher abstinence rates in the naltrexone groups,[74,75] and one reported non-significant differences in abstinence rates.[65,66] These three studies were all non-randomized studies.

In relation to other treatment modalities, one non-randomized study found that naltrexone and treatment in a therapeutic community both produced similar improvements in abstinence.[76] Another non-randomized comparison of naltrexone with psychotherapy revealed significantly more naltrexone clients than those in psychotherapy were opiate-free.[77] The only randomized trial which compared naltrexone with behavior therapy[78] demonstrated at 12 months post-treatment that 49% of naltrexone participants contacted were opiate-free compared to 27% of those clients in the behavior therapy group. At 5-year follow-up, 20% of naltrexone participants remained abstinent while only 8% of those who participated in behavior therapy were abstinent.[78]

Opioid abstinence outcomes are substantially improved while subjects remain in naltrexone treatment, and accordingly opioid abstinence rates are highest in highly motivated subjects with good treatment retention.

In comparisons of abstinence between naltrexone and either placebo or agonist maintenance treatments, the results are equivocal and limited by heterogeneity in design and measurement of outcomes.[3,71]

Psychosocial outcomes

Psychosocial adjustment is also an important measure of treatment outcome. A number of studies reported post-treatment improvement in employment and psychosocial adjustment after naltrexone treatment.[18,42,61,62,79] Five studies compared psychosocial treatment outcomes in naltrexone with placebo or no treatment control groups.[27,30,44,55,80] In every case, psychosocial improvements were significantly greater for those clients from the naltrexone group. In a meta-analysis, subjects treated with both naltrexone and behavior therapy had a significantly reduced risk of re-incarceration compared to subjects treated with behavior therapy only (odds ratio [OR]=0.30, 95% confidence interval [CI] 0.12–0.76).[3]

In contrast, Krupistky and colleagues reported improvements in depression, anxiety, anhedonia, and overall adjustment in participants who stayed in treatment, irrespective of allocation to placebo or naltrexone.[49] A study randomizing subjects to three different doses of naltrexone reported that those retained in naltrexone treatment at 3 months did not have significantly different depression scores from those not receiving naltrexone.[32]

Only two studies could be located which directly compared psychosocial outcomes between naltrexone treatment and other forms of intervention. O'Brien and colleagues observed that naltrexone-treated participants reported greater satisfaction with the program and more treatment benefits than the participants treated with methadone and propoxyphene.[74] Arndt and colleagues' naltrexone-treated participants showed significant improvements on psychiatric symptoms, employment status, and legal status, compared to those participants treated within a therapeutic community.[76]

Naltrexone combined with psychosocial therapy

Whilst ancillary support and therapy will provide benefit to any treatment modality, as an opiate antagonist, naltrexone appears to have a greater need for these services due to its lack of reinforcing opiate effects.[81] Various psychosocial treatments have been used successfully with naltrexone, including supportive counseling (individual, group, and family),[20,74,81] behavioral therapy,[74,81] and cognitive behavioral therapy.[82]

Studies specifically examining the additional benefit of psychotherapeutic interventions have found that the combined use of naltrexone and psychosocial therapy proved more effective than psychosocial therapy alone,[3,83–85] and more effective than naltrexone treatment alone, in improving post-treatment outcome.[23,84,86]

Recent randomized controlled trials have investigated outcomes for standard naltrexone treatment compared to naltrexone plus adjunctive therapy, including: enhanced versus standard counseling treatment;[31] low-value contingency management or high-value contingency management;[87] structured group counseling;[46] contingency management and contingency management plus family involvement;[88] and voucher incentives.[70]

In the vast majority of cases, retention and opioid abstinence were reported to be higher for those participants receiving the enhanced or additional psychosocial protocols in conjunction with naltrexone maintenance therapy. Rawson and colleagues reported participants in the enhanced naltrexone maintenance group were retained significantly longer in treatment than participants in the standard naltrexone group, 14.7 weeks compared to 9.1 weeks.[31] A greater percentage of the enhanced naltrexone treatment group were opioid-free (86.2%) compared to the standard naltrexone treatment group (74.6%); however by the 6-month follow-up there was no significant difference in abstinence rates between the two groups.[31] Carroll and colleagues reported higher treatment retention and a significant reduction in opiate use for participants who were involved in naltrexone plus contingency management compared to standard naltrexone maintenance treatment.[87] Preston and colleagues compared three groups: a contingent group (who earned vouchers for each naltrexone dose), a non-contingent group (who earned vouchers independently of naltrexone); and a no voucher control group. Significantly higher retention was found for participants in the contingent group, and while the contingent group tended to have a lower proportion of opiate-positive specimens, this difference was non-significant.[70] Tucker and colleagues found no significant differences in retention between those who received standard naltrexone treatment and those participants who received naltrexone plus group counseling.[46] All participants in this study significantly reduced their level of heroin use across the study.[46]

The above studies represent the randomized controlled trials. Behavioral naltrexone therapy (BNT) combines pharmacotherapy with efficacious behavioral interventions such as contingency management, network therapy, and components of the community reinforcement approach.[45] Developed to encourage higher retention, a randomized controlled trial has yet to be reported in the literature. In the pilot study, retention at 6 months was poor (19%) with the predictable early drop-out being most problematic.[45] Additional analysis on these participants demonstrated that at least three quarters of the participants were also taking non-opiate drugs during treatment.[89] In a naturalistic study of 981 consecutive admissions there was no significant difference in retention between those clients voluntarily receiving additional psychosocial support and those who chose not to have additional support.[57] Unfortunately, the quality of the psychosocial support was not assessed, thus the interpretation and generalizability of the findings are questionable.

The role of families has been noted as an important feature of effective naltrexone maintenance treatment. In a randomized trial of naltrexone maintenance treatment with behavioral family counseling or individually based treatment, the behavioral family counseling group had fewer drug-related legal and family problems at 12-month follow-up.[90] In studies of naltrexone maintenance in Italy and Russia, the importance of families in successful treatment outcomes was noted. The majority of families showed strong support for the naltrexone maintenance treatment program, and the authors hypothesize that family participation contributed to high retention and good clinical outcomes.[49,50,63] Likewise, Hulse and Basso evaluated the role of vigilant supervision of dosing by 'salient others' and reported that supervision of naltrexone dosing predicted better outcomes, both in terms of treatment retention and relapse.[91] On the other hand, Bartu and colleagues found no association between the presence of a partner and improved retention in treatment.[57]

Other attempts to improve retention and outcomes from naltrexone maintenance have included combination pharmacotherapies, such as the use of both naltrexone and antidepressant medication. A pilot trial comparing naltrexone plus a selective serotonin reuptake inhibitor and naltrexone plus placebo in 13 abstinent opiate-dependent clients demonstrated a reduction in opiate craving, as measured by an opiate craving questionnaire, but no significant difference in retention over the 12 weeks of the study.[92] While adding fluoxetine to naltrexone treatment did not improve retention or opioid relapse outcomes in a large Russian study, 6-month relapse-free retention rates in the naltrexone plus fluoxetine and naltrexone plus placebo groups were 43% and 36%, respectively.[50] A small study investigating treatment with both naltrexone and the benzodiazepine prazepam found a significantly lower percentage of opioid-positive urine samples in the group treated with naltrexone and prazepam than in groups treated with naltrexone alone or placebo.[13]

A number of studies have examined the relationship between client characteristics and treatment outcome.[18,19,42,59,62,64–66,69,75] Clients with personality disorders and polydrug users were more likely to relapse.[93] Being employed and having family or social support are two of the characteristics associated with successful outcome across a number of studies. There also appears to be a trend towards greater success being associated with being older, more heavily heroin dependent, and having a greater number of previous treatment attempts. External motivators, such as criminal charges or the threat of losing employment, also appear to be associated with a greater likelihood of successful treatment.[45] Those participants who had been using methadone at baseline had significantly poorer retention rates than those using heroin at baseline.[45]

Serious adverse events

One important outcome from pharmacotherapy treatment is the rate of adverse and serious adverse events. Adverse events are defined as any reaction, side-effect, or untoward event that occurs during the course of the clinical trial, whether or not the event is considered to be drug related. Side-effects for naltrexone were outlined earlier in the chapter. Here we concentrate upon serious adverse events (SAEs) as any fatal or immediately life-threatening clinical experience, any permanently or severely disabling event, an event that requires hospitalization, or a congenital anomaly.[94]

The most pertinent SAE is opiate overdose – both non-fatal and fatal. The first evidence of increased rates of overdose in a sample of naltrexone clients was reported by Miotto and colleagues.[28] Thirteen of 81 participants in a naltrexone study overdosed within a 12-month period of study participation. Rates of non-fatal overdose across three studies (LAAM, buprenorphine, and naltrexone) revealed a significantly higher non-fatal overdose rate for participants of the naltrexone study. Ritter reported that 16.5% of the naltrexone study participants had experienced a non-fatal overdose, compared to only 5% of participants in a concurrent buprenorphine maintenance study, and no overdoses were recorded for a concurrent LAAM maintenance study.[95] In a naltrexone treatment study from the same center, 24 non-fatal overdoses in a sample of 97 were reported within a 6-month follow-up period.[46] In a study of 66 patients randomized to different doses of naltrexone, two patients completed suicide and one patient took a deliberate (non-fatal) opioid overdose.[32]

In a comprehensive analysis of rates of SAEs across both withdrawal and maintenance treatments with methadone, buprenorphine, LAAM, and naltrexone, Digiusto and colleagues calculated both in-treatment and out-of-treatment SAE rates. After leaving treatment, the overdose rate for naltrexone participants was eight times that recorded for participants who had ceased agonist pharmacotherapy treatment. SAEs other than overdose were similar between the pharmacotherapies, both during and after treatment.[96] Of the 5 deaths reported after treatment, 3 were from the naltrexone group, the remaining 2 from the opioid agonist treatment groups.[96]

Death rates of clients after naltrexone treatment has ceased are generally reported to be elevated when compared to other treatments for heroin dependence. Estimates of mortality rates are complicated, but may vary 10-fold between 0.8% and 8% per annum.[97–99] Methadone maintenance clients have an estimated mortality rate of less than 1% per annum.[99] The mortality rates from published naltrexone outcome studies indicate a higher rate (3–5%).[28,32,100] An uncontrolled study examined Australia-wide death rates in methadone, buprenorphine, and naltrexone maintenance treatment over a 4-year period. During the highest risk time of both naltrexone treatment (shortly after treatment cessation) and methadone maintenance treatment (during treatment induction), the relative risk of death in oral naltrexone-treated subjects was 7.4 times higher than in methadone maintenance subjects ($p < 0.0001$).[101]

The distinction between in-treatment overdose risk and post-treatment overdose risk is an important one. Naltrexone is protective against overdose whilst the client remains on the medication,[2,102] but the primary cause of naltrexone-related death is by opioid overdose after the cessation of naltrexone treatment.[6] Such deaths are poorly monitored,[103] as only a mention of recently ceased or non-compliant naltrexone treatment in coronial records identifies the death as naltrexone-related.[101] The data so far indicate that the rate of overdose after treatment is significantly higher for naltrexone treatment compared to other pharmacotherapy treatments.

Sustained-release naltrexone formulations

Sustained-release naltrexone formulations such as implants or depots were primarily developed to overcome the common problem of poor compliance and low retention with oral naltrexone treatment,[104–107] and have been in development for many years. At least nine different sustained-release formulations are available, examples include the Vivitrol and Depotrex depot formulations and the GoMedical, Prodetoxone, and Wedgewood implant formulations.[40] Of these, only the Prodetoxone implant is approved for the treatment of heroin dependence in Russia,[108] and no sustained-release preparation is approved for the treatment of heroin dependence in either the European Union, US, or Australia.[40]

Effective blood concentrations of naltrexone

There is evidence to suggest that there are marked individual variations in plasma concentrations of naltrexone resulting from sustained-release formulations and, further, that there is considerable intraindividual variation in plasma levels.[109] This suggests that different individuals, when given the same dose of naltrexone, may have different levels of protection against opioid agonists. It also suggests that, at different times, the same individual may have different levels of protection, an issue of concern given the risk faced by patients if they relapse to opioid use.

A case study of blood naltrexone levels in 5 patients receiving sequential naltrexone implants also demonstrated great intra- and interpersonal variability.[110] In this study, blood levels of above 2 ng/ml naltrexone, and 10 ng/ml 6-β-naltrexol, were considered 'adequate implant coverage'. Naltrexone levels dropped below 2 ng/ml for two subjects, and over half of the samples tested for 6-β-naltrexol were below 10 ng/ml. As the blood sampling frequency in this study was not consistent between subjects, additional instances of low blood naltrexone could have been missed.

Opioid use during treatment was not reported, but participants remained 'non heroin dependent.'[110]

The criterion for 'adequate coverage' was lower than others have suggested: levels of 10–30 ng/ml blood naltrexone are considered fully effective in antagonizing the euphoric effects of 25 mg intravenous heroin; 2 ng/ml only has 87% efficacy.[111] If 10 ng/ml blood naltrexone was taken as the criterion, only 4 of 46 samples (9%) in the previous study provided adequate coverage.[110]

The first randomized controlled study of sustained-release naltrexone in the treatment of heroin dependence used two doses of depot naltrexone. The 192 mg naltrexone depot resulted in mean plasma naltrexone levels between 0.4 and 1.9 ng/ml, and the 384 mg naltrexone depot gave plasma naltrexone levels between 1.3 and 3.2 ng/ml.[112] The authors noted that blood naltrexone levels tended to decrease in the fourth week after administration, but further details on this decline were not provided.

Brewer reported on an opiate challenge using 100 mg of intravenous diamorphine in a client with a naltrexone implant 3 weeks after insertion. No objective agonist effects were observed. Naltrexone blood level was 5 ng/ml and 6-β-naltrexol was 12 ng/ml.[113] The second client was challenged with 500 mg of intranasal pure pharmaceutical diamorphine. The client had serum naltrexone levels at 2.8 ng/ml and serum 6-β-naltrexol at a concentration of 9 ng/ml. No objective opiate response to this dose was observed.[113]

Based on their results of 34 clients (10 clients received a '1.7 g' naltrexone implant and 24 clients received a '3.4 g' naltrexone implant) Hulse and colleagues ascribed blood concentrations of 2 ng/ml for naltrexone and 10 ng/ml for 6-β-naltrexol as being the therapeutically active levels for naltrexone maintenance treatment.[110] The authors calculated the time intercept for naltrexone and 6-β-naltrexol blood levels for a person with an average body weight of 70 kg. They then calculated that the '1.7 g' naltrexone implant can be regarded as therapeutically active for 90 days and the '3.4 g' implant for 188 days.[110] Due to a miscalculation by the naltrexone implant manufacturer (Go Medical), it was later found that the '1.7 g' and '3.4 g' implants actually contained 1.1 g and 2.2 g naltrexone, respectively.[114]

In further testing of the Go Medical naltrexone implants, a 3.3 g implant resulted in blood naltrexone levels above 2 ng/ml for 145 days (95% CI 125–167 days), which did not result in a significantly longer period of blood naltrexone levels above 2ng/ml than the 2.2g naltrexone implant (136 days, 95% CI 114–158 days). The smallest 1.1g naltrexone implant provided blood naltrexone levels of about 2ng/ml for 95 days (95% CI 69–121 days).[115] This study by Ngo and colleagues (2008) found the 1.1g and 2.2g implants produced shorter periods of blood naltrexone levels greater than 2ng/ml than previously reported.[110]

Olsen and colleagues studied 10 opioid-dependent clients who received between one and four 1g implants simultaneously.[109] The study found considerable variations between individual concentration profiles. Inter-individual variation was noted for the duration naltrexone concentrations were above 1ng/ml, with a range between 30 and 80 days (median, 55 days). Considerable intraindividual variation in naltrexone concentrations for some clients who received more than one implant was also observed. For example, for one client, the maximum plasma concentration of naltrexone varied from 10.8 to 22.1ng/ml. For another client the length of time that the concentration of naltrexone was above 1ng/ml varied from 52 to 80 days.[109]

Comer and colleagues reported on 12 heroin-dependent individuals who participated in an 8-week inpatient study of depot naltrexone.[116] After a 1-week detoxification period, 6 clients received a depot of 192mg naltrexone and 6 clients received a depot of 384mg naltrexone. The effects of intravenous heroin (0, 6.25, 12.5, 18.75, 25mg) were studied for the next 6 weeks. One dose was tested per weekday and a placebo could be administered on any day. The doses of heroin were administered in ascending order. The primary findings from this study were that low (192mg) and high (384mg) doses of depot naltrexone both antagonized heroin-induced subjective effects for 3 and 5 weeks respectively, and plasma levels of naltrexone remained above 1ng/ml for 22 days for the low dose and 29 days for the high dose.[116] Another inpatient study of 5 heroin-dependent individuals supported this work; 384mg depot naltrexone antagonized both the reinforcing and subjective effects of heroin for 4 to 5 weeks.[117]

Foster and colleagues reported on two clients who claimed to have injected 50mg of methadone and 300mg of morphine at 40 and 21 days post implantation of a 1g implant, respectively, without experiencing opiate effects, and a third client who was challenged in the laboratory with 1000 μg of intravenous fentanyl (equivalent to 1000mg of pethidine) 2 weeks after the implant with no observable opiate response.[106]

More research is needed to investigate minimum levels of naltrexone and its metabolite needed to block all opiate effects and the degree of intra- and interindividual variation in these blood levels. While the 2ng/ml plasma therapeutic level of naltrexone is used by several research groups,[112,113,118–120] other researchers believe that there is presently insufficient evidence to establish the plasma naltrexone level needed to block the effects of heroin doses commonly used by heroin-dependent people.[121]

Considering reports of fatal and non-fatal opioid overdose in patients with active naltrexone implants,[108,122] further research would assist in determining the dose of heroin capable of overriding the naltrexone blockade during the initial weeks post administration.

Serious adverse events of sustained-release naltrexone

The chronic administration of antagonists such as naltrexone increases the density of opioid receptors in the central nervous system in a type of homeostatic compensation.[123,124] Rodent models have demonstrated that this 'upregulation' is accompanied by an increase in opioid agonist potency, or functional supersensitivity.[124,125] In humans, upregulation of opioid receptors has been suggested to have the potential to enhance the risk of opioid overdose in people receiving naltrexone treatment;[28] however, it is unclear whether the receptor upregulation actually has any discernible clinical impact. One study found no effects of 2 weeks of oral naltrexone treatment upon the effects of a small dose of morphine on respiratory depression (in normal volunteers), and concluded that naltrexone maintenance was unlikely to induce hypersensitivity to opioids.[126] This study has not yet been replicated.

Mortality rates in patients treated with sustained-release naltrexone are not a commonly reported outcome, although it is clear that both fatal and non-fatal opioid overdose in a patient with an active naltrexone implant is possible.[108,122] In both of these case reports, a large dose of heroin was used to overcome the naltrexone blockade.[108,122]

A non-randomized pre–post design was also used to examine hospital presentations for opioid overdose in 361 naltrexone implant recipients, 40% of whom had previously received oral naltrexone treatment for heroin dependence. While no opioid overdoses occurred in the 6 months post implant treatment, there was a significant increase in sedative overdoses, some occurring within 10 days of implant treatment.[127]

Design flaws are particularly evident in two non-randomized, pre–post studies comparing naltrexone implant and methadone maintenance treatment in terms of mortality[128] and hospital admissions.[129] Uncontrolled differences between the study cohorts make comparisons between the treatment groups unreliable,[128] and make it difficult to attribute causality of any changes to the treatment type.[129] Differences in motivation level, situational influences, socioeconomic background, and pre-existing illnesses between the two treatment groups were not controlled for.[128,129] These design flaws notwithstanding, a mortality rate of 3.76 deaths per 1,000 person years was reported in 341 new entrants to naltrexone implantation treatment.[128] In 314 new recipients of naltrexone implants there was also a significant increase in risk of admission for overdose on non-opioid drugs (OR=16.31, 95% CI 3.07–86.53) between the 6 months pre and post treatment, and no significant change in opioid overdose in the 6 months pre and post either treatment.[129] One death (opioid-related) in a naltrexone implant treated patient was noted, however details of 12 non-drug-related deaths in the study participants were not provided.[129]

Various SAEs have been recorded following use of naltrexone implants. These include pulmonary edema, drug toxicity, withdrawal, aspiration pneumonia, variceal rupture, and death. A case series (n=6) from New York and Pennsylvanian emergency departments in a 2-year period included two fatalities.[111] Over a 3-year period, the US Food and Drug Administration noted an additional 10 deaths in patients with a recent naltrexone pellet implantation.[111]

The development of naltrexone implants is still in progress by several companies to overcome difficulties such as high initial burst releases of naltrexone[130] and tissue inflammatory reactions. Marked tissue irritation, in some cases sufficient to warrant naltrexone implant removal, has been noted in a number of clinical studies.[106,107,109,121,131–134] In one study a degree of inflammation was noted in subjects up to 2 years post implant.[135] In another case series, 2 patients had their implants removed due to infection and were prescribed oral naltrexone, tragically to die from opioid overdose within a fortnight after implant removal.[136]

Some authors have commented that local tissue reactions may preclude the clinical use of naltrexone implants,[131] or that repeated implants had the potential to cause tissue reaction problems[121] and so limit the number of implants a patient would want to receive.[133,134]

Outcomes from sustained-release naltrexone

There are few high-quality efficacy data of sustained-release naltrexone in the treatment of heroin dependence, and the great majority of the literature consists of small case studies, pre and post implantation studies, and non-controlled trials. A meta-analysis of sustained-release naltrexone in the treatment of opioid dependence found that there was insufficient evidence to evaluate the effectiveness of this naltrexone formulation, and particularly that more data on side-effects and adverse events are needed.[40]

There has been one small randomized controlled trial of the use of depot naltrexone for the treatment of heroin dependence, and this was the only trial meeting inclusion criteria for efficacy data in the recent Cochrane review.[40] Sixty heroin-dependent subjects were randomized to either placebo, 192 mg depot naltrexone, or 384 mg depot naltrexone in an 8-week study.[112] Treatment involved twice-weekly therapy sessions and depot administration at the beginning of weeks 1 and 5. Retention in treatment during the 8-week study showed a dose-dependent effect. There was a significant difference between mean number of days to drop-out between placebo (27 days) and 384 mg naltrexone (48 days), $p \leq 0.001$, as well as between the 384 mg naltrexone and 192 mg naltrexone depot groups (36 days), $p = 0.046$. At the final 8-week follow-up, 39%, 60%, and 68% of subjects remained in treatment in the placebo, 192 mg, and 384 mg depot naltrexone groups, respectively. When all missing urine tests were considered positive for opioids, the 384 mg depot naltrexone group had significantly more opioid-negative urine samples than the placebo group.[112] While this study reports a promising dose-dependent effect for treatment retention, it should be noted that the study may have some selection bias. Of the original 98 patients assessed for study entry, 38 were excluded before study randomization for reasons including: left against medical advice ($n = 16$), administrative discharges ($n = 8$), left at own request ($n = 3$) and 'other reasons' ($n = 11$).[137] Outcomes for the subjects beyond the 8-week study period were not reported.

Mental health hospital admissions were the focus of a study using record linkage to examine comparative levels of pre- and post-implantation admissions in 359 (82%) of 437 patients receiving their first naltrexone implant treatment between 2001 and 2002.[114] The risk of hospitalization for mental conditions was not statistically significant pre and post naltrexone implantation treatment. The study used an indirect measure of mental health status (hospital admissions) and did not include a control group so a causal relationship between naltrexone implantation and these outcomes cannot be imputed.[114]

A paper discussing two cohorts of British patients receiving naltrexone implants (n=101) reported heroin use outcomes at 1 and 3 months post implantation, which were confirmed by telephone self report from patients, and their families in 66% of cases.[106] At 3 months, 23% of subjects had relapsed to regular opioid use and 'several' had tested out the blockade of naltrexone by using opioids,[106] although details of this opioid use were not explored systematically.

In a non-randomized, non-controlled study, 156 Spanish patients received naltrexone implants and psychosocial support therapy following a rapid opioid detoxification procedure. Of the 101 clients who completed detoxification treatment, 55% presented opiate-free at 6 months, and 21% presented opiate-free at 12 months.[107] Outcomes for those lost to follow-up were not reported.

Small cases studies of heroin-dependent pregnant women, adolescents, and physicians have been specifically targeted for investigation of the effectiveness of naltrexone implants. These studies have given preliminary evidence that pregnant heroin users can be managed by naltrexone implant without obvious risk (as determined by the study authors) to the mother or developing fetus.[138] A review of medical records in 8 high-risk dependent heroin-using adolescents showed that hospital presentations for accidental opiate overdose were much lower post naltrexone implant treatment than pre treatment.[139] Successful maintenance of naltrexone blood levels through sequential implant treatment in a single opioid-dependent anesthetist has been reported.[105] A response to this case study warned of an undue reliance upon naltrexone implants in the overall management of opioid abuse and dependence.[140]

It is too early to draw any conclusions regarding the efficacy of naltrexone implants in comparison with oral naltrexone.[40] While mortality and hospital admissions have been compared between sustained-release naltrexone and the gold standard methadone maintenance treatment,[128,129] retention and opioid use outcomes have not been examined between these treatments.[40]

The ongoing development of sustained-release naltrexone attempts to overcome the problems of low retention in oral naltrexone treatment. Blood naltrexone levels required to block commonly administered doses of opioids are still subject to debate, and important queries concerning treatment safety (particularly opioid overdose risk) remain. There are few high-quality efficacy data of sustained-release naltrexone in the treatment of heroin dependence, but the first small randomized controlled study has shown promising evidence of a dose-dependent relationship with retention outcomes. The efficacy of sustained-release naltrexone in terms of treatment retention and opioid use has not been adequately compared with placebo and agonist maintenance treatments. Until such trials are completed, sustained-release naltrexone remains experimental.

Future directions

Much of the published naltrexone maintenance literature in the last decade has been concerned with monitoring clinical outcomes in large client cohorts, and the development of practice guidelines rather than randomized controlled trials testing hypotheses regarding naltrexone maintenance efficacy. The evidence of this can be seen in the Cochrane reviews of both oral and sustained-release naltrexone, where the quality of randomized controlled studies available is not yet sufficient to evaluate the efficacy of these forms of treatment in heroin-dependent subjects.[3,40]

Critical issues for naltrexone have been acceptability, uptake, and early retention in treatment. A number of papers have outlined key reasons for the poor acceptability of naltrexone. These included a fear of, or inability to withdraw from opiates, the necessity of an opiate-free period which is a high-risk time for relapse, inability to cope with depression during the opiate-free period, fear of a new drug, and fear of aversive reactions or residual dependence.[17,36,42,43]

Retention and compliance remain problematic for naltrexone maintenance programs, and the agonist pharmacotherapies with their higher retention remain the preferred treatments. In those studies with higher retention in treatment, whether due to well-developed family support, the negative consequences of ceasing treatment, or comprehensive psychosocial therapy, opioid use and psychiatric outcomes tend to be better.[54]

Naltrexone treatment, whether oral or sustained-release formulations, carries with it a significant risk of opioid overdose. The evidence so far suggests that this overdose risk may be higher and more difficult to monitor than risk associated with the agonist pharmacotherapies.[101,103] It is hoped that further studies will provide more information.

The development of depot and implantable naltrexone remains in its infancy and still requires substantial research before clinicians can confidently engage with this form of treatment.[40] We look forward to new research in this area.

References

1. Kleber HD. Pharmacologic treatments for opioid dependence: detoxification and maintenance options. Dialogues Clin Neurosci 2007; 9: 455–70.
2. Gutstein HB, Akil H. Chapter 21: Opioid Analgesics, in Goodman and Gilman's The Pharmacological Basis of Therapeutics, 11th edition, Brunton LL, Parker KL, Buxton ILO, et al., eds. 2006, McGraw-Hill: New York.
3. Kirchmayer U, Davoli M, Verster A. Naltrexone maintenance treatment for opioid dependence. Cochrane Database Syst Rev 2004; 4.
4. Arnold-Reed DE, Hulse GK, Hansson RC, et al. Blood morphine levels in naltrexone-exposed compared to non-naltrexone-exposed fatal heroin overdoses. Addict Biol 2003; 8: 343–50.
5. Lee MC, Wagner HN Jr, Tanada S, et al. Duration of occupancy of opiate receptors by naltrexone. J Nucl Med 1988; 29(7): 1207–11.
6. Bell J, Kimber J, Lintzeris N, et al. Clinical Guidelines and Procedures for the Use of Naltrexone in the Management of Opioid Dependence. 2003, Australian Government Department of Health and Ageing: Canberra.
7. O'Brien CP, Greenstein RA, Mintz J, Woody GE. Clinical experience with naltrexone. Am J Drug Alcohol Ab 1975; 2(3–4): 365–77.
8. Altman JL, Meyer RE, Mirin SM, et al. Opiate antagonists and the modification of heroin self-administration behavior in man: an experimental study. Int J Addict 1976; 11(3): 485–99.
9. Mello NK, Mendelson JH, Kuehnle JC. Operant analysis of human heroin self-administration and the effects of naltrexone. J Pharmacol Exp Ther 1981; 216(1): 45–54.
10. Judson BA, Carney TM, Goldstein A. Naltrexone treatment of heroin addiction: efficacy and safety in a double-blind dosage comparison. Drug Alcohol Depen 1981; 7(4): 235–46.
11. Resnick R, Volauka J, Freedman AM, Thomas M. Studies of EN-1639A (Naltrexone): a new narcotic antagonist. Am J Psychiat 1974; 131: 646–50.

12. Gonzalez JP, Brogden RN. Naltrexone: a review of its pharmacodynamic and pharmacokinetic properties and therapeutic efficacy in the management of opioid dependence. Drugs 1988; 35: 192–213.
13. Stella L, D'Ambra C, Mazzeo F, et al. Naltrexone plus benzodiazepine aids abstinence in opioid-dependent patients. Life Sci 2005; 77: 2717–22.
14. Atkinson RL, Berke LK, Drake CR, et al. Effects of long-term therapy with naltrexone on body weight in obesity. Clin Pharmacol Ther 1985; 38: 419–22.
15. Garcia-Alonso F, Gutierrez M, San L, et al. A multicentre study to introduce naltrexone for opiate dependence in Spain. Drug Alcohol Depen 1989; 23(2): 117–21.
16. Greenstein RA, Arndt IC, McLellan AT, et al. Naltrexone: a clinical perspective. J Clin Psychiat 1984; 45(9, Part 2): 25–8.
17. Hollister LE, Johnson K, Boukhabza D, Gillespie HK. Adversive effects of naltrexone in subjects not dependent on opiates. Drug Alcohol Depen 1981; 8: 37–41.
18. Ling W, Wesson DR. Naltrexone treatment for addicted health-care professionals: a collaborative private practice experience. J Clin Psychiat 1984; 45(9 Pt 2): 46–8.
19. Resnick RB, Washton AM, Thomas MA, Kestenbaum RS. Naltrexone in the treatment of opiate dependence. In: The international challenge of drug abuse. NIDA Research Monograph Series, Petersen RC, ed. 1978, US Department of Health, Education, and Welfare: Rockville, Maryland, 321–32.
20. Tennant FS Jr, Rawson RA, Cohen AJ, Mann A. Clinical experience with naltrexone in suburban opioid addicts. J Clin Psychiat 1984; 45(9 Pt 2): 42–5.
21. Brewer C, Wong VS. Naltrexone: report of lack of hepatotoxicity in acute viral hepatitis, with a review of the literature. Addict Biol 2004; 9(1): 81–7.
22. Sullivan MA, Nunes EV. New-onset mania and psychosis following heroin detoxification and naltrexone maintenance. Am J Addict 2005; 14: 486–7.
23. O'Brien CP. A new approach to the management of opioid dependence: naltrexone, an oral antagonist. J Clin Psychiat 1984; 45(9, Section 2): 1–59.
24. Tucker TK, Ritter AJ. Naltrexone in the treatment of heroin dependence: a literature review. Drug Alcohol Rev 2000; 19: 73–82.
25. Hollister LE. Clinical evaluation of naltrexone treatment of opiate-dependent individuals. Report of the National Research Council Committee on Clinical Evaluation of Narcotic Antagonists. Arch Gen Psychiat 1978; 35: 335–40.
26. San L, Pomarol G, Peri JM, et al. Follow-up after a six-month maintenance period on naltrexone versus placebo in heroin addicts. Brit J Addict 1991; 86: 983–90.
27. Shufman EN, Porat S, Witztum E, et al. The efficacy of naltrexone in preventing reabuse of heroin after detoxification. Biol Psychiat 1994; 35(12): 935–45.
28. Miotto K, McCann MJ, Rawson RA, et al. Overdose, suicide attempts and death among a cohort of naltrexone-treated opioid addicts. Drug Alcohol Depen 1997; 45: 131–4.
29. Rawlins M, Randall M, Meyer R, et al. Aftercare on narcotic antagonists: prospects and problems. Int J Addict 1976; 11(3): 501–11.

30. Gerra G, Marcato A, Caccavari R, et al. Clonidine and opiate receptor antagonists in the treatment of heroin addiction. J Subst Abuse Treat 1995; 12(1): 35–41.
31. Rawson RA, McCann MJ, Shoptaw SJ, et al. Naltrexone for opioid dependence: evaluation of a manualized psychosocial protocol to enhance treatment response. Drug Alcohol Rev 2001; 20: 67–78.
32. Rea F, Bell JR, Young MR, Mattick RP. A randomised, controlled trial of low dose naltrexone for the treatment of opioid dependence. Drug Alcohol Depen 2004; 75: 79–88.
33. Dean AJ, Saunders JB, Jones RT, et al. Does naltrexone treatment lead to depression? Findings from a randomized controlled trial in subjects with opioid dependence. J Psychiat Neurosci 2006; 31(1): 38–45.
34. Miotto K, McCann M, Basch J, et al. Naltrexone and dysphoria: fact or myth? Am J Addict 2002; 11(2): 151–60.
35. Kleber HD. Naltrexone. J Subst Abuse Treat 1985; 2(2): 117–22.
36. Schecter A. The role of narcotic antagonists in the rehabilitation of opiate addicts: a review of naltrexone. Am J Drug Alcohol Ab 1980; 7(1): 1–18.
37. Forman RF, Bovasso G, Woody G. Staff beliefs about addiction treatment. J Subst Abuse Treat 2001; 21: 1–9.
38. Roman PM, Johnson JA. Adoption and implementation of new technologies in substance abuse treatment. J Subst Abuse Treat 2002; 22: 211–18.
39. Thomas C, Wallack S, Swift R, et al. Adoption of naltrexone in alcoholism treatment. J Addict Dis 2001; 20: 180.
40. Lobmaier P, Kornor H, Kunoe N, Bjorndal A. Sustained-release naltrexone for opioid dependence. Cochrane Database Syst Rev 2008 (Issue 2).
41. Fram DH, Marmo J, Holden R. Naltrexone treatment: the problem of patient acceptance. J Subst Abuse Treat 1989; 6(2): 119–22.
42. Lewis DC, Mayer J, Hersch RG, Black R. Narcotic antagonist treatment: clinical experience with naltrexone. Int J Addict 1978; 13(6): 961–73.
43. Singleton EG, Sherman MF, Bigelow GE. The index of choice: indications of methadone patients' selection of naltrexone treatment. Am J Drug Alcohol Ab 1984; 10(2): 209–21.
44. National Research Council Committee on Clinical Evaluation of Narcotic Antagonists. Clinical evaluation of naltrexone treatment of opiate-dependent individuals. Report of the National Research Council Committee on clinical evaluation of narcotic antagonists. Arch Gen Psychiat 1978; 35(3): 335–40.
45. Rothenberg JL, Sullivan MA, Church SH, et al. Behavioral naltrexone therapy: an integrated treatment for opiate dependence. J Subst Abuse Treat 2002; 23(4): 351–60.
46. Tucker T, Ritter A, Maher C, Jackson H. A randomized control trial of group counseling in a naltrexone treatment program. J Subst Abuse Treat 2004; 27: 277–88.
47. Shearer J, Wodak A, Dolan K. Evaluation of a prison-based naltrexone program. Int J Prisoner Health 2007; 3(3): 214–24.
48. Sullivan MA, Garawi F, Bisaga A, et al. Management of relapse in naltrexone maintenance for heroin dependence. Drug Alcohol Depen 2007; 91: 289–92.

49. Krupitsky EM, Zvartau EE, Masalov DV, et al. Naltrexone for heroin dependence treatment in St. Petersburg, Russia. J Subst Abuse Treat 2004; 26: 285–94.
50. Krupitsky EM, Zvartau EE, Masalov DV, et al. Naltrexone with or without fluoxetine for preventing relapse to heroin addiction in St. Petersburg, Russia. J Subst Abuse Treat 2006; 31: 319–28.
51. Gibson AE, Doran CM, Bell JR, et al. A comparison of buprenorphine treatment in clinic and primary care settings: a randomised trial. Med J Australia 2003; 179: 38–42.
52. Lintzeris N, Bell J, Bammer G, et al. A randomized controlled trial of buprenorphine in the management of short-term ambulatory heroin withdrawal. Addiction 2002; 97: 1395–404.
53. Mattick RP, Digiusto E, Doran CM, et al. National Evaluation of Pharmacotherapies for Opioid Dependence: Report of Results and Recommendations. 2004, National Drug and Alcohol Research Centre: Sydney.
54. Johansson BA, Berglund M, Lindgren A. Efficacy of maintenance treatment with naltrexone for opioid dependence: a meta-analytical review. Addiction 2006; 101: 491–503.
55. Cornish JW, Metzger D, Woody GE, et al. Naltrexone pharmacotherapy for opioid dependent federal probationers. J Subst Abuse Treat 1997; 14(6): 529–34.
56. Tucker TK, Ritter AJ, Maher C, Jackson H. Naltrexone maintenance for heroin dependence: uptake, attrition and retention. Drug Alcohol Rev 2004; 23(3): 299–309.
57. Bartu A, Freeman NC, Gawthorne GS, et al. Characteristics, retention and readmissions of opioid-dependent clients treated with oral naltrexone. Drug Alcohol Rev 2002; 21: 335–40.
58. Schifano E, Marra R. Naltrexone for heroin addiction: encouraging results from Italy. Int J Clin Pharmacol Ther Toxicol 1990; 28: 144–6.
59. Capone T, Brahen L, Condren R, et al. Retention and outcome in a narcotic antagonist treatment program. J Clin Psychol 1986; 42(5): 825–33.
60. Gutiérrez M, Ballesteros J, Gonzalez Oliveros R, de Apodaka JR. Retention rates in two naltrexone programmes for heroin addicts in Vitoria, Spain. Eur Psychiat 1995; 10(4): 183–8.
61. Brahen LS, Henderson RK, Capone T, Kordal N. Naltrexone treatment in a jail work-release program. J Clin Psychiat 1984; 45(9, Sec 2): 49–52.
62. Washton AM, Pottash AC, Gold MS. Naltrexone in addicted business executives and physicians. J Clin Psychiat 1984; 45: 39–41.
63. Loffreda A, Falcone G, Motola G, et al. Use of naltrexone for the treatment of opiate addiction in Campania, Italy: the role of family. J Subst Use 2003; 8(3): 182–5.
64. Lerner A, Sigal M, Bacalu A, et al. A naltrexone double blind placebo controlled study in Israel. Israel J Psychiat 1992; 29(1): 36–43.
65. Grey CC, Osborn E, Reznikoff M. Psychosocial factors in outcome in two opiate addiction treatments. J Clin Psychol 1986; 42(1): 185–9.

66. Osborn E, Grey C, Reznikoff M. Psychosocial adjustment, modality choice, and outcome in naltrexone versus methadone treatment. Am J Drug Alcohol Ab 1986; 12: 383–8.
67. Ahmadi J, Ahmadi K. Controlled trial of maintenance treatment of intravenous buprenorphine dependence. Iranian J Med Sci 2003; 172(4): 171–3.
68. Rounsaville BJ. Can psychotherapy rescue naltrexone treatment of opioid addiction? In: Integrating behavioural therapies with medications in the treatment of drug dependence. NIDA Research Monograph Series, Onken LS, Blaine JD, Boren JJ, eds. 1995, US Department of Health and Human Services: Rockville, MD, 37–52.
69. Greenstein RA, Evans BD, McLellan AT, O'Brien CP. Predictors of favourable outcome following naltrexone treatment. In: NIDA Research Monograph Series. 1982, National Institute on Drug Abuse: Rockville, MD, 294–301.
70. Preston KL, Silverman K, Umbricht A, et al. Improvement in naltrexone treatment compliance with contingency management. Drug Alcohol Depen 1999; 54(2): 127–35.
71. Hulse G, Basso M. Reassessing naltrexone maintenance as a treatment for illicit heroin users. Drug Alcohol Rev 1999; 18: 263–9.
72. Hensel M, Kox WJ. Safety, efficacy, and long-term results of a modified version of rapid opiate detoxification under general anaesthesia: a prospective study in methadone, heroin, codeine and morphine addicts. Acta Anaesth Scand 2000; 44(3): 326–33.
73. Judson B, Goldstein A. Naltrexone treatment of heroin addiction: one-year follow-up. Drug Alcohol Depen 1984; 13(4): 357–65.
74. O'Brien CP, Greenstein R, Woody GE. Update on naltrexone treatment. In: The international challenge of drug abuse. NIDA Research Monograph Series, Petersen RC, ed. 1978, Department of Health, Education, and Welfare: Rockville, Maryland, 315–20.
75. Greenstein R, O'Brien C, Mintz J, et al. Clinical experience with naltrexone in a behavioural research study: an interim report. In: Narcotic antagonists: Naltrexone. NIDA Research Monograph Series, Julius D, Renault P, eds. 1976, National Institute on Drug Abuse: Rockville, MD.
76. Arndt I, McLellan AT, O'Brien CP. Abstinence treatments for opiate addicts: therapeutic community or naltrexone? 45th Annual Scientific Meeting of the Committee on Problems of Drug Dependence, Inc. In: Problems of drug dependence. NIDA Research Monograph Series, Harris LS, ed. 1984, US Department of Health and Human Services, Public Health Service, National Institutes of Health: Rockville, MD, 275–81.
77. Rawson RA, Washton AM, Resnick RB, Tennant FS. Clonidine hydrochloride detoxification from methadone treatment – the value of naltrexone aftercare. Advan Alcohol Subst Ab 1984; 3: 41–9.
78. Rawson RA, Tennant FS. Five-year follow-up of opiate addicts with naltrexone and behavior therapy. 45th Annual Scientific Meeting of the Committee on Problems of Drug Dependence, Inc. In: Problems of drug dependence. NIDA Research Monograph Series, Harris LS, ed. 1984, US Department of Health and

Human Services, Public Health Service, National Institutes of Health: Rockville, MD, 289–95.

79. Foy A, Sadler C, Taylor A. An open trial of naltrexone for opiate dependence. Drug Alcohol Rev 1998; 17: 167–74.
80. Thomas M, Kauders F, Harris M, et al. Clinical experiences with naltrexone in 370 detoxified addicts. In: Narcotic antagonists: Naltrexone. NIDA Research Monograph Series, Julius D, Renault P, eds. 1976, National Institute on Drug Abuse: Rockville, MD, 88–92.
81. Christie MJ, Harvey AI. Pharmacological options for management of opioid dependence. Drug Alcohol Rev 1993; 12(1): 71–80.
82. Onken LS, Blaine JD, Boren JJ, eds. Integrating behavioural therapies with medications in the treatment of drug dependence. NIDA Research Monograph Series. Vol. 150; 1995, US Department of Health and Human Services: Rockville, MD.
83. Rawson R, Glazer M, Callahan E, Liberman R. Naltrexone and behaviour therapy for heroin addiction. In: Behavioural analysis and treatment of substance abuse. NIDA Research Monograph Series, N. Krasnegor, ed. 1979, National Institute on Drug Abuse: Rockville, MD, 26–43.
84. Callahan E, Rawson R, McCleave B, et al. The treatment of heroin addiction: naltrexone alone and with behaviour therapy. Int J Addict 1980; 15: 795–807.
85. Anton R, Hogan I, Jalali B, et al. Multiple family therapy and naltrexone in the treatment of opiate dependence. Drug Alcohol Depen 1981; 8: 157–68.
86. Callahan E, Rawson R, Glazer M, et al. Comparison of two naltrexone treatment programs: naltrexone alone versus naltrexone plus behaviour therapy. In: Narcotic antagonists: Naltrexone. NIDA Research Monograph Series, Julius D, Renault P, eds. 1976, National Institute on Drug Abuse: Rockville, MD, 150–7.
87. Carroll KM, Sinha R, Nich C, et al. Contingency management to enhance naltrexone treatment of opioid dependence: a randomized clinical trial of reinforcement magnitude. Exp Clin Psychopharmacol 2002; 10(1): 54–63.
88. Carroll KM, Ball SA, Nich C, et al. Targeting behavioral therapies to enhance naltrexone treatment for opioid dependence: efficacy of contingency management and significant other involvement. Arch Gen Psychiat 2001; 58(8): 755–61.
89. Church SH, Rothenberg JL, Sullivan MA, et al. Concurrent substance use and outcome in combined behavioral and naltrexone therapy for opiate dependence. Am J Drug Alcohol Ab 2001; 27(3): 441–52.
90. Fals-Stewart W, O'Farrell TJ, Behavioral family counseling and naltrexone for male opioid-dependent patients. J Consult Clin Psychol 2003; 71(3): 432–42.
91. Hulse G, Basso M. The association between naltrexone compliance and daily supervision. Drug Alcohol Rev 2000; 19: 41–8.
92. Farren CK, O'Malley S. A pilot double blind placebo controlled trial of sertraline with naltrexone in the treatment of opiate dependence. Am J Addict 2002; 11(3): 228–34.
93. Roozen HG, Kerkhof AJ, van den Brink W. Experiences with an outpatient relapse program (community reinforcement approach) combined with naltrexone in the treatment of opioid-dependence: effect on addictive

behaviors and the predictive value of psychiatric comorbidity. Eur Addict Res 2003; 9(2): 53–8.

94. Therapeutic Goods Administration, Note for guidance on clinical safety data management: definitions and standards for expedited reporting. Commonwealth Department of Health and Aged Care: Canberra, 2000.
95. Ritter AJ. Naltrexone in the treatment of heroin dependence: relationship with depression and risk of overdose. Aust NZ J Psychiat 2002; 36(2): 224–8.
96. Digiusto E, Shakeshaft A, Ritter A, et al. Serious adverse events in the Australian National Evaluation of Pharmacotherapies for Opioid Dependence (NEPOD). Addiction 2004; 99: 450–60.
97. Warner-Smith M, Lynskey M, Hall W, Monteiro M. Challenges and approaches to estimating mortality attributable to the use of selected illicit drugs. Eur Addict Res 2001; 7: 104–16.
98. Hall W, Ross J, Lynskey M, et al. How many dependent opioid users are there in Australia? In NDARC Monograph No.44. 2000, National Drug and Alcohol Research Centre: Sydney.
99. Caplehorn JRM, Dalton MSYN, Halder F, et al. Methadone maintenance and addicts' risk of fatal heroin overdose. Subst Use Misuse 1996; 31: 177–96.
100. Bell JR, Young MR, Masterman SC, et al. A pilot study of naltrexone-accelerated detoxification in opioid dependence. Med J Australia 1999; 171: 26–30.
101. Gibson A, Degenhardt L. Mortality related to pharmacotherapies for opioid dependence: a comparative analysis of coronial records. Drug Alcohol Rev 2007; 26: 405–10.
102. Krupitsky E, Masalov D, Didenko T, et al. Prevention of suicide by naltrexone in a recently detoxified heroin addict. Eur Addict Res 2001; 7(2): 87–8.
103. Hall W, Wodak A. Is naltrexone a cure for heroin dependence? The evidence so far is not promising. Medical J Australia 1999; 171: 9–10.
104. Hulse G, O'Neil G. Using naltrexone implants in the management of the pregnant heroin user. Aust NZ J Obstet Gynaecol 2002; 42(5): 569–73.
105. Hulse GK, O'Neil G, Hatton M, Paech MJ. Use of oral and implantable naltrexone in the management of the opioid impaired physician. Anaesth Intens Care 2003; 31(2): 196–201.
106. Foster J, Brewer C, Steele T. Naltrexone implants can completely prevent early (1-month) relapse after opiate detoxification: a pilot study of two cohorts totalling 101 patients with a note on naltrexone blood levels. Addict Biol 2003; 8: 211–17.
107. Carreno JE, Alvarez CE, San Narciso GI, et al. Maintenance treatment with depot opioid antagonists in subcutaneous implants: an alternative in the treatment of opioid dependence. Addict Biol 2003; 8: 429–38.
108. Krupitsky EM, Burakov AM, Tsoy MV, et al. Overcoming opioid blockade from depot naltrexone (Prodetoxon). Addiction 2007; Online publication 11 May 2007.
109. Olsen L, Christopherson A, Frogopsahl G, et al. Plasma concentrations during naltrexone implant treatment of opiate-dependent patients. Brit J Clin Pharmacol 2004; 58(2): 219–22.

110. Hulse G, Arnold-Reed DE, O'Neil G, et al. Achieving long-term continuous blood naltrexone and 6-ß-naltrexol coverage following sequential naltrexone implants. Addict Biol 2004; 9: 67–72.
111. Hamilton R, Olmedo R, Shah S, et al. Complications of ultrarapid opioid detoxification with subcutaneous naltrexone pellets. Acad Emerg Med 2002; 9(1): 63–8.
112. Comer SD, Sullivan MA, Yu E, et al. Injectable, sustained-release naltrexone for the treatment of opioid dependence: a randomized, placebo-controlled trial. Arch Gen Psychiat 2006; 63: 210–18.
113. Brewer C. Serum naltrexone and 6-beta-naltrexol levels from naltrexone implants can block very large amounts of heroin: a report of two cases. Addict Biol 2002; 7: 321–3.
114. Ngo HTT, Tait RJ, Arnold-Reed DE, Hulse GK. Mental health outcomes following naltrexone implant treatment for heroin-dependence. Prog Neuro-Psychoph 2007; 31: 605–12.
115. Ngo HTT, Arnold-Reed DE, Hansson RC, et al. Blood naltrexone levels over time following naltrexone implant. Prog Neuro-Psychoph 2008; 32: 23–8.
116. Comer SD, Collins ED, Kleber HD, et al. Depot naltrexone: long-lasting antagonism of the effects of heroin in humans. Psychopharmacology 2002; 159: 351–60.
117. Sullivan MA, Vosburg SK, Comer SD. Depot naltrexone: antagonism of the reinforcing, subjective, and physiological effects of heroin. Psychopharmacology 2006; 189: 37–46.
118. Hulse GK, Arnold-Reed DE, O'Neil G, et al. Blood naltrexone and 6-ß-naltrexol levels following naltrexone implant: comparing two naltrexone implants. Addict Biol 2004; 9: 59–65.
119. Navaratnam V, Jamaludin A, Raman N, et al. Determination of naltrexone dosage for narcotic agonist blockade in detoxified Asian addicts. Drug Alcohol Depen 1994; 34: 231–6.
120. Kranzler HR, Modesto-Lowe V, Nuwayser ES. Sustained-release naltrexone for alcoholism treatment: a preliminary study. Alcohol Clin Exp Res 1998; 22(5): 1074–9.
121. Waal H, Frogopsahl G, Olsen L, et al. Naltrexone implants – duration, tolerability and clinical usefulness. Eur Addict Res 2006; 12: 138–44.
122. Gibson A, Degenhardt L, Hall W. Opioid deaths can occur in patients with naltrexone implants. Med J Australia 2007; 186(3): 152–3.
123. Parkes JH, Sinclair JD. Reduction of alcohol drinking and upregulation of opioid receptor by oral naltrexone in AA rats. Alcohol 2000; 21: 215–21.
124. Lesscher HM, Bailey A, Burbach JP, et al. Receptor-selective changes in mu-, delta- and kappa-opioid receptors after chronic naltrexone treatment in mice. Eur J Neurosci 2003; 17(5): 1006–12.
125. Hyytia P, Ingman K, Soini SL, et al. Effects of continuous opioid receptor blockade on alcohol intake and up-regulation of opioid receptor subtype signalling in a genetic model of high alcohol drinking. N-S Arch Pharmacol 1999; 360: 391–401.
126. Cornish JW, Henson D, Levine S, et al. Naltrexone maintenance: effect on morphine sensitivity in normal volunteers. Am J Addict 1993; 2(1): 34–8.

127. Hulse GK, Tait RJ, Comer SD, et al. Reducing hospital presentations for opioid overdose in patients treated with sustained release naltrexone implants. Drug Alcohol Depen 2005; 79(3): 351–7.
128. Tait RJ, Ngo HTT, Hulse GK. Mortality in heroin users 3 years after naltrexone implant or methadone maintenance treatment. J Subst Abuse Treat 2008; 35: 116–24.
129. Ngo HTT, Tait RJ, Hulse GK. Comparing drug-related hospital morbidity following heroin dependence treatment with methadone maintenance or naltrexone implantation. Arch Gen Psychiat 2008; 65(4): 457–65.
130. Liu Y, Sunderland VB, O'Neil AG. In vitro and in vivo release of naltrexone from biodegradable depot systems. Drug Dev Ind Pharm 2006; 32: 85–94.
131. Chiang CN, Hojlister LE, Kishimoto A, Barnett G. Kinetics of a naltrexone sustained-release preparation. Clin Pharmacol Ther 1984; 36(5): 704–8.
132. Chiang CN, Hollister LE, Gillespie HK, Foltz RL. Clinical evaluation of a naltrexone sustained-release preparation. Drug Alcohol Depen 1985; 16: 1–8.
133. Galloway GP, Koch M, Cello R, Smith DE. Pharmacokinetics, safety, and tolerability of a depot formulation of naltrexone in alcoholics: an open-label trial. BMC Psychiat 2005; 5(18).
134. Johnson BA, Ait-Daoud N, Aubin HJ, et al. A pilot evaluation of the safety and tolerability of repeat dose administration of long-acting injectable naltrexone (Vivitrex) in patients with alcohol dependence. Alcohol Clin Exp Res 2004; 28(9): 1356–61.
135. Hulse GK, Stalenberg V, McCallum D, et al. Histological changes over time around the site of sustained release naltrexone-poly (dl-lactide) implants in humans. J Control Release 2005; 108: 43–55.
136. Oliver P. Fatal opiate overdose following regimen changes in naltrexone treatment. Addiction 2005; 100: 560–3.
137. Comer SD, Sullivan MA, Yu E, et al. Response to: lack of information in naltrexone study. Arch Gen Psychiat 2007; 64(7): 865.
138. Hulse GK, Arnold-Reed DE, O'Neil G, Hansson RC. Naltrexone implant and blood naltrexone levels over pregnancy. Aust NZ J Obstet Gynaecol 2003; 43: 386–8.
139. Hulse GK, Tait RJ. A pilot study to assess the impact of naltrexone implant on accidental opiate overdose in 'high-risk' adolescent heroin users. Addict Biol 2003; 8: 337–42.
140. Warhaft N. Response to use of oral and implantable naltrexone in the management of the opioid impaired physician. Anaesth Intens Care 2003; 31(5): 592–3.

chapter 9

Pharmacotherapies and pregnancy

Adrian Dunlop, Dimitra Petroulias, Dolly Marope, Katie Khoo, Jo Kimber, Alison Ritter, Tracey Burrell, and David Osborn

Introduction

Gender is an important factor in the treatment of opiate dependence. Co-existing pregnancy and opiate dependence raise multiple important issues, for the pregnant women and her baby. Women respond differently to opiate substitution treatment compared to men, both in terms of effectiveness and adverse effects.[1] As pregnancy advances, the pharmacokinetics and pharmacodynamics of medications can change, necessitating careful monitoring of pregnant women to ensure adequate treatment.[2] Substance use also has a significant potential to affect the developing embryo and fetus. Critically, a range of environmental issues can negatively impact on the health of pregnant women who use heroin, as well as on the health of their babies.

The prevalence of regular heroin use in the Australian population has increased steadily since the late 1960s, particularly during the decade of the 1990s, peaking at 10.0 per 1000 population in the late 1990s and decreasing to 4.0 per 1000 by 2002, with the latest estimate being approximately 45,000 users in 2002.[3–6] The majority of people using heroin are in the 15–39 age group.[4]

Gender differences in the epidemiology of heroin use are noticeable. The 2007 Australian National Household Survey reported that 1.0% of women aged above 14 had ever used heroin in their lifetime, compared to 2.1% of men (i.e. approximately 90,000 women and 180,000 men). In the previous 12 months, 0.1% of women reported heroin use, compared to 0.3% of men.[7] Data from the National Minimum Data Set for Alcohol and other Drug Treatment Services for 2006–07 showed that of the 14,870 treatment episodes delivered for the treatment of heroin dependence (predominately withdrawal, counseling, case management, and rehabilitation), 35% were received by women, of median age 29 years.[8] A report on Australian methadone and buprenorphine treatment for 2006–07 showed that of the 38,568 clients on opiate pharmacotherapy, 35% were female (13,754 women).[9]

Given this prevalence of heroin use, clinicians across a range of treatment services are likely to have contact with and may manage an opioid-dependent woman during pregnancy. The exact proportion of opioid-dependent women of child-bearing age in Australia being treated for their opioid dependence is unknown, however in Europe and the US it has been estimated to be approximately one third.[10] A New South Wales study found that in babies exposed to substance use and admitted to neonatal intensive care units, a high proportion of mothers (86%) were enrolled in opiate substitution programs.[11] A cohort study of 89,080 pregnancies in South Australia found that in 0.8% of pregnancies, substance use was reported; of this group 12% reported using heroin.[12] While there are no reliable estimates of the number of infants born each year with the neonatal withdrawal syndrome in Australia,[13] Burns et al described 129 cases of neonatal abstinence syndrome (NAS) of 454 women on methadone during pregnancy in New South Wales in 2002, although this is likely to be an underestimate of NAS prevalence.[14]

This chapter aims to provide information regarding the available evidence for current pharmacotherapy treatments for opioid dependence during pregnancy, with particular regard to the effect such treatments have on the developing embryo, fetus, and the neonate. It begins by examining the health problems associated with heroin use during pregnancy and how these may affect the developing embryo, fetus, and infant. A discussion of pharmacotherapy management of opioid-dependent pregnant women follows, which focuses on the evidence that may improve antenatal and consequently neonatal outcomes.

While this chapter focuses on the literature on the treatment of opioid dependence in pregnancy, key authors in the field have stressed the importance of considering the range of problems that frequently affect this population, including use of substances in addition to opioids, mental health diagnoses, medical and social problems including homelessness, exposure to violence, and lack of support.[2,15,16]

Method

The studies reported were identified using:

- the Medline and Cochrane database (search January 1966 to June 2008); keywords included heroin, buprenorphine, methadone, naltrexone, levo-alpha-acetylmethadol hydrochloride (LAAM), opioid/s, pregnant/pregnancy, neonatal/neonates, development;
- hand searching, from product manufacturers and from experts in the field.

Heroin use during pregnancy

The management of drug-using pregnant women can be complex, difficult, and require considerable resources across health and welfare disciplines. It is paramount for the wide range of care providers to be aware of the unique medical, psychologic, and social needs of this group of pregnant women. Pregnant women dependent on heroin are at risk of experiencing medical and obstetric complications during pregnancy, due to a variety of factors in addition to heroin exposure itself.[2,17,18] These may include:

- other substance use including tobacco, benzodiazepine, amphetamine, cocaine, alcohol, cannabis, and other drug use;
- repeated maternal cycles of opioid intoxication and withdrawal that are reflected in the physiology of the neonate;
- physical factors including poor nutrition; blood-borne virus exposure including human immunodeficiency virus (HIV), and hepatitis B and C viruses (HCV, HBV); and opiate overdose;
- psychological factors including depression, anxiety, post-traumatic stress disorder, and other mental health problems;
- social factors including exposure to abuse and violence, financial stress, homelessness, relationship problems, and legal problems;
- poor attendance for antenatal care.

These factors confound our understanding of the relationship between heroin dependence and the manner in which it complicates pregnancy.[2,17,19] The majority of studies that have been conducted on opiate dependence (in combination with other substance use) and pregnancy have not been able to take into consideration these multiple confounders. Controlled studies have only been conducted relatively recently in the field of pregnancy and addictions.[20,21]

Early reports of poor outcomes among neonates born to heroin-dependent women coincide with increased use of heroin in the 1950s and 1960s.[22–24] There is a greater risk of morbidity and mortality for neonates exposed to heroin than for non-drug-exposed infants.[25–28] Major causes of neonatal mortality include respiratory distress syndrome, asphyxia neonatorum, hyaline membrane disease, anoxia and central nervous system (CNS) hemorrhage, broncho/aspiration pneumonia, and congenital abnormalities. Other obstetric and neonatal complications associated with the heroin dependence include miscarriage, amnionitis, intrauterine growth reduction (IUGR), placental insufficiency, premature labor, placental abruption, intracranial hemorrhage, meconium aspiration, and other conditions.[2,17,29,30] Heroin dependence during pregnancy is also associated with a reduction in birth weight and premature births compared to infants born to women who were not using heroin during pregnancy.[30–34]

There are a small number of studies reporting multiple congenital anomalies that varied with no discrete patterns or causal relationship identified.[35–37] The incidence of sudden infant death syndrome (SIDS) associated with opioid dependence during pregnancy has been reported to be between 3 and 9 times higher than the general population.[38,39] Others have found this association only in infants with very low birthweight. A 2-year follow-up study of infant mortality of infants born to heroin-dependent women compared to non-drug-using controls found an increased risk of infant mortality of 5.9 times (95% confidence interval [CI] 1.4–24) in opioid-exposed infants of low birthweight.[40]

Confounding factors such as polydrug use are highly likely to have a significant effect on obstetric and neonatal outcomes. Tobacco use, for example, is common in heroin users and can have a profound effect on birthweight, prematurity, and neonatal morbidity. In non-opioid-dependent pregnant women, smoking has been associated with low birthweight (<2,500 g), preterm birth (<32 weeks), intrauterine growth reduction, and perinatal death.[41–44] Poor antenatal care attendance is also common among heroin-dependent pregnant women,[25,27] which may have a significant negative impact on obstetric and neonatal health.

It should be noted that since neonatal data on heroin effects were first collected in the 1960s and 1970s there has been a significant positive effect on birth outcomes of infants born to heroin-dependent women.[45] This may have been due to several factors, including an increase in capacity to manage premature low-birthweight neonates as well as the development of specialized drugs and pregnancy services.

Neonatal abstinence syndrome

Chronic intrauterine exposure to opioids may result in the development of physical dependence by the fetus. Opioids cross the placental barrier and are readily bound to opioid receptors in the fetal brain and other organs in the body, creating the potential for the development of fetal neuroadaptation to the opioids. At birth, the supply of opioids via the placenta ceases and symptoms of neonatal withdrawal (the NAS) may manifest as opioid central nervous system levels drop.[46–48] NAS is described as a generalized disorder characterized by multiple behavioral and physiologic signs and symptoms that are indicators of non-specific central and autonomic nervous system instability, gastrointestinal dysfunction, and respiratory distress.[2,17] These symptoms include irritability, hyperreflexia, hyperactivity, abnormal cry, diarrhea, fever, vomiting, and tachypnea. If untreated the syndrome can progress to include fluid loss, respiratory instability, aspiration, apnea, seizures, coma, and death. The onset, duration, and severity of NAS can vary based on such factors as the timing and amount of the mother's last opioid maintenance dose, other drug use by the mother, and the rate of elimination of the drug by the newborn. NAS often requires medical intervention and prolonged hospitalization, and for infants that experience moderate to severe NAS the risk of developing mother–infant attachment disorder may be increased.[2,17] Recovery occurs when the infant's metabolism has adjusted to the absence of exogenous opioids.[49] Significant neonatal withdrawal is an indication for pharmacologic management.[50] For infants born to heroin-dependent mothers the incidence of NAS has been reported as between 55 and 95%.[26,27,51,52]

NAS is often used to describe neonatal withdrawal resulting from a mother's opioid use during pregnancy, but the use of other substances by the mother may also contribute to the syndrome. Most are psychoactive substances that have the potential for physical dependence:[2]

- alcohol
- barbiturates
- benzodiazepines
- nicotine.

Neurobehavioral abnormalities may also be seen in the newborn after fetal exposure to the following substances:[53,54]

- cocaine
- amphetamines.

The literature on substance use in pregnancy does not describe in detail the effects of combinations of substances on fetal development, including neonatal abstinence. Nicotine dependence alone, even at moderate to low-level dependence, may be associated with a NAS.[44] A prospective study of 27 nicotine-exposed and 29 non-nicotine-exposed full-term newborn infants found that tobacco-exposed infants were more excitable and hypertonic, required more handling, and showed more stress/abstinence signs than non-nicotine-exposed newborns.[44] Nicotine use in conjunction with opioid pharmacotherapy maintenance may also affect the timing and severity of NAS in prenatally exposed infants. Choo et al found that the NAS of neonates of methadone-maintained mothers smoking more than 20 cigarettes daily was more severe than for neonates of mothers smoking 10 or less cigarettes.[55] An Australian data linkage study by Burns et al showed women who smoked, as well as indigenous women, were more likely to have infants with NAS.[14] Burns and colleagues also showed an association of smoking with prematurity using data linkage of pregnant patients on methadone maintenance.[56] Consideration of, and an appropriate treatment response to the use of any or all of psychoactive substances is important in managing not only the pregnant woman but also their newborn.

Management of the pregnant opioid-dependent woman

Pregnancy is an ideal time for health professionals to engage a heroin-dependent woman to manage her heroin dependence and other problems. Women are more likely to be motivated during pregnancy to make important health and lifestyle changes. Use of pharmacotherapies such as methadone or buprenorphine maintenance to manage a pregnant women's opioid dependence is the main focus of this chapter. However, a range of health and welfare services must work collaboratively to ensure optimal outcomes for both the mother and newborn during pregnancy, but importantly in the longer term. These services include, but are not limited to, drug and alcohol treatment (pharmacologic and counseling), psychoeducation, social interventions such as access to accommodation, adequate responses to violence from partners or others, and financial welfare, as well as the management of other physical or medical problems such as blood-borne virus infections and poor diet.[57,58] Antenatal care is an important component of the optimal management of pregnancy, more so for opioid-dependent pregnant women as it has been found to improve the pregnancy outcomes for both the mother and the child.[27,59–62] Discussion of all these services is beyond the scope of this chapter.

Antenatal care

When considering the four decades of studies that have examined the effects of maternal methadone maintenance on the neonates, it is not possible to determine the degree to which improvements in obstetric and neonatal outcomes such as higher birthweights, longer gestations, and decreased perinatal mortality rates[27,63–66] are due to the effects of opiate substitution or enhanced antenatal care. Opioid-dependent pregnant women on maintenance programs are more likely to receive comprehensive medical and obstetric care than those not in a treatment program. Further, continuous methadone maintenance has been shown to be associated with earlier presentation for antenatal care and reduced prematurity.[67]

Generally, studies that have examined the association between level of antenatal care and neonatal outcomes in women receiving opioid substitution treatment have shown better neonatal outcomes with more antenatal care. In the Connaughton et al study, for example, 82% of neonates born to methadone-maintained women with inadequate antenatal care suffered neonatal morbidity, whereas the incidence of neonatal morbidity was less (69%) for neonates born to methadone-maintained women receiving adequate antenatal care.[27] Chang et al found that pregnant women who received an intensive treatment program including weekly antenatal care, relapse prevention groups, thrice-weekly urine drug screens, and child care during treatment had newborns with higher birthweights than women receiving the usual treatment of daily methadone medication, counseling, and random urine drug screens.[60]

An evaluation of a comprehensive care program for pregnant women with opioid dependence also found that improved gestational age and birthweight was associated with longer and more frequent antenatal care. Premature birth occurred for 18% of women on drug treatment who had poor antenatal care, twice as high as that for women on drug treatment who received good antenatal care.[61] Carroll et al reported on a randomized controlled trial comparing standard care to enhanced treatment (midwife antenatal care, child care, and contingency management) for methadone-maintained women, and found trends towards longer gestation, with a mean increase of 1.4 weeks, and a small increase in birthweight in those receiving enhanced care.[62]

In summary, the level of antenatal care received by drug-dependent women may impact on gestational age, birthweight of the neonate, and obstetric complications. Therefore, the level of antenatal care is an important variable to measure when examining the relative effect of opioid substitution treatment use by pregnant women on neonatal outcomes.

Treatments for opioid dependence during pregnancy

Withdrawal

Withdrawal from opioids during pregnancy is not routinely encouraged as evidence of safety is limited, and the risk of relapse to dependent heroin use with associated harm is very high.

The few reports on the effect of opioid withdrawal during pregnancy have found that opioid withdrawal in the first trimester can precipitate uterine contractions, and thus increase the risk of spontaneous abortion,[49,68] and withdrawal in the third trimester is associated with an increased risk of intrauterine growth reduction, premature labor, or fetal death.[68–71] It has been shown that opioid withdrawal is associated with fetal stress, in utero meconium aspiration, and an increase in the oxygen requirement of the infant.[69,70,72] Hypoxia is thought to be the principal cause of fetal death.[69]

There are no data to suggest that the risk of relapse is reduced per se by pregnancy. Relapse rates for pregnant opioid-dependent women who have undergone withdrawal treatment range from 29% to 96%.[27,68,72,73] In addition, there is minimal success with withdrawal treatment during pregnancy, with only 30 to 60% completing the withdrawal treatment itself.[68,71,73] Relapse to illicit heroin use and its complications is more likely to pose a significant risk of morbidity and mortality to the mother and infant than NAS, which, once identified, can be managed. A prospective study of 34 pregnant women that monitored outcomes during withdrawal noted that 20 women underwent detoxification without relapsing to heroin use, 4 women chose methadone maintenance treatment, and the remaining 10 women resumed opioid use. Two infants with fetal growth reduction were delivered by mothers who resumed heroin use.[71]

In summary, due to the increased risk of relapse into heroin use, it is important for pregnant opioid-dependent women to be stabilized and maintained on opioids such as methadone or buprenorphine.

Opioid maintenance therapies during pregnancy

Methadone maintenance is recommended for use during pregnancy, as there are four decades of experience with this treatment during pregnancy. Despite limited experience with buprenorphine maintenance during pregnancy, there is an interest in the use of buprenorphine during pregnancy as the NAS is hypothesized to be milder than that observed with methadone.

Substitution maintenance for an opioid-dependent pregnant woman is based on a risk assessment and is recommended for several reasons: substitution of illicit drugs of unknown quality and dose with a prescribed pharmacotherapy stabilizes the mother's illicit opioid-dependency behavior; stabilization of erratic serum opioid levels in the mother protects the fetus from repeated episodes of intoxication and withdrawal;[74,75] and engagement in opioid substitution facilitates pregnant women receiving adequate antenatal care and advice.[57,58]

Overall the objectives of opioid substitution treatment during pregnancy should include:[76]

- reducing the harmful effects of heroin and other drug use including tobacco;
- reducing maternal and infant morbidity and mortality associated with heroin use;
- improving physical, psychologic, and social health for pregnant women;
- appropriately identifying the need for long-term support to pregnant women and their families until their children reach school age.

Methadone maintenance

Of the opioid substitution pharmacotherapies used for the management of heroin dependence, methadone is the only one recommended for use in pregnancy due to the substantial literature that exists regarding effectiveness, safety, and reduction in neonatal and maternal harm.[2,77–79] Guidelines in the UK, USA, and Australia recommend methadone maintenance as appropriate treatment of opiate dependence in pregnancy.[80–82]

Preclinical studies of methadone in pregnancy show that neonatal withdrawal appears to be the most significant sequela of antenatal methadone exposure.[83,84] Exposure to methadone does not appear to be associated with increased birth defects[85] or abnormal effects in terms of structural brain development.[86] The adverse events of methadone exposure do not appear to recur over several generations.[87]

Clinical studies

The use of methadone as a maintenance agent for pregnant opioid-dependent women was developed in Philadelphia by Dr Loretta Finnegan in the early 1970s, principally because opioid substitution treatment held the potential to facilitate access across general medical, social, and obstetric services for this group,[88] despite the lack of comprehensive knowledge of the safety of methadone in pregnancy at that time. Since that time, methadone has become accepted as a first-line agent in the treatment of opioid dependence in pregnancy. A total of over 5000 births of neonates to pregnant women have been reported in the medical literature; however, the majority of these studies are observational studies, with randomized controlled studies only appearing more recently in the literature, in particular since there has been more than one possible opioid substitute that could feasibly be used during pregnancy.[15]

Serious adverse events

Early reports of perinatal death rates in heroin users were particularly high, for example a US study in the 1970s reported a perinatal death rate of 107/1000 births in 149 heroin users.[30] This contrasts markedly with the current Australian perinatal mortality rate of 5.3/1000 births for the general population.[89] Comparative studies that report on perinatal mortality in heroin- and methadone-maintained groups range in mortality rates for heroin from 22 to 106 per 1000, and in methadone from 0 to 42 per 1000, the incidence being less in methadone pregnancies in the majority of studies and equal in one study. Many medical complications seen in the neonates of heroin-dependent pregnant women are related to low birthweight and prematurity.[90] These conditions are associated with multiple causes of perinatal death reported including: stillbirth, placental abruption, respiratory distress syndrome and asphyxia, meconium aspiration syndrome, hydrops, congenital abnormalities, hyaline membrane disease, anoxia, CNS hemorrhage, meningocele and hydrocephalus, SIDS, sickle cell anemia, and several undetermined cases, all seen in heroin-exposed pregnancies.[25,27,29,33,91–94]

Congenital abnormalities have been reported in neonates born to pregnant women maintained on methadone, including hydrocephalus, gastroschisis, anencephaly, microcephaly, polydactyly, and hydrocele,[27,29,33,95] without any clear causal relationship related to methadone.

A range of neonatal morbidities has been reported of infants exposed to heroin or methadone. The etiology of these adverse events is likely to be multifactorial and not solely related to opioid exposure alone but due to other substance use (including tobacco), poor nutrition, poor mental health, social factors including homelessness and violence, and poor antenatal care. Obstetric morbidities reported in pregnant women who use heroin include respiratory distress, asphyxia, hyperbilirubinemia, sepsis, IUGR, placental abruption, placenta previa, cerebral palsy, and hyaline membrane disease.[25,27,33,61,91,95] Many of these are clearly related to, or exacerbated by prematurity. Further, prematurity is increased in pregnant women with inadequate antenatal care. Adequate access to antenatal care that can be provided through methadone maintenance allows the capacity for in utero screening, and early diagnosis and management of pregnancy complications. More recently, blood-borne viruses including HIV, HCV, and HBV have been reported amongst pregnant opioid-dependent women.[34,60,92,94,96–99]

Gestational age and birth size

Methadone has been associated with an increase in birthweight compared to heroin.[63,100–103] In some studies the improvement in birthweight in the methadone-maintained group is similar to non-drug-using comparison populations.[104,105]

Kandall et al reported a positive dose–response relationship between methadone dose and birthweight.[63] Hagiopan et al reported on a positive relationship between head circumference, gestational age, and higher methadone doses.[106] However, the protective effect of methadone varies across studies; some studies have not shown an increase in birthweight in methadone-maintained pregnancies compared to heroin-dependent pregnant women;[25,91,107,108] length at birth may also not be improved in this group.[109] Many of these studies have smaller sample sizes than those studies that have found a protective effect.

The prevalence of low birthweight (<2,500 g) in neonates born to methadone-maintained pregnant women varies from 19% to 41%.[27,29,61,93,108,110] In addition, one study has reported longer periods on methadone at higher doses to be associated with improved birthweight in methadone-maintained pregnancies compared to controls.[111]

There are a number of reasons for the variation in effect including different study designs and sample sizes, different populations studied, different approaches to methadone dosing and dose levels, and maternal use of other drugs including nicotine, benzodiazepines, and cocaine. A meta-analysis has compared neonatal birth weight of a group of women typically stabilized on methadone late in the third trimester who continued to use heroin with a group of women stabilized on methadone earlier and not using heroin. This meta-analysis showed the late stabilizing/heroin-using group to have a 4-fold increased risk of low birthweight (95% CI 2.8–7.7) compared to the group stabilized on methadone who did not have an increased risk of low birthweight (risk ratio 1.4; confidence interval [CI] 0.8–2.2).[112] However, even this analysis was not able to take into account all of the other factors that would impact on birthweight. In addition, any protective effect of pregnant women being in methadone treatment may be diminished in a population using other drugs, particularly benzodiazepines.[29,113]

Neonatal abstinence syndrome

NAS is seen in neonates born to methadone-maintained pregnant women as in heroin-dependent women. An important outcome measure is the proportion requiring pharmacologic treatment, as this is an index of the requirement for longer periods of hospitalization and possible admission to neonatal special or intensive care units. The prevalence of NAS in infants born to methadone-maintained pregnant women ranges from 59 to 100%.[25,61,93,95,101,114] The proportion of infants born to methadone-maintained pregnant women overall requiring pharmacologic treatment for NAS has been reported at being from 18 to 77%.[25,61,91,95,99,115–119]

Several studies comparing NAS prevalence in neonates born to methadone-maintained pregnant women compared to heroin-dependent women have shown a similar proportion of infants experiencing NAS.[25,91,120] However, one study found a higher proportion in neonates born to methadone-maintained women requiring treatment for NAS.[91] Infants born to methadone-maintained pregnant women may require a longer period of treatment for NAS.[25] In contrast, another study has shown a shorter period of treatment for neonates born to methadone-maintained women compared to neonates born to heroin-dependent women.[92] A recent study that randomized pregnant heroin users attending antenatal care to continue illicit heroin use or receive methadone maintenance found that 89% of newborns from the heroin groups experienced NAS, compared to 100% of those in the methadone group. Mean Finnegan scores were higher in the methadone group, and duration of NAS also appeared longer.[121]

Some authors have demonstrated an association between higher methadone doses and increased prevalence of NAS,[61,94,99,103,114,118,122–124] while others have not found a methadone dose–response relationship with NAS incidence or severity,[25,93,98,120,125,126] nor an increased duration of NAS in methadone-exposed infants compared to heroin-exposed infants.[25,92] There is some evidence that benzodiazepines prolong NAS[125,127] and may be related to decreased birthweight in exposed infants.[113] Again, there may be a wide range of reasons for the difference in outcomes reported, including different population studies, and varying levels of other drug use, including benzodiazepines and possibly nicotine, that may contribute to the abstinence syndrome.

Further, the relationship between maternal methadone dose level, in utero exposure, and NAS risk or severity is unclear. Firstly, maternal serum levels may not correlate with maternal methadone dose levels as there is significant interindividual variation in methadone pharmacokinetics.[128] Secondly, maternal serum levels may not correlate with neonatal plasma levels or NAS severity. While a relationship between maternal dose and neonatal plasma levels post delivery has been reported,[119] others have not found a relationship between neonatal serum levels of methadone and NAS severity.[129–131] Vagal tone has been suggested as a predictor of the development of NAS.[132] Clearly the etiology of NAS is complex and dependent on both maternal and neonatal factors.

In severe NAS, neonates may experience seizures. A higher proportion of seizures in neonatal withdrawal in infants born to pregnant women on methadone substitution compared to infants born to pregnant women using heroin has been reported.[25,91] However, a 1-year follow-up on infants with seizures post withdrawal showed all infants followed up had normal neurologic examination results.[133]

Higher doses of methadone may be required in pregnancy,[134,135] as increasing opioid withdrawal symptoms can occur in pregnant women with increasing gestational age[136] and metabolism may be increased in pregnant women.[135,137] Split dosing of methadone is an approach that can be used.[138,139] Normalization of fetal activity on ultrasound when methadone was spilt dosed has been reported.[140]

Recently, effects of peak methadone doses on fetal neurobehavior have been reported. Peak methadone doses affect both fetal heart rate and motor activity.[141] This impact appears to be diminished when methadone is split dosed.[142]

The therapeutic goal of substitution treatment for opioid-dependent pregnant women is a crucial issue. Some authors have suggested a primary goal of treatment to be maintenance on the lowest possible dose to minimize neonatal exposure,[99] including offering withdrawal from methadone, particularly in highly motivated pregnant women. However, accurate assessment of levels of motivation is complex and not well supported in the literature and may vary during the course of pregnancy depending on the wide range of psychosocial pressures pregnant women may experience. In contrast, other authors have suggested that methadone is most efficacious when provided in adequate doses to suppress additional opioid use as part of a comprehensive treatment program, and that NAS, when adequately identified, is not life-threatening and can be safely managed.[15,21,143,144] More recently, guidelines from the UK, USA, and Australia support the use of individual titration to effective doses of methadone in pregnancy.[80–82]

Behavioral incentives

The recent development of experimental studies has demonstrated that behavioral incentives have an important role in the management of substance use in pregnancy. Voucher rewards may be particularly promising with regard to smoking cessation in pregnancy. Voucher-based rewards have been shown to be effective in a non-opiate group of tobacco-dependent pregnant women in reducing tobacco use.[145,146] Given the high prevalence of tobacco dependence, and the known harmful effects of tobacco on the developing fetus, these studies are of significant importance. The understanding of voucher-based rewards in opioid-dependent groups is in an earlier stage of development. Escalating voucher-based incentives have been trialled in a pregnant methadone group and found to have a modest effect in promoting treatment attendance.[147]

Developmental outcomes

The results of studies investigating the long-term development of infants exposed to methadone in utero show a consistent pattern of appropriate motor and cognitive development during the first 2 years of life.[61,75,114,148–152] However, motor development in methadone-exposed infants generally lagged behind infants born to non-opioid-dependent mothers from comparable socioeconomic and racial backgrounds.[114,148,149,151] The treatment or severity of NAS has not been found to be associated with developmental outcomes.[114,133,150]

With regard to the cognitive development, some reported poorer cognitive development among methadone-exposed children compared to non-drug-exposed children,[114,152] while others reported no differences.[75,148,149] Kaltenbach et al found infants exposed to methadone in utero had lower mental development scores at 12 months than non-drug-exposed infants born to mothers matched for socioeconomic, racial, and medical backgrounds, yet no difference at 24 months.[150] Similarities of mental scores between the methadone-exposed and non-exposed children at 24 months may be due to the low socioeconomic status of the non-exposed children impacting on mental development, resulting in decreases in mental scores between 1 and 2 years for these children. Suffet and Brotman also found a decrease of cognitive development through to 2 years of age for methadone-exposed infants from low socioeconomic backgrounds.[61] A recent review article has shown that, when compared to drug-free controls, there is a consistent pattern of neurodevelopment impairment of opiate-exposed neonates.[153]

However, case control studies show a pattern of the effect of impaired neurodevelopment largely being accounted for by socioeconomic factors. Steinhused et al reported on impaired performance IQ on a group of children born to methadone-maintained mothers; this effect, though small in size, persisted after adjusting for socioeconomic state.[154] In contrast, Ornoy's adoption studies suggest developmental delay may be largely due to environmental deprivation rather than drug exposure in utero.[155,156] Messinger's prospective cohort study of opioid- and cocaine-exposed neonates did not find mental, motor, or behavioral deficits after controlling for birthweight and environmental risks.[157]

Two studies have shown that the rate of the development of strabismus in infants of methadone- or opioid-dependent mothers has been found to be approximately 10 times greater than in the general population,[158,159] although the reason for this is not well understood. It should be noted, however, that these studies did not control for other drug use such as alcohol or nicotine, found also to be associated with this ophthalmologic condition.[160,161]

The inconsistency of findings regarding developmental outcomes associated with methadone maintenance may be attributable to a number of factors. Differences in the daily methadone dose, length of maintenance during pregnancy, and amount of antenatal care and other drug use may impact on the child's long-term development. However, one study found no associations between perinatal factors such as mother's age, length of methadone treatment, methadone dose, and polydrug use and obstetric complications or developmental outcome.[162]

Environmental factors occurring postnatally, such as birth complications, health, and nutrition, and a wide range of social factors may have more of an impact on the child's developmental progress. A review of a number of studies on high-risk infants suggested that newborn status is a very poor predictor of developmental outcome and rather is highly dependent on environmental factors via an ongoing reciprocal interaction between the child and its environment.[163] Genetic effects are also thought to influence the development of children.[164] For an opioid-dependent mother regardless of whether she is in treatment for her dependence, the effects of antenatal drug exposure on a child's development may be confounded by postnatal health factors such as malnutrition; similarly, social factors like maternal depression, inadequate social support, lower maternal education, maternal polydrug use, and less optimal caretaking environments can also have an impact.[114,149,165] Although most of the developmental studies controlled for socioeconomic status, other environmental risk factors such as those aforementioned need to be taken into consideration when studying the effect of antenatal drug exposure on developmental outcomes.

Other methodologic issues with neonatal developmental and drug exposure research include the conduct of assessments at only one point in time as well as not assessing multiple areas of functioning (including perceptual, cognitive, and motor skills; speech and language abilities; and behavior). Repeating assessments over time is useful to determine whether identified developmental effects are permanent or transient.[165]

In summary, further research is required to better understand the effects of a maternal methadone maintenance treatment on the developmental outcomes of children. A child's development is dependent upon a multitude of factors including antenatal conditions, the postnatal environment, and genetic factors, making it all the more difficult to understand the direct effect of in utero methadone exposure.

Buprenorphine maintenance

Buprenorphine, alone or in combination with naloxone (as buprenorphine–naloxone), is the most recent opioid maintenance pharmacotherapy approved for use in Australia, Europe, and the US for the treatment of opioid dependence. Since its introduction into Australia the proportion of substitution maintenance treated patients on buprenorphine has increased significantly to approximately 28%.[9] One consequence of such an increase in the availability of buprenorphine is an increase in the number of women becoming pregnant while being treated with buprenorphine. Women who become pregnant on buprenorphine are faced with two options: to discontinue buprenorphine and transfer to methadone maintenance or to continue on buprenorphine.

Pharmacologically, buprenorphine differs from methadone in several ways. The effects of buprenorphine on the developing fetus have been postulated to be different from the effects of methadone. Unlike methadone, a full μ agonist, buprenorphine is a partial μ opioid receptor agonist with low intrinsic activity and high receptor affinity, and also a potent μ opioid receptor antagonist.[166–168] Due to its partial μ -agonist low intrinsic activity, buprenorphine appears to possess a markedly greater safety profile than methadone with regard to opioid overdose as buprenorphine produces relatively limited respiratory depression.[169,170] In particular, pre-clinical and clinical studies have shown that buprenorphine produces a 'ceiling effect' above which further increases in dose have no further effect[171,172] nor a decreased effect.[173] The limited respiratory depression and the ceiling on buprenorphine's agonist activity limit the possibility of overdose. However, as stated in Chapter 6, the risk of overdose is increased with the concomitant use of buprenorphine and respiratory depressant drugs such as benzodiazepines. Buprenorphine is also associated with a milder withdrawal syndrome in dependent adults upon abrupt cessation after chronic dosing compared to methadone.[174–176]

The greater safety profile and milder withdrawal syndrome upon abrupt cessation suggest that buprenorphine maintenance during pregnancy may be safer for the neonate than methadone. It is postulated to have a reduced potential for respiratory depression in the neonate. Additionally, it is possible that buprenorphine maintenance during pregnancy may be associated with less frequent and less severe NAS in the newborn.[174,177]

Overall, pre-clinical studies have shown that buprenorphine exposure antenatally appears to lack teratogenicity,[178,179] has little maternal or offspring toxicity,[179] and no mutagenic action.[180] In particular, the effects of buprenorphine antenatally do not seem to be greater than exposure to methadone.[178,181–186] Any potential adverse effects of buprenorphine in utero seem more likely to occur at higher than recommended doses for the treatment of opioid dependence (Reckitt Benckiser Pharmaceuticals, Inc, personal communication 2002, cited in Johnson et al[10]).

Clinical studies

The body of evidence from the clinical research literature regarding the use of buprenorphine in pregnancy is rapidly evolving. Table 9.1 provides a summary of 21 published studies of original cases documenting the exposure of buprenorphine in pregnancy.

Eleven studies published between 1995 and 2008 were from France, 4 were from Austria, 2 were from the US, and one was from each of Italy, Belgium, Australia, and the Czech Republic. Ten reports are retrospective case studies or case series (reports 1–10), 3 are prospective observational studies (reports 12–14), 1 report is both a retrospective and prospective study (report 11), 2 are case comparison studies of methadone and buprenorphine (reports 15 and 16), 2 are open label, single arm studies designed as pilot studies for future clinical trials (reports 17 and 18), and 3 are randomized controlled studies (reports 19–21). A total of 425 pregnant women maintained on buprenorphine have been reported in these studies (113 retrospectively, 312 prospectively) compared to over 5000 in the methadone literature.

The discussion of the effect of buprenorphine in utero in the human studies will focus where possible on the following outcome variables: serious adverse events, gestational age and birth size at delivery, and the NAS and developmental outcomes.

Serious adverse events

A total of four fetal deaths not related to planned terminations were reported for women on buprenorphine maintenance therapy.[187,188] Lacroix et al[188] reported two malformations in a neonate exposed to sulfamethoxazole,

Table 9.1 Summary of published clinical studies on the use of buprenorphine for opiate dependence in pregnancy

Authors	*Year*	*Country*	*Buprenorphine (n)*	*Methadone (n)*	*Retro studies (n^1)*	*Pros studies (n^2)*	*Live births (n)*	*NAS (n)*	*Births requiring treatment for NAS (%)*
Retrospective case-studies or case-series/prospective observational studies									
1. Herve and Quernum[193]	1998	France	1		1		1	1	100
2. Regini et al[191]	1998	Italy	1		1		1	1	100
3. Ross194	2004	Australia	1		1		1	0	0
4. Reisinger[205,254]	1996	Belgium	4		4		4	1	0
5 Mazurier et al[255]	1996	France	6		6		6	6	100
6. Dos Santos[195]	1998	France	12		12		12	11	92
7. Kayemba-Kay's and Laclyde[206]	2003	France	13		13		13	11	77
8. Burlet et al[256]	1999	France	14		14		14	9	57
9. Marquet et al[238,257,258]	1997, 1998, 2002	France	21		21		21	13	48
10. Noblett et al[196]	2000	France	27		27		27	18	89[3]
11. Jernite et al[190,259]	1998, 1999	France	24		13	11	24	16	67
12. Schindler et al[199]	2003	Austria	2			2	2	2	0

(Continued)

Table 9.1 Summary of published clinical studies on the use of buprenorphine for opiate dependence in pregnancy

Authors	*Year*	*Country*	*Buprenorphine (n)*	*Methadone (n)*	*Retro studies (n¹)*	*Pros studies (n²)*	*Live births (n)*	*NAS (n)*	*Births requiring treatment for NAS (%)*
13 Loustauneau et al.[187,260]	1999, 2000	France	18			18	14	8	36
14 Lacroix et al[188]	2004	France	34			34	31	13	26
Prospective observational case-comparison studies									
15 Ebner et al[250]	2007	Austria	14	22		36[5]	14; 22[4]	NR	21; 68
16 Lejeune et al[192]	2006	France	159	101		260[5]	159;101[4]	200[5]	52; 49
Open-label non-randomized controlled studies									
17 Johnson et al[198]	2001	USA	3			3	3	3	0
18 Fischer et al[197]	2000	Austria	15			15	15	7	20
Randomized controlled trials									
19 Jones et al[201]	2005	USA	10	11		21	21	NR	20; 46
20 Fischer et al[202]	2006	Austria	8	6		14	14	8; 6[4]	63; 50
21 Binder[121]	2008	Czech Rep	38	32		70	70	34; 32[4]	NR
Total			425	172	113	484			

[1]Retro: retrospective collection; [2]Pros: prospective collection; [3](17 cases were treated independent of Finnegan score); [4](buprenorphine, methadone); [5]includes buprenorphine and methadone cases; NR: not reported; NAS: neonatal abstinence syndrome.

trimethoprim (category C in pregnancy, using the Australian Drug Evaluation Committee classification system[189]), lamividine, and zidovudine (category B3 in pregnancy) for HIV therapy in utero; and in a neonate exposed to aspirin and cannabis in utero. Jernite et al reported on three neonates who experienced acute fetal stress. One neonate exposed to high doses of benzodiazepines in combination with high doses of buprenorphine in utero experienced convulsions.[190]

Regini et al reported on a single case of cerebral palsy in the neonate.[191] The authors commented that maternal epilepsy, with possible other drug use, problems with adherence to buprenorphine treatment, profound neonatal narcosis with naloxone reversal, and possible hypoxia, may all have been associated with the development of this condition.

IUGR was reported by 4 studies. Fischer et al[77] and Jernite et al[190] reported IUGR in 1 (7%) and 7 (29%)[77,190] neonates, respectively, however it is unlikely buprenorphine was the principal etiologic agent as growth reduction could be associated with nicotine addiction, malnutrition, and other socioeconomic factors. Of the studies where there is a comparison, Lejune et al[121] reported IUGR in 49 (31%) buprenorphine neonates compared to 38 methadone neonates (38%), while Binder et al[192] reported IUGR in 4 (11%) buprenorphine compared to 3 (9%) methadone neonates.[121,192] Neither difference between groups was statistically significant.

Neonatal abstinence syndrome and birth size

A common outcome measure across published studies was the prevalence of the NAS that required pharmacologic treatment; this ranged from 0 to 100% of neonates. The difference in reported rates of NAS requiring treatment across studies cannot be compared for several reasons: there is a difference in the type of studies; there are differences in the measurement of the severity of NAS; and there are different thresholds that different centers use for instigating NAS treatment. Further, inclusion and exclusion criteria vary across studies and study types, and the underlying populations may vary considerably in terms of opioid and other substance use and other health problems described above, all of which may contribute to the propensity for a neonate to develop NAS. Not all studies reported on other maternal drug use.[187,190,191,193–196]

More recent studies have attempted to account or control for potential confounding factors such as other drug use by excluding women using other substances[77,121,197–201] and/or by reporting additional drug use.[192,200,201] Johnson et al reported on 3 cases treated as hospital inpatients for the duration of the pregnancies, thereby reducing the risk of additional drug use or other factors that may affect maternal health. Buprenorphine doses of 8–12 mg sublingual tablets were used. Neonatal abstinence syndrome was observed in all three cases; however, none required pharmacotherapy for neonatal withdrawal.[198]

Fischer et al reported on 15 cases of women maintained on buprenorphine as outpatients during pregnancy.[202] Mothers were maintained on buprenorphine for a mean period of 11.7 weeks with a mean daily dose of 7.4 mg buprenorphine at delivery. One woman was HIV positive; all women were nicotine and cannabis dependent on entry. Average gestational age was 39.6 weeks with a mean birthweight of 3,049 g. NAS was observed in 7/15 cases (47%), for a mean duration of 1.1 days. Three required pharmacotherapy for NAS. The mothers of neonates requiring treatment for NAS reported a higher mean number of cigarettes smoked per day (17.5 per day) compared to mothers of neonates who had mild or no NAS (9.44 per day). Schindler et al reported on two women who conceived whilst taking buprenorphine. Both women delivered well infants, both of whom experienced NAS but did not require pharmacotherapy management of NAS.[197] In summary, buprenorphine combined with minimal additional substance use would appear to present a reduced risk of NAS requiring treatment.

Comparison between buprenorphine and methadone

Two case comparison and three randomized controlled trials have compared outcomes between methadone and buprenorphine. Lejeune et al[192] and Ebner et al[199] have published case comparison studies. The former study is a multicenter case comparison observational study comparing the outcomes of 100 patients on methadone and 159 on buprenorphine. The methadone group was typically treated in a specialist treatment center (74% in a specialist center vs 25% in general practice), whereas the buprenorphine group was more likely to be treated in general practice settings (74% in general practice vs 20% in a specialist center). Those on buprenorphine also tended to be on substitution treatment before pregnancy was diagnosed (82% vs 72%) and were more likely to have a partner. Six percent were HIV positive.[192]

Significant drug use occurred in both groups with no significant difference between the groups. No neonatal deaths occurred across either group. There was no difference in attendance for antenatal care or the type of delivery intervention, mean birthweight, low head circumference or length, prevalence of fetal distress, or IUGR. There was no difference in mean gestational age at delivery, however there was a difference in the proportions of premature delivery (<37 weeks) in the methadone group (18% vs 9%). The prevalence of the NAS (65%), mean time to onset of the NAS, mean maximal withdrawal score, proportion requiring pharmacotherapy treatment (50%), mean duration of treatment, proportion requiring transfer to a higher level of care setting, and age at regaining birthweight was not significantly different between the groups. A significant difference was seen in the age at maximum withdrawal scores (92 hours vs 70 hours) and a trend for longer hospital stays was seen in the methadone group. The authors reported some association between buprenorphine or methadone dose at delivery and intensity of neonatal withdrawal, however there was a marked overlap of the data between groups. Mean doses of buprenorphine and methadone per day were not reported.

The participants in Ebner et al's study were recruited from an interdisciplinary, multiprofessional treatment center in Vienna.[199] Women with a positive drug urine test at birth (other than nicotine or cannabis) were excluded from the study. Fourteen women were prescribed buprenorphine and 22 were prescribed methadone. No difference was found between groups in neonatal birthweight or length and head circumference. In the methadone group, 68% of neonates experienced NAS requiring treatment, while in the buprenorphine group, only 21% required treatment.

Three randomized controlled trials, including two pilot studies and one larger study, have been published comparing buprenorphine to methadone in pregnancy.[121,200,201] A large-scale, multisite trial spanning three countries, the MOTHER study (maternal opiate treatment – human experimental research), is currently under way.[203]

Jones et al reported on a randomized trial comparing 21 women on opiate substitution: 11 on methadone and 10 on buprenorphine (including one twin pregnancy). Behavioral incentives (voucher payments for negative urine screens) were used in both groups. Adequate maintenance doses were achieved (mean doses: methadone 79 mg, buprenorphine 19 mg). There was no statistical difference between rates of NAS requiring treatment, however the sample size was small. Length of neonatal hospital stay was shorter for the buprenorphine group compared to the methadone group.[205] Jones et al also reported on the use of short-acting morphine as an intermediate step to transition women between methadone and buprenorphine during the second trimester.[204]

Fischer et al reported on a randomized trial comparing the outcomes of 14 women: 8 on buprenorphine and 6 on methadone. Maternal mean maintenance doses of 48 mg methadone and 15 mg buprenorphine were achieved. Again there was no difference between rates of NAS requiring treatment. There was a lower rate of additional opioid use seen in the methadone group, but better retention in the buprenorphine group.[201] While both studies have demonstrated that experimental research is feasible in opioid dependence and pregnancy, both studies had to screen large numbers of opioid-dependent pregnant women to find a group who were eligible and wanted to remain in the study.

Binder et al reported on a trial that randomized women either to receive methadone or buprenorphine treatment or to remain on 'street' heroin while receiving antenatal care. Forty-seven women remained on heroin, 32 received methadone, and 38 received buprenorphine treatment. Low birthweight and IUGR were particularly seen in the group who remained on heroin. The profile of NAS, in duration and severity, appeared significantly longer for the group on methadone compared to the group who received buprenorphine. Unfortunately, exact rates of NAS requiring treatment and the details of treatment (including maternal maintenance doses) are not discretely described in this study. There are also several unusual features of this study: participants could only be low-level tobacco smokers (less than 10 cigarettes per day), aged less than 30, have 3 to 4 years of opioid dependence, be HCV and HIV negative, and be diagnosed in the first trimester of pregnancy. These features combined make generalization of this particular finding difficult; however, it may remain the only published study comparing a group who remained on heroin during pregnancy to opiate substitution treatment groups.[121]

Developmental outcomes

Data on the long-term outcomes of children born to women taking buprenorphine during pregnancy are extremely limited. Reisinger reported on 4 children exposed to buprenorphine during pregnancy and followed them up from ages 3 to 5 years old; all were found to be 'well'. One infant was breastfed while the mother was taking buprenorphine for 6 weeks with no reported adverse event.[205] Schindler et al reported on normal developmental assessment of 2 infants in that study at 6 and 12 months.[197]

A study by Kayemba-Kay's and Laclyde followed up 13 children exposed to buprenorphine in utero (as well as some level of heroin, benzodiazepine, and cannabis exposure): 7 experienced transient lower limb hypertonia, jerky movements, and jitteriness, from the ages of 3 to 9 months. The symptoms resolved spontaneously in 2 children while 3 required intensive physiotherapy and 2 required specialized care. The 2 children who required specialized care for their symptoms were found to have abnormal developmental outcomes and milestone acquisitions. The rest were found to have milestone acquisitions and neurodevelopmental tests within normal limits. The author suggested hypertonia may be part of a post-acute withdrawal syndrome and expressed a need for more long-term follow-up studies of children born to mothers on substitution therapy, particularly buprenorphine.[206] The methodologic issues associated with studying the effect on the development of the child due to buprenorphine exposure in utero are comparable to those discussed for methadone.

Poisonings

Concern has been raised regarding child methadone poisonings.[207] A review of over 75,000 opioid child poisonings in the US (predominantly codeine, oxycodone, and morphine poisonings) found 102 cases of methadone (liquid and tablet) poisoning, including 21 deaths. The authors commented that of all opioids, methadone may be the most lethal for children aged less than 6 years.[208] In contrast, buprenorphine may be associated with a reduced risk of overdose in pediatric poisoning, due to the partial agonist effects of the medication and poor oral absorption (as children are less likely to leave buprenorphine sublingually). While the need for mechanical ventilation in child buprenorphine poisonings has been reported,[209] a report on 53 children exposed to buprenorphine using the US poisons centers data showed no fatalities, with severe respiratory depression occurring only in a small minority (7%).[210,211]

Buprenorphine–naloxone

Buprenorphine–naloxone was introduced to Australia and listed under the pharmaceutical benefits scheme in 2006. The safety of naloxone is not known in pregnancy. There are no studies of buprenorphine–naloxone in pregnancy. If used by injection, naloxone may induce a withdrawal state in a pregnant woman, thus putting the embryo or fetus at risk of abortion or premature labor. Pregnancy and breastfeeding are listed as contraindications to the use of buprenorphine–naloxone; the medication is listed as category C by the Australian Drug Evaluation Committee.[212]

Levo-alpha-acetylmethadol hydrochloride

LAAM, a synthetic opioid analgesic, is a μ opioid receptor agonist and so has pharmacodynamic actions qualitatively similar to both morphine and methadone. It has a long duration of action due to the metabolites nor-LAAM and dinor-LAAM also being active. LAAM was only marketed briefly in the US (from 1993) and several countries in the European Union (from 1997). However, due to 10 cases of life-threatening arrhythmias in association with QT prolongation, the European Agency for the Evaluation of Medicinal Products recommended that marketing authorization be withdrawn in Europe in 2001. While the US Food and Drug Administration (FDA) still lists LAAM as an approved agent, in 2003 the manufacturers stopped sale of the medication and it remains unavailable in the US.[213,214]

Teratogenic studies carried out in naïve and tolerant rabbits and in tolerant rats have revealed no embryotoxic or teratogenic effects.[215] LAAM was not found to affect fetal skeletal development, number of implementation sites, resorption sites, or live young.[215] The only abnormality was found at high doses (6 and 12 mg/kg/day), with an increased incidence of angulated ribs among fetuses. Reproduction, perinatal, and lactation performance studies found that tolerant rats exposed to LAAM showed an increased number of stillbirths, a decrease in survival of offspring during lactation, and lower body weight of the offspring, although these results are reported to be similar to studies with methadone.[215,216] Exposure to LAAM in utero in tolerant rats found evidence of developmental toxicity in the form of post-implantation losses at all doses of LAAM up to 15 mg/kg/day.[217] However, there was no evidence of selective fetal toxicity or teratogenic activity.[217]

There are no clinical trial data and only a few case reports available on the safety and efficacy of LAAM during pregnancy. In one multisite study on LAAM in the US headed by Fudala and colleagues, three female subjects became pregnant while receiving LAAM (Fudala et al, unpublished data). One was given LAAM during the first 4 weeks of gestation before being transferred to methadone maintenance therapy for the remainder of the pregnancy. Twins were delivered at 27 weeks' gestation and died soon after birth. The causes of death were disorders which may occur in very early stages of pregnancy, thus the investigators indicated that the possibility that LAAM may have contributed to these abnormalities could not be excluded. The other two females who became pregnant during the study chose to have their pregnancies terminated and there is no information regarding the aborted embryo or fetuses.

Newborn rats exposed to LAAM in utero experience withdrawal.[218] Respiratory studies found the possibility of prolonged exposure to LAAM in utero influenced the respiratory control in newborn puppies.[219] There is a possibility that NAS could be of greater frequency and severity in infants born to LAAM-maintained mothers compared with infants exposed to methadone in utero. The half-lives of LAAM and its metabolites are of significantly longer duration than for methadone and may lead to accumulation in utero and possibly delayed emergence of NAS.

Naltrexone

Naltrexone is a pure opioid antagonist at the μ opioid receptors and does not lead to dependence. It is registered as a category B3 agent by the Australian Therapeutic Goods Administration.[220] It is expected that infants born to naltrexone-maintained mothers will not be born with physical opioid dependence or other agonist-like side-effects and therefore will not exhibit any abstinence signs and symptoms. Naltrexone treatment is contraindicated in patients dependent on opioids, as it will induce severe withdrawal symptoms. This would also apply to pregnant women who have not completely withdrawn from opioids, both from the perspective of preventing withdrawal in pregnant women and to prevent withdrawal in the fetus or embryo which may be associated with spontaneous abortion or premature labor.

Pre-clinical trials report that when naltrexone was administered to rats and rabbits during pregnancy at doses 32 and 59 times the recommended therapeutic doses, there was no evidence of teratogenicity (Orphan Product Information, 2002).[221] Naltrexone (50 mg/kg) was found to have no effect on the length of gestation, course of pregnancy, litter size, or the viability of the mother rats and offspring.[222] The offspring were found to be larger in body weight and length than controls, which the authors hypothesized to suggest that endogenous opioids are important growth-inhibiting hormones.[222] At doses 5 and 18 times the recommended therapeutic dose in rats and rabbits there was an increased incidence of early fetal loss (Orphan Product Information, 2002). It should be noted that rats do not produce appreciable quantities of the major human metabolite, 6-β-naltrexone, thus the potential reproductive toxicity of this metabolite in rats is unknown (Orphan Product Information, 2002).

There are no adequate and well-controlled studies of naltrexone in pregnant women (Orphan Product Information, 2002). In an oral naltrexone program in Western Australia, 26 women become pregnant. The exposure to oral naltrexone varied between the women, with some pregnant women ceasing and recommencing naltrexone use due to relapse. It was reported by the authors that, for the 7 women who delivered while on naltrexone, the obstetric and neonatal outcomes were 'good'.[223] A subsequent publication by the same group found no serious adverse events in a group of 17 women maintained on naltrexone implants. This group had no differences in prematurity or low birthweight when compared to a group of 90 women maintained on methadone during pregnancy.[224] However, the safety of naltrexone implants has been questioned[225,226] as adequate clinical trials have not yet been conducted to demonstrate safety and efficacy.[227,228] A Cochrane review of sustained release has demonstrated the need for further information on side-effects and adverse events to conduct a harm–benefit analysis.[229]

Postnatal care

Breastfeeding

There are numerous advantages to breastfeeding infants, ranging from increased maternal–infant bonding to improvements in infant health during the early part of life.[230,231] However, breastfeeding may expose an infant to drugs and thereby the risk of adverse effects. Levels of methadone excreted in milk have been reported to be low (ranging between 0.02 and 0.57 μg/ml), and may not have any significant effect in neonates and babies.[232–237] Breastfeeding has not been found to affect the blood concentrations of methadone in the neonate.[129,236]

The literature on buprenorphine is less extensive. Buprenorphine is poorly absorbed orally, and infants whose mothers were maintained on buprenorphine would therefore absorb minimal amounts. It is not known if LAAM is excreted in human milk in sufficient concentrations to have an effect on an infant. However, an animal study found that LAAM administered to lactating rats caused hepatic metabolic induction in the offspring, suggesting that LAAM and/or its metabolites passed to the pups via the milk.[238] In animal studies, it was found that naltrexone and 6-β-naltrexone were excreted in the milk of lactating rats dosed orally with naltrexone. It is unknown whether naltrexone is excreted in human milk (Orphan Product Information, 2002). With regards breastfeeding and buprenorphine, Marquet et al reported on one infant breastfed while the mother was taking buprenorphine for 8 weeks post delivery. Breastfeeding was abruptly ceased at 8 weeks and the infant did not develop a withdrawal syndrome.[239]

Levels of methadone both in the short and long term are low in breast milk.[240,241] A review article of 8 studies of women on methadone maintenance who were breastfeeding recommended breastfeeding for this group, provided women were stable on methadone maintenance.[237] As a general principle, breastfeeding should be encouraged among pregnant opioid-dependent women maintained on methadone. Breastfeeding for stable HIV-negative women on methadone is supported by US, UK, and Australian guidelines.[80–82] Asymptomatic hepatitis C is generally not a contraindication to breastfeeding, provided they do not have cracked or bleeding nipples.[237,242]

Management of neonatal abstinence syndrome

There are several screening tools designed to assess the presence and severity of NAS attributed to opioid withdrawal.[243–246] The Neonatal Abstinence Scoring System (otherwise commonly known as the Finnegan scale), and modified versions, is currently the most commonly used method in the identification and rating of the severity of NAS in many clinical settings, particularly in Australia. It is also the one most often used in clinical trials including those investigating the mother's opioid maintenance and the effect on NAS, and those investigating different pharmacologic treatment for NAS.

Supportive methods of management of NAS such as cuddling, settling, massage, relaxation baths, pacifiers, or waterbeds and minimal stimulation may suffice if symptoms are mild or non-progressive. However, more severe symptoms require adequate pharmacotherapy to prevent complications. Many pharmacologic agents have been used to ameliorate symptoms in infants with NAS including a variety of opioids, clonidine, chloral hydrate, chlorpromazine, diazepam, and phenobarbitone. However, evidence for the most optimal treatment is limited. To date, two systematic reviews have been conducted to examine the effectiveness and safety of using opioids compared to sedative or non-pharmacologic treatments for the treatment of NAS[247] and the use of sedatives compared to non-opiate control.[248] The reviews found substantial methodologic concerns including the lack of standardization of outcome variables, problems with randomization and blinding, and lack of standardization of treatment initiation, dosage alterations, and termination of treatment.

From the available evidence it seems that for infants whose mothers are using opioids, the use of opioids such as morphine or paregoric is appropriate for the initial treatment of NAS with better outcomes than with the use of symptomatic treatments alone or supportive care alone.[199,247,249,250] However, the use of paregoric is generally not recommended in Australia because of the potentially toxic additive substances such as camphor and ethanol. Further studies are required to determine the optimal regimen and dose for morphine. With regard to symptomatic treatments, one study supports the use of phenobarbitone in addition to morphine for severe NAS.[251] There is insufficient evidence for the use of clonidine or chlorpromazine.[248]

Australian guidelines for the management of drug use in pregnancy recommend morphine as the medication of choice for the management of opioid-dependent infants. Sublingual buprenorphine has been trialled for the treatment of neonatal withdrawal and appears safe.[252] When doses of morphine reach 'ceiling levels' and NAS is not controlled then the addition of phenobarbitone is recommended.[253] Phenobarbitone is the recommended medication for withdrawal from non-opioid drugs of addiction.

Conclusion

Regular heroin use is associated with a range of immediate and long-term adverse consequences to the health and psychologic and social well-being of an individual. Women who use heroin during pregnancy are at particularly high risk of medical, obstetric, and social ill health. The risks to pregnant women and their babies include risks from multiple substances being used (including tobacco and other drugs), poor mental health, poor medical health (including inadequate nutrition and exposure to blood-borne viruses), and serious social problems including homelessness, experiencing violence, and lack of support. Impaired obstetric and neonatal health outcomes such as prematurity, miscarriage, intrauterine growth reduction, and perinatal death are some of the consequences reported as a result of heroin use during pregnancy.

Treatment for heroin dependence during pregnancy should aim to:

- reduce the harmful effects of heroin and other drug use including tobacco;
- reduce maternal and infant morbidity and mortality associated with heroin use;
- improve physical, psychologic, and social health for pregnant women; and
- provide an opportunity to identify and provide long-term support to pregnant women and their families.

The wide range of issues raised in providing appropriate care to pregnant women who use heroin underlines the need for multidisciplinary input into their care. Expertise is required across substance use, obstetric, mental health, midwife, and social and welfare domains.

Opiate substitution treatment for heroin dependence is an ideal intervention to reduce the risks of adverse outcomes during pregnancy, for both the mother and newborn child. Pregnancy provides an opportunity to offer a range of interventions to address the needs of heroin-dependent pregnant women, including antenatal care, substance abuse treatment, treatment of mental health and medical problems, and a range of social interventions.

While numerous studies of the effects of heroin and other drug use on pregnant women and their babies have been reported, relatively few have been able to account for the wide range of substance use and medical, mental, and social health issues that confound our understanding of the relationship between substance use in pregnancy and short- and long-term birth outcomes. Experimental studies and more robust observational studies have been published recently, adding significantly to knowledge and understanding in this field.

Methadone is recommended as the first-line treatment for opioid-dependent pregnant women around the world. An advanced evidence base has been developed over four decades regarding use of this treatment in pregnancy. Methadone is associated with increased antenatal care attendance and reduced risk of low birthweight, prematurity, and neonatal death. Therapeutic doses of methadone should be used in pregnancy. The most significant adverse event associated with methadone treatment in pregnancy at birth is NAS, which can be managed safely provided it is identified early. The proportion of infants born to methadone-maintained pregnant women overall requiring pharmacologic treatment for NAS is between 18 and 77%. Key issues still to be resolved with methadone include a more advanced understanding of the role of split dosing in pregnancy. While still in an early stage of development, behavioral incentives to reduce substance use during pregnancy show some promise, particularly if they can be used to assist tobacco cessation.

Buprenorphine has been reported for the management of heroin dependence in pregnancy for over a decade. During this period of time the evidence on safety of the medication has developed significantly. There does not appear to be evidence of increased risk of severe adverse events in pregnancy compared to methadone. While definitive experimental research has not yet been completed, from available research that compares buprenorphine to methadone in pregnancy, the prevalence of NAS requiring pharmacologic treatment and the duration and severity of NAS may be less with buprenorphine. In terms of safety, in studies where a prospective comparison with methadone exists, the prevalence of severe adverse events with buprenorphine is not greater than 1 in 82. Overall, preliminary data suggest that neonatal outcomes of buprenorphine during pregnancy are comparable to methadone, in terms of reduced risk of severe NAS. Epidemiologic data suggest a reduced risk of fatal child poisonings with buprenorphine compared to methadone.

References

1. Jones HE, Fitzgerald H, Johnson RE. Males and females differ in response to opioid agonist medications. Am J Addict 2005; 14(3): 223–33.
2. Finnegan LP, Kandall SR. Maternal and neonatal effects of alcohol and drugs. In: Lowinson JH, Ruiz P, Millman R, Langrod JG, eds. Substance Abuse: A comprehensive textbook. 3 edn. 513–534. Baltimore, Maryland: Williams & Wilkins, 1997.
3. Kaya CY, Tugai Y, Filar JA, et al. Heroin users in Australia: population trends. Drug Alcohol Rev 2004; 23(1): 107–16.
4. Law MG, Lynskey M, Ross J, Hall W. Back-projection estimates of the number of dependent heroin users in Australia. Addiction 2001; 96(3): 433–43.
5. Hall WD, Ross JE, Lynskey MT, et al. How many dependent heroin users are there in Australia? Med J Australia 2000; 173(10): 528–31.
6. Degenhardt L, Rendle V, Hall W, et al. Estimating the number of current regular heroin users in NSW and Australia 1997–2002. Technical Report Number 198. Sydney: National Drug and Alcohol Research Centre, University of New South Wales, 2004.
7. Australian Institute of Health and Welfare. 2007 National drug strategy household survey: first results. Canberra: AIHW (Drug Statistics Series No. 20), 2002.
8. Australian Institute of Health and Welfare. Alcohol and other drug treatment services in Australia 2006–07: Report on the National Minimum Data Set. Drug Treatment Series Number 8. Cat. no. HSE 59. Canberra: Australian Institute of Health and Welfare 2008.
9. Australian Institute of Health and Welfare. National Opioid Pharmacotherapy Statistics Annual Data collection: 2007 report. Bulletin 62. Canberra: Australian Government, 2008.
10. Johnson RE, Jones HE, Fischer G. Use of buprenorphine in pregnancy: patient management and effects on the neonate. Drug Alcohol Depen 2003; 70(2 Suppl): S87–S101.
11. Abdel-Latif ME, Bajuk B, Lui K, et al. Short-term outcomes of infants of substance-using mothers admitted to neonatal intensive care units in New South Wales and the Australian Capital Territory. J Paediatr Child H 2007; 43(3): 127–33.
12. Kennare R, Heard A, Chan A, et al. Substance use during pregnancy: risk factors and obstetric and perinatal outcomes in South Australia. Aust NZ J Obstet Gyn 2005; 45(3): 220–5.

13. Oei J, Lui K. Management of the newborn infant affected by maternal opiates and other drugs of dependency. J Paediatr Child H 2007; 43(1–2): 9–18.
14. Burns L, Mattick RP. Using population data to examine the prevalence and correlates of neonatal abstinence syndrome. Drug Alcohol Rev 2007; 26(5): 487–92.
15. Winklbaur B, Kopf N, Ebner N, et al. Treating pregnant women dependent on opioids is not the same as treating pregnancy and opioid dependence: a knowledge synthesis for better treatment for women and neonates. Addiction 2008; 103(9): 1429–40.
16. Jones H, Tuten M, Keyser-Marcus L, Svikis D. Speciality Treatment for Women. In: Strain EC, Stitzer ML, eds. The Treatment of Opioid Dependence. Baltimore: The Johns Hopkins University Press, 2006.
17. Finnegan LP. Drug dependence in pregnancy: Clinical management of mother and child. Prepared for The National Institute on Drug Abuse. London: Castle House Publications Ltd, 1978.
18. Soby JM. Prenatal Exposure to Drugs/Alcohol. Springfield, Illinois: Charles C. Thomas, 2006.
19. Glantz JC, Woods JRJ. Cocaine, heroin, and phencyclidine: obstetric perspectives. Clin Obstet Gynecol 1993; 36(2): 279–301.
20. Minozzi S, Amato L, Vecchi S, et al. Maintenance agonist treatments for opiate dependent pregnant women. Cochrane Database Sys Rev 2008(2): CD006318.
21. Winklbaur B, Jung E, Fischer G, et al. Opioid dependence and pregnancy. Curr Opin Psychiatr 2008; 21(3): 255–9.
22. Krause SO, Murray PM, Holmes JB, Burch RE. Heroin addiction among pregnant women and their newborn babies. Am J Obstet Gynecol 1958; 75(4): 754–8.
23. Claman AD, Strang RI. Obstetric and gynecologic aspects of heroin addiction. Am J Obstet Gynecol 1962; 83: 252–7.
24. Hill RM, Desmond MM. Management of the narcotic withdrawal syndrome in the neonate. Pediatr Clin N Am 1963; 10: 67–86.
25. Kandall SR, Albin S, Gartner LM, et al. The narcotic-dependent mother: fetal and neonatal consequences. Early Hum Dev 1977; 1(2): 159–69.
26. Zelson C, Rubio E, Wasserman E. Neonatal narcotic addiction: 10 year observation. Pediatrics 1971; 48(2): 178–89.
27. Connaughton JF, Reeser D, Schut J, Finnegan LP. Perinatal addiction: Outcome and management. Am J Obstet Gynecol 1977; 129: 679–86.
28. Fajemirokun-Odudeyi O, Sinha C, Tutty S, et al. Pregnancy outcome in women who use opiates. Eur J Obstet Gyn R B 2006; 126(2): 170–5.
29. Ellwood DA, Sutherland P, Kent C, O'Connor M. Maternal narcotic addiction: pregnancy outcome in patients managed by a specialized drug-dependency antenatal clinic. Aust NZ J Obstet Gyn 1987; 27(2): 92–8.
30. Fricker HS, Segal S. Narcotic addiction, pregnancy, and the newborn. Am J Dis Child 1978; 132(4): 360–6.
31. Whiting M, Whitman S, Bergner L, Patrick S. Addiction and low birth weight: a quasi-experimental study. Am J Public Health 1978; 68(7): 676–8.

32. Little BB, Snell LM, Klein VR, et al. Maternal and fetal effects of heroin addiction during pregnancy. J Reprod Med 1990; 35(2): 159–62.
33. Stimmel B, Adamsons K. Narcotic dependency in pregnancy. Methadone maintenance compared to use of street drugs. JAMA 1976; 235(11): 1121–4.
34. Thornton L, Clune M, Maguire R, et al. Narcotic addiction: the expectant mother and her baby. Irish Med J 1990; 83(4): 139–42.
35. Amarose AP, Norusis MJ. Cytogenetics of methadone-managed and heroin-addicted pregnant women and their newborn infants. Am J Obstet Gynecol 1976; 124(6): 635–40.
36. Abrams CA. Cytogenetic risks to the offspring of pregnant addicts. Addict Dis 1975; 2(1–2): 63–77.
37. Ostrea EM, Chavez CJ. Perinatal problems (excluding neonatal withdrawal) in maternal drug addiction: a study of 830 cases. J Pediatr 1979; 94(2): 292–5.
38. Rajegowda BK, Kandall SR, Falciglia H. Sudden unexpected death in infants of narcotic-dependent mothers. Early Hum Dev 1978; 2(3): 219–25.
39. Kandall SR, Gaines J, Habel L, et al. Relationship of maternal substance abuse to subsequent sudden infant death syndrome in offspring. J Pediatr 1993; 123(1): 120–6.
40. Ostrea EM Jr, Ostrea AR, Simpson PM. Mortality within the first 2 years in infants exposed to cocaine, opiate, or cannabinoid during gestation. Pediatrics 1997; 100(1): 79–83.
41. Kramer MS. Determinants of low birth weight: methodological assessment and meta-analysis. B World Health Organ 1987; 65(5): 663–737.
42. Kleinman JC, Kopstein A. Smoking during pregnancy, 1967–80. Am J Public Health 1987; 77(7): 823–5.
43. England LJ, Kendrick JS, Wilson HG, et al. Effects of smoking reduction during pregnancy on the birth weight of term infants. Am J Epidemiol 2001; 154(8): 694–701.
44. Law KL, Stroud LR, LaGasse LL, et al. Smoking during pregnancy and newborn neurobehavior. Pediatrics 2003; 111(6 Pt 1): 1318–23.
45. Finnegan LP. Drug addiction and pregnancy: The newborn. In: Chasnoff IJ, ed. Drugs, Alcohol, Pregnancy and Parenting, 59–71. Dordrecht, Netherlands: Kluwer Academic Publishers, 1988.
46. Herzlinger RA, Kandall SR, Vaughan HG Jr. Neonatal seizures associated with narcotic withdrawal. J Pediatr 1977; 91(4): 638–41.
47. Kaltenbach KA, Finnegan LP. Prenatal narcotic exposure: perinatal and developmental effects. Neurotoxicology 1989; 10(3): 597–604.
48. Finnegan LP, Kaltenbach K. Neonatal abstinence syndrome. In: Hoekelman RA, Friedman SB, Nelson N, Seidel HM, eds. Primary Pediatric Care. 2 edn. 1367–78. St Louis: CT Mosby, 1992.
49. Finnegan LP. Neonatal abstinence syndrome: assessment and pharmacotherapy. In: Rubatelli F, Granati B, eds. Neonatal therapy: an update. 22–46. Amsterdam: Excepta Medica, 1986.
50. Finnegan LP. Drug Dependence in Pregnancy. London: Castle House Publications, 1980.

51. Perlmutter JF. Drug addiction in pregnant women. Am J Obstet Gynecol 1967; 99(4): 569–72.
52. Reddy AM, Harper RG, Stern G. Observations on heroin and methadone withdrawal in the newborn. Pediatrics 1971; 48(3): 353–8.
53. Smith LM, Lagasse LL, Derauf C, et al. Prenatal methamphetamine use and neonatal neurobehavioral outcome. Neurotoxicol Teratol 2008; 30(1): 20–8.
54. Lester BM, Tronick EZ, LaGasse L, et al. The maternal lifestyle study: effects of substance exposure during pregnancy on neurodevelopmental outcome in 1-month-old infants. Pediatrics 2002; 110(6): 1182–92.
55. Choo RE, Huestis MA, Schroeder JR, et al. Neonatal abstinence syndrome in methadone-exposed infants is altered by level of prenatal tobacco exposure. Drug Alcohol Depen 2004; 75: 253–60.
56. Burns L, Mattick RP, Cooke M, et al. The use of record linkage to examine illicit drug use in pregnancy. Addiction 2006; 101(6): 873–82.
57. Finnegan LP, Hagan T, Kaltenbach KA. Scientific foundation of clinical practice: opiate use in pregnant women. B New York Acad Med 1991; 67(3): 223–39.
58. Finnegan LP. Treatment issues for opioid-dependent women during the perinatal period. J Psychoactive Drugs 1991; 23(2): 191–201.
59. Bergsjo P, Villar J. Scientific basis for the content of routine antenatal care. II. Power to eliminate or alleviate adverse newborn outcomes; some special conditions and examinations. Acta Obstet Gyn Scan 1997; 76(1): 15–25.
60. Chang G, Carroll KM, Behr HM, Kosten TR. Improving treatment outcome in pregnant opiate-dependent women. J Subst Abuse Treat 1992; 9(4): 327–30.
61. Suffet F, Brotman R. A comprehensive care program for pregnant addicts: obstetrical, neonatal, and child development outcomes. Int J Addict 1984; 19(2): 199–219.
62. Carroll K, Chang G, Behr H. Improving treatment outcome in pregnant, methadone-maintained women. Am J Addiction 1995; 4: 56–9.
63. Kandall SR, Albin S, Lowinson J, et al. Differential effects of maternal heroin and methadone use on birthweight. Pediatrics 1976; 58(5): 681–5.
64. Davis MM, Shanks B. Neurological aspects of perinatal narcotic addiction and methadone treatment. Addict Dis 1977; 2(1–2): 213–26.
65. Zelson C, Lee SJ, Casalino M. Neonatal narcotic addiction. Comparative effects of maternal intake of heroin and methadone. New Engl J Med 1973; 289(23): 1216–20.
66. Finnegan LP. Women, pregnancy and methadone. Heroin Addiction Related Clinical Problems 2000; 2(1): 1–8.
67. Burns L, Mattick RP, Lim K, et al. Methadone in pregnancy: treatment retention and neonatal outcomes. Addiction 2007; 102(2): 264–70.
68. Luty J, Nikolaou V, Bearn J. Is opiate detoxification unsafe in pregnancy? J Subst Abuse Treat 2003; 24(4): 363–7.
69. Rementeria JL, Nunag NN. Narcotic withdrawal in pregnancy: stillbirth incidence with a case report. Am J Obstet Gynecol 1973; 116(8): 1152–6.
70. Zuspan FP, Gumpel JA, Mejia-Zelaya A, et al. Fetal stress from methadone withdrawal. Am J Obstet Gynecol 1975; 122(1): 43–6.

71. Dashe JS, Jackson GL, Olscher DA, et al. Opioid detoxification in pregnancy. Obstet Gynecol 1998; 92(5): 854–8.
72. Blinick G, Wallach RC, Jerez E. Pregnancy in narcotics addicts treated by medical withdrawal. The methadone detoxification program. Am J Obstet Gynecol 1969; 5(7): 997–1003.
73. Maas U, Kattner E, Weingart-Jesse B, et al. Infrequent neonatal opiate withdrawal following maternal methadone detoxification during pregnancy. J Perinat Med 1990; 18(2): 111–18.
74. Blinick G, Jerez E, Wallach RC. Methadone maintenance, pregnancy, and progeny. JAMA 1973; 225(5): 477–9.
75. Kaltenbach K, Finnegan LP. Perinatal and developmental outcome of infants exposed to methadone in-utero. Neurotoxicol Teratol 1987; 9(4): 311–13.
76. Dunlop AJ, Panjari M, O' Sullivan H, et al. Clinical Guidelines for the use of Buprenorphine in Pregnancy. Fitzroy, Australia: Turning Point Alcohol and Drug Centre 2003.
77. Fischer G, Johnson RE, Eder H, et al. Treatment of opioid-dependent pregnant women with buprenorphine. Addiction 2000; 95(2): 239–44.
78. Wang EC. Methadone treatment during pregnancy. J Obstet Gynaecol Neonat Nurs 1999; 28(6): 615–22.
79. Kandall SR. Treatment strategies for drug-exposed neonates. Clin Perinatol 1999; 26(1): 231–43.
80. Department of Health (England) and the devolved administrations. Drug Misuse and Dependence: UK Guidelines on Clinical Management: Department of Health (England), The Scottish Government, Welsh Assembly Government, Northern Ireland Executive, 2007.
81. Center for Substance Abuse Treatment. Medication-Assisted Treatment for Opioid Addiction in Opioid Treatment Programs. (Treatment Improvement Protocol Series 43). Rockville, Maryland: Substance Abuse and Mental Health Services Administration, U.S. Department of Health and Human Services, 2005.
82. NSW Department of Health. National clinical guidelines for the management of drug use during pregnancy, birth and the early development years of the newborn. North Sydney: Commonwealth of Australia, 2006.
83. Hutchings DE. Methadone and heroin during pregnancy: a review of behavioral effects in human and animal offspring. Neurobehav Toxicol Ter 1982; 4(4): 429–34.
84. Hutchings DE. Issues of risk assessment: lessons from the use and abuse of drugs during pregnancy. Neurotoxicol Teratol 1990; 12(3): 183–9.
85. Hutchings DE, Dow-Edwards D. Animal models of opiate, cocaine, and cannabis use. Clin Perinatol 1991; 18(1): 1–22.
86. Nassogne MC, Gressens P, Evrard P, Courtoy PJ. In contrast to cocaine, prenatal exposure to methadone does not produce detectable alterations in the developing mouse brain. Brain Res Dev Brain Res 1998; 110(1): 61–7.
87. Walz MA, Davis WM, Pace HB. Parental methadone treatment: a multigenerational study of development and behavior in offspring. Dev Pharmacol Therap 1983; 6(2): 125–37.

88. Kandall SR, Doberczak TM, Jantunen M, Stein J. The methadone-maintained pregnancy. Clin Perinatol 1999; 26(1): 173–83.
89. AIHW National Perinatal Statistics Unit. Australia's mothers and babies 2005. AIHW Cat. No. PER 21. Sydney: AIHW National Perinatal Statistics Unit (Perinatal Statistics Series no. 20), 2007.
90. Ruiz P, Strain E, Langrod J. Maternal and neonatal effects of alcohol and drugs. In: Ruiz P, Strain E, Langrod J, eds. The Substance Abuse Handbook. Philadelphia, PA: Lippincott Williams & Wilkins, 2007.
91. Zelson C. Infant of the addicted mother. New Engl J Med 1973; 288(26): 1393–5.
92. Sinha C, Ohadike P, Carrick P, et al. Neonatal outcome following maternal opiate use in late pregnancy. Int J Gynecol Obstet 2001; 74(3): 241–6.
93. Newman RG, Bashkow S, Calko D. Results of 313 consecutive live births of infants delivered to patients in the New York City Methadone Maintenance Treatment Program. Am J Obstet Gynecol 1975; 121(2): 233–7.
94. Scully M, Geoghegan N, Corcoran P, et al. Specialized drug liaison midwife services for pregnant opioid dependent women in Dublin, Ireland. J Subst Abuse Treat 2004; 26(1): 27–3.
95. Morrison CL, Siney C, Ruben SM, Worthington M. Obstetric liaison in drug dependency. Eur Addict Res 1995; 3(2): 93–101.
96. Keenan E, Dorman A, O'Connor J. Six year follow up of forty five pregnant opiate addicts.[see comment]. Irish J Med Sci 1993; 162(7): 252–5.
97. O'Neill K, Baker A, Cooke M, et al. Evaluation of a cognitive-behavioural intervention for pregnant injecting drug users at risk of HIV infection. Addiction 1996; 91(8): 1115–25.
98. Fischer G, Jagsch R, Eder H, et al. Comparison of methadone and slow-release morphine maintenance in pregnant addicts. Addiction 1999; 94(2): 231–9.
99. Dashe JS, Sheffield JS, Olscher DA, et al. Relationship between maternal methadone dosage and neonatal withdrawal. Obstet Gynecol 2002; 100(6): 1244–9.
100. Giles W, Patterson T, Sanders F, et al. Outpatient methadone programme for pregnant heroin using women. Aust NZ J Obstet Gyn 1989; 29(3 Pt 1): 225–9.
101. Olofsson M, Buckley W, Andersen GE, Friis-Hansen B. Investigation of 89 children born by drug-dependent mothers. I. Neonatal course. Acta Paediatr 1983; 72(3): 403–6.
102. Ramer CM, Lodge A. Neonatal addiction: a two-year study. Part I. Clinical and developmental characteristics of infants of mothers on methadone maintenance. Addict Dis 1975; 2(1–2): 227–34.
103. Ostrea EM, Chavez CJ, Strauss ME. A study of factors that influence the severity of neonatal narcotic withdrawal. J Pediatr 1976; 88(4 Pt. 1): 642–5.
104. Finnegan LP, Reeser DS, Connaughton JF. The effects of maternal drug dependence on neonatal mortality. Drug Alcohol Depen 1977; 2: 131–40.
105. Ostrea EM Jr, Chavez CJ, Strauss ME. A study of factors that influence the severity of neonatal narcotic withdrawal. Addict Dis 1975; 2(1–2): 187–99.

106. Hagopian GS, Wolfe HM, Sokol RJ, et al. Neonatal outcome following methadone exposure in utero. J Matern-Fetal Neonat Med 1996; 5(6): 348–54.
107. Edelin KC, Gurganious L, Golar K, et al. Methadone maintenance in pregnancy: consequences to care and outcome. [see comment]. Obstet Gynecol 1988; 71(3 Pt 1): 399–404.
108. Lam SK, To WK, Duthie SJ, Ma HK. Narcotic addiction in pregnancy with adverse maternal and perinatal outcome. Aust NZ J Obstet Gyn 1992; 32(3): 216–21.
109. Lifschitz MH, Wilson GS, Smith EO, Desmond MM. Fetal and postnatal growth of children born to narcotic-dependent women. J Pediatr 1983; 102(5): 686–91.
110. Brown HL, Britton KA, Mahaffey D, et al. Methadone maintenance in pregnancy: a reappraisal. Am J Obstet Gynecol 1998; 179: 459–63.
111. Doberczak TM, Thornton JC, Bernstein J, Kandall SR. Impact of maternal drug dependency on birth weight and head circumference of offspring. Am J Dis Child 1987; 141(11): 1163–7.
112. Hulse GK, Milne E, English DR, Holman CDJ. The relationship between maternal use of heroin and methadone and infant birth weight. Addiction 1997; 92(11): 1571–9.
113. McCarthy JE, Siney C, Shaw NJ, Ruben SM. Outcome predictors in pregnant opiate and polydrug users. European J Pediatr 1999; 158(9): 748–9.
114. Rosen TE, Johnson HL, Long-term effects of prenatal methadone maintenance. In: Pinkert TM, ed. Current Research on the Consequences of Maternal Drug Abuse: NIDA Monograph 59. 73–83. Rockville, MD: National Institute on Drug Abuse; U.S. Department of Health and Human Services, 1985.
115. Rohrmeister K, Bernert G, Langer M, et al. Opiate addiction in gravidity – consequences for the newborn. Results of an interdisciplinary treatment concept. Z Geburtshilfe Neonatol 2001; 205(6): 224–30.
116. Shaw NJ, McIvor L. Neonatal abstinence syndrome after maternal methadone treatment. Arch Dis Child. Fetal Neonat Ed 1994; 71(3): F203–5.
117. Sharpe C, Kuschel C. Outcomes of infants born to mothers receiving methadone for pain management in pregnancy. Arch Dis Child Fetal Neonatl Ed 2004; 89(1): F33–6.
118. Malpas TJ, Darlow BA, Lennox R, Horwood LJ. Maternal methadone dosage and neonatal withdrawal. Aust NZ J Obstet Gyn 1995; 35(2): 175–7.
119. Doberczak TM, Kandall SR, Friedmann P. Relationship between maternal methadone dosage, maternal-neonatal methadone levels, and neonatal withdrawal. Obstet Gynecol 1993; 81(6): 936–40.
120. Stimmel B, Goldberg J, Reisman A, et al. Fetal outcome in narcotic-dependent women: the importance of the type of maternal narcotic used. Am J Drug Alcohol Ab 1982; 9(4): 383–95.
121. Binder T, Vavrinkova B. Prospective randomised comparative study of the effect of buprenorphine, methadone and heroin on the course of pregnancy, birthweight of newborns, early postpartum adaptation and course of the neonatal abstinence syndrome (NAS) in women followed up in the outpatient department. Neuroendocrinol Lett 2008; 29(1): 80–6.

122. Harper RG, Solish G, Feingold E, et al. Maternal ingested methadone, body fluid methadone, and the neonatal withdrawal syndrome. Am J Obstet Gynecol 1977; 129(4): 417–24.
123. Madden JD, Chappel JN, Zuspan F, et al. Observation and treatment of neonatal narcotic withdrawal. Am J Obstet Gynecol 1977; 127(2): 199–201.
124. Doberczak TM, Kandall SR, Wilets I. Neonatal opiate abstinence syndrome in term and preterm infants. J Pediatr 1991; 118(6): 933–7.
125. Berghella V, Lim PJ, Hill MK, et al. Maternal methadone dose and neonatal withdrawal. Am J Obstet Gynecol 2003; 189(2): 312–17.
126. Strauss ME, Andresko M, Stryker JC, Wardell JN. Relationship of neonatal withdrawal to maternal methadone dose. Am J Drug Alcohol Ab 1976; 3(2): 339–45.
127. Sutton LR, Hinderliter SA. Diazepam abuse in pregnant women on methadone maintenance. Implications for the neonate. Clin Pediatr 1990; 29(2): 108–11.
128. Lugo RA, Satterfield KL, Kern SE. Pharmacokinetics of methadone. J Pain Palliative Care Pharmacotherapy 2005; 19(4): 13–24.
129. Mack G, Thomas D, Giles W, Buchanan N. Methadone levels and neonatal withdrawal. J Paediatr Child Health 1991; 27(2): 96–100.
130. Blinick G, Inturrisi CE, Jerez E, Wallach RC. Methadone assays in pregnant women and progeny. Am J Obstet Gynecol 1975; 121(5): 617–21.
131. Rosen TS, Pippenger CE. Disposition of methadone and its relationship to severity of withdrawal in the newborn. Addict Dis 1975; 2(1–2): 169–78.
132. Jansson LM, Dipietro JA, Elko A, et al. Maternal vagal tone change in response to methadone is associated with neonatal abstinence syndrome severity in exposed neonates. J Matern-Fetal Neonat Med 2007; 20(9): 677–85.
133. Doberczak TM, Shanzer S, Cutler R, et al. One-year follow-up of infants with abstinence-associated seizures. Arch Neurol 1988; 45(6): 649–53.
134. Drozdick J, 3rd, Berghella V, Hill M, Kaltenbach K. Methadone trough levels in pregnancy. Am J Obstet Gynecol 2002; 187(5): 1184–8.
135. Pond SM, Kreek MJ, Tong TG, et al. Altered methadone pharmacokinetics in methadone-maintained pregnant women. J Pharmacol Exp Ther 1985; 233(1): 1–6.
136. McLellan AT, Woody GE, Evans BD, O'Brien CP. Treatment of mixed abusers in methadone maintenance: role of psychiatric factors. Ann NY Acad Sci 1982; 398: 65–78.
137. Jarvis MA, Wu-Pong S, Kniseley JS, Schnoll SH. Alterations in methadone metabolism during late pregnancy. J Addict Dis 1999; 18(4): 51–61.
138. DePetrillo PB, Rice JM. Methadone dosing and pregnancy: impact on program compliance. Int J Addict 1995; 30(2): 207–17.
139. Swift RM, Dudley M, DePetrillo P, et al. Altered methadone pharmacokinetics in pregnancy: implications for dosing. J Subst Ab 1989; 1(4): 453–60.
140. Wittmann BK, Segal S. A comparison of the effects of single- and split-dose methadone administration on the fetus: ultrasound evaluation. Int J Addict 1991; 26(2): 213–18.
141. Jansson LM, Dipietro J, Elko A, et al. Fetal response to maternal methadone administration. Am J Obst Gynecol 2005; 193(3 Pt 1): 611–17.

142. Jansson LM, DiPietro JA, Velez M, et al. Maternal Methadone Dosing Schedule and Fetal Neurobehavior. The College of Problems of Drug Dependence 70th Annual General Meeting; Puerto Rico, 2008.
143. Berghella V. Improving the management of opioid-dependent pregnancies – reply to Dashe et al. Am J Obstet Gynecol 2004; 190(6): 1806–7.
144. Bell J, Harvey-Dodds L. Pregnancy and injecting drug use. BMJ 2008; 336: 1303–5.
145. Higgins ST, Heil SH, Solomon LJ, et al. A pilot study on voucher-based incentives to promote abstinence from cigarette smoking during pregnancy and postpartum. Nicotine & Tobacco Research 2004; 6(6): 1015–20.
146. Heil SH, Higgins ST, Bernstein IM, et al. Effects of voucher-based incentives on abstinence from cigarette smoking and fetal growth among pregnant women. Addiction 2008; 103(6): 1009–18.
147. Jones HE, Haug N, Silverman K, et al. The effectiveness of incentives in enhancing treatment attendance and drug abstinence in methadone-maintained pregnant women. Drug Alcohol Depen 2001; 61(3): 297–306.
148. Strauss ME, Lessen-Firestone JK, Chavez CJ, Stryker JC. Children of methadone-treated women at five years of age. Pharmacol Biochem Behav 1979; (11 Suppl): 3–6.
149. Hans SL. Developmental consequences of prenatal exposure to methadone. Ann NY Acad Sci 1989; 562: 195–207.
150. Kaltenbach K, Graziani LJ, Finnegan LP. Methadone exposure in utero: developmental status at one and two years of age. Pharmacol Biochem Behav 1979; (11 Suppl): 15–17.
151. Wilson GS, Desmond MM, Wait RB. Follow-up of methadone-treated and untreated narcotic-dependent women and their infants: health, developmental, and social implications. J Pediatr 1981; 98(5): 716–22.
152. Chasnoff IJ. Effects of Maternal Narcotic vs. Nonnarcotic Addiction on Neonatal Neurobehavior and Infant Development. In: Pinkert TM, ed. Current Research on the Consequences of Maternal Drug Abuse: NIDA Monograph 59. 84–95. Rockville, MD: National Institute on Drug Abuse; U.S. Department of Health and Human Services, 1985.
153. Hunt RW, Tzioumi D, Collins E, et al. Adverse neurodevelopmental outcome of infants exposed to opiate in-utero. Early Hum Dev 2008; 84(1): 29–35.
154. Steinhausen HC, Blattmann B, Pfund F, et al. Developmental outcome in children with intrauterine exposure to substances. Eur Addict Res 2007; 13(2): 94–100.
155. Ornoy A, Michailevskaya V, Lukashov I, et al. The developmental outcome of children born to heroin-dependent mothers, raised at home or adopted. Child Abuse Neglect 1996; 20(5): 385–96.
156. Ornoy A, Segal J, Bar-Hamburger R, Greenbaum C. Developmental outcome of school-age children born to mothers with heroin dependency: importance of environmental factors. Dev Med Child Neurol 2001; 43(10): 668–75.
157. Messinger DS, Bauer CR, Das A, et al. The maternal lifestyle study: cognitive, motor, and behavioral outcomes of cocaine-exposed and opiate-exposed infants through three years of age. Pediatrics 2004; 113(6): 1677–85.

158. Gill AC, Oei J, Lewis NL, et al. Strabismus in infants of opiate-dependent mothers. Acta Paediatr 2003; 92(3): 379–85.
159. Nelson LB, Ehrlich S, Calhoun JH, et al. Occurrence of strabismus in infants born to drug-dependent women. Am J Dis Child 1987; 141(2): 175–8.
160. Hakim RB, Tielsch JM. Maternal cigarette smoking during pregnancy. A risk factor for childhood strabismus. Arch Ophthalmol 1992; 110(10): 1459–62.
161. Stromland K, Hellstrom A. Fetal alcohol syndrome – an ophthalmological and socioeducational prospective study. Pediatrics 1996; 97(6 Pt 1): 845–50.
162. Rosen TS, Johnson HL. Children of methadone-maintained mothers: follow-up to 18 months of age. J Pediatr 1982; 101(2): 192–6.
163. Sameroff A, Chandler M. Reproductive risk and the continuum of caretaking casualty. In: Horowitz FD, ed. Review of Child Development Research, 187–244. Chicago: University of Chicago Press, 1975.
164. Falek A, Madden JJ, Shafer DA, Donahoe RM. Individual differences in opiate-induced alterations at the cytogenetic, DNA repair, and immunologic levels: opportunity for genetic assessment. In: Braude MC, Helen M. Chao, eds. Genetic and Biological Markers in Drug Abuse and Alcoholism: NIDA Research Monograph 66. 11–24. Rockville, MD: National Institute on Drug Abuse; U.S. Department of Health and Human Services, 1986.
165. Zuckerman B. Developmental Consequences of Maternal Drug Use During Pregnancy. In: Pinkert TM, ed. Current Research on the Consequences of Maternal Drug Abuse: NIDA Monograph 59. 96–106. Rockville, MD: National Institute on Drug Abuse; U.S. Department of Health and Human Services, 1985.
166. Dum JE, Herz A. In vivo receptor binding of the opiate partial agonist, buprenorphine, correlated with its agonistic and antagonistic actions. Brit J Pharmacol 1981; 74(3): 627–33.
167. Cowan A. Update on the general pharmacology of buprenorphine. In: Cowan A, Lewis JW, eds. Buprenorphine: Combacting Drug Abuse with a Unique Opioid. 31–47. New York: Wiley-Liss, 1995.
168. Richards ML, Sadee W. In vivo opiate receptor binding of oripavines to mu, delta and kappa sites in rat brain as determined by an ex vivo labeling method. Eur J Pharmacol 1985; 114(3): 343–53.
169. Walsh SL, Eissenberg T. The clinical pharmacology of buprenorphine: extrapolating from the laboratory to the clinic. Drug Alcohol Depen 2003; 70: S13–S27.
170. Davids E, Gastpar M. Buprenorphine in the treatment of opioid dependence. Eur Neuropsychopharm 2004; 14(3): 209–16.
171. Cowan A, Lewis JW, Macfarlane IR. Agonist and antagonist properties of buprenorphine, a new antinociceptive agent. Brit J Pharmacol 1977; 60(4): 537–45.
172. Walsh SL, Preston KL, Stitzer ML, et al. Clinical pharmacology of buprenorphine: Ceiling effects at high doses. Clin Pharm Th 1994; 55: 569–80.
173. Lizasoain I, Leza JC, Lorenzo P. Buprenorphine: bell-shaped dose-response curve for its antagonist effects. Gen Pharmacol 1991; 22(2): 297–300.

174. Jasinski DR, Pevnick JS, Griffith JD. Human pharmacology and abuse potential of the analgesic buprenorphine: a potential agent for treating narcotic addiction. Arch Gen Psychiat 1978; 35(4): 501–16.
175. Seow SSW, Quigley AJ, Ilett KF, et al. Buprenorphine: a new maintenance opiate? Med J Australia 1986; 144: 407–11.
176. Fudala PJ, Jaffe JH, Dax EM, Johnson RE. Use of buprenorphine in the treatment of opioid addiction. II. Physiologic and behavioral effects of daily and alternate-day administration and abrupt withdrawal. Clin Pharm Th 1990; 47(4): 525–34.
177. Schottenfeld RS. Clinical trials of pharmacologic treatments in pregnant women methodologic considerations. In: Chiang CN, Finnegan LP, eds. Medications Development for the Treatment of Pregnant Addicts and Their Infants: NIDA Research Monograph 149. 201–23. Rockville, MD: National Institute on Drug Abuse; U.S. Department of Health and Human Services, 1995.
178. Mori N, Sakanoue M, Kamata S, et al. Toxicological studies of buprenorphine (II) teratogenicity in rat. Iyakuhin Kenkyu 1982; 13(2): 509–31.
179. Mori N, Sakanoue M, Kamata S, et al. Toxicological studies of buprenorphine (III) teratogenicity in rat. Iyakuhin Kenkyu 1982; 13(2): 532–45.
180. Lewis JW, Rance MJ, Sanger DJ. The pharmacology and abuse potential of buprenorphine: a new antagonist analgesic. In: Mello NK, ed. Advan Subst Ab 103–154. Greenwich: Jessica Kingsley Publishers, 1983.
181. Hutchings DE, Zmitrovich AC, Hamowy AS, Liu PYR. Prenatal administration of buprenorphine using the osmotic minipump – a preliminary study of maternal and offspring toxicity and growth in the rat. Neurotoxicol Teratol 1995; 17(4): 419–23.
182. Evans RG, Olley JE, Rice GE, Abrahams JM. Effects of subacute opioid administration during late pregnancy in the rat on the initiation, duration and outcome of parturition and maternal levels of oxytocin and arginine vasopressin. Clin Exp Pharmacol Physiol 1989; 16(3): 169–78.
183. Robinson SE, Wallace MJ. Effect of perinatal buprenorphine exposure on development in the rat. J Pharmacol Exp Ther 2001; 298(2): 797–804.
184. Robinson SE. Effect of prenatal opioid exposure on cholinergic development. J Biomed Sci 2000; 7(3): 253–7.
185. Wu VW, Mo Q, Yabe T, et al. Perinatal opioids reduce striatal nerve growth factor content in rat striatum. Eur J Pharmacol 2001; 414(2–3): 211–14.
186. Barron S, Chung VM. Prenatal buprenorphine exposure and sexually dimorphic nonreproductive behaviors in rats. Pharmacol Biochem Behav 1997; 58(2): 337–43.
187. Loustauneau A, Auriacombe M, Franques P, et al. A report of 18 pregnancies among buprenorphine-treated women. Drug Alcohol Depen 2000; 60 (suppl1): S132.
188. Lacroix I, Berrebi A, Chaumerliac C, et al. Buprenorphine in pregnant opioid-dependent women: first results of a prospective study. Addiction 2004; 99(2): 209–14.

189. Therapeutic Goods Administration. Prescribing medicines in pregnancy. An Australian categorisation of risk of drug use in pregnancy. 4th Edition. Canberra: Commonwealth Department of Health and Aged Care, 1999.
190. Jernite M, Viville B, Escande B, et al. Buprenorphine and pregnancy. Analysis of 24 cases. Arch Pediatr 1999; 6(11): 1179–85.
191. Regini P, Cutrone M, Donzelli F, et al. Buprenorphine neonatal withdrawal syndrome, which therapy? Med Sur Pediatr 1998; 20(1): 67–9.
192. Lejeune C, Simmat-Durand L, Gourarier L, et al. Prospective multicenter observational study of 260 infants born to 259 opiate-dependent mothers on methadone or high-dose buprenorphine substitution. Drug Alcohol Depen 2006; 82(3): 250–7.
193. Herve F, Quenum S. [Buprenorphine (Subutex) and neonatal withdrawal syndrome.] Arch Pediatrie 1998; 5(2): 206–7.
194. Ross D. High dose buprenorphine in pregnancy – case report. Aust NZ J Obstet Gyn 2004; 44: 80.
195. Dos Santos A. Neonatal abstinence syndrome after prenatal exposure to drugs. A report of 41 observations. Universite Victor Segalen Bordeaux 2; 1998.
196. Noblett C, Burtin N, Guillemant Y, et al. Management of neonatal withdrawal syndrome to Subutex: a 3-year retrospective study of 27 exposed pregnancies. Therapie 2000; 55(3): 422.
197. Schindler SD, Eder H, Ortner R, et al. Neonatal outcome following buprenorphine maintenance during conception and throughout pregnancy. Addiction 2003; 98(1): 103–10.
198. Johnson RE, Jones HE, Jasinski DR, et al. Buprenorphine treatment of pregnant opioid-dependent women: maternal and neonatal outcomes. Drug Alcohol Depen 2001; 63: 97–103.
199. Ebner N, Rohrmeister K, Winklbaur B, et al. Management of neonatal abstinence syndrome in neonates born to opioid maintained women. Drug Alcohol Depend 2007; 87(2–3): 131–8.
200. Jones HE, Johnson RE, Jasinski DR, et al. Buprenorphine versus methadone in the treatment of pregnant opioid-dependent patients: effects on the neonatal abstinence syndrome. Drug Alcohol Depend 2005; 79(1): 1–10.
201. Fischer G, Ortner R, Rohrmeister K, et al. Methadone versus buprenorphine in pregnant addicts: a double-blind, double-dummy comparison study. Addiction 2006; 101(2): 275–81.
202. Fischer G, Johnson RE, Eder H, et al. Treatment of opioid-dependent pregnant women with buprenorphine. Addiction 2000; 95(2): 239–344.
203. Kaltenbach K, Jones H, Fischer G, Selby P. New approaches in the treatment of opioid dependency during pregnancy. Heroin Addict Relat Clin Probl 2007; 9(3): 9–20.
204. Jones HE, Johnson RE, Jasinski DR, et al. Randomized controlled study transitioning opioid-dependent pregnant women from short-acting morphine to buprenorphine or methadone. Drug Alcohol Depend 2005; 78(1): 33–8.
205. Reisinger M. Use of buprenorphine during pregnancy. Res Clin Forums 1997; 19(2): 43–5.

206. Kayemba-Kay's S, Laclyde JP. Buprenorphine withdrawal syndrome in newborns: a report of 13 cases. Addiction 2003; 98(11): 1599–604.
207. NSW Ombudsman. Report of Reviewable Deaths in 2005; Volume 2: Child Deaths. Sydney: NSW Ombudsman, 2006.
208. Sachdeva DK, Stadnyk JM. Are one or two dangerous? Opioid exposure in toddlers. J Emerg Med 2005; 29(1): 77–84.
209. Geib A-J, Babu K, Ewald MB, Boyer EW. Adverse effects in children after unintentional buprenorphine exposure. Pediatrics 2006; 118(4): 1746–51.
210. Schwarz KA, Cantrell FL, Vohra RB, Clark RF. Suboxone (buprenorphine/naloxone) toxicity in pediatric patients: a case report. Pediatr Emerg Care 2007; 23(9): 651–2.
211. Hayes BD, Klein-Schwartz W, Doyon S. Toxicity of buprenorphine overdoses in children. Pediatrics 2008; 121(4): e782–6.
212. Reckitt Benckiser. Suboxone Product Information. West Ryde, New South Wales: Reckitt Benckiser, 2005.
213. Clark N, Lintzeris N, Gijsbers A, et al. LAAM maintenance vs methadone maintenance for heroin dependence. (Cochrane Review). The Cochrane Library, Issue 3. Chichester, UK: John Wiley & Sons, Ltd, 2004.
214. Jaffe JH. Can LAAM, like Lazarus, come back from the dead? [comment]. Addiction 2007; 102(9): 1342–3.
215. Wolven A, Archer S. Toxicology of LAAM. In: Blaine JD, Renault PF, eds. Px: 3 x/week LAAM Alternative to Methadone NIDA Research Monograph 8. 29–38. Rockville, MD: National Institute on Drug Abuse; U.S. Department of Health, Education and Welfare, 1976.
216. Lichtblau L, Sparber SB. Outcome of pregnancy in rats chronically exposed to 1-alpha-acetylmethadol (LAAM). J Pharmacol Exp Ther 1981; 218(2): 303–8.
217. York RG, Denny KH, Moody DE, Alburges ME. Developmental toxicity of levo-alpha-acetylmethadol (LAAM) in tolerant rats. Int J Toxicol 2002; 21(2): 147–59.
218. Sparber SB, Lichtblau L. Postnatal abstinence or acute toxicity can account for morbidity in developmental studies with opiates. Life Sci 1983; 33(12): 1135–40.
219. McGillkiard KL, Jones SE, Robertson GE, Olsen GD. Altered respiratory control in newborn puppies after chronic prenatal exposure to alpha-1-acetylmethadol (LAAM). Resp Physiol 1982; 47(3): 299–311.
220. Australian Drug Evaluation Committee Therapeutic Good Administration. Prescribing medicines in pregnancy. 4 ed. Woden, ACT: Publications Unit TGA, 1999.
221. Orphan Australia. Revia Product Information. Melbourne: Orphan Australia, 2002.
222. McLaughlin PJ, Tobias SW, Lang CM, Zagon IS. Chronic exposure to the opioid antagonist naltrexone during pregnancy: maternal and offspring effects. Physiol Behav 1997; 62(3): 501–8.
223. Hulse GK, O'Neill G, Pereira C, Brewer C. Obstetric and neonatal outcomes associated with maternal naltrexone exposure. Aust NZ J Obstet Gyn 2001; 41(4): 424–8.

224. Hulse GK, O'Neil G, Arnold-Reed DE. Methadone maintenance vs. implantable naltrexone treatment in the pregnant heroin user. Int J Gynaecol Obstet 2004; 85(2): 170–1.
225. Lintzeris N, Lee S, Scopelliti L, et al. Unplanned admissions to two Sydney public hospitals after naltrexone implants [see comment]. Med J Australia 2008; 188(8): 441–4.
226. Gibson AE, Degenhardt LJ, Hall WD. Opioid overdose deaths can occur in patients with naltrexone implants [see comment]. Med J Australia 2007; 186(3): 152–3.
227. Wodak AD, Ali R, Henry D, Sansom L. Ensuring the safety of new medications and devices: are naltrexone implants safe? [comment] Med J Australia 2008; 188(8): 438–9.
228. Degenhardt L, Gibson A, Mattick RP, Hall W. Depot naltrexone use for opioid dependence in Australia: large-scale use of an unregistered medication in the absence of data on safety and efficacy. Drug Alcohol Rev 2008; 27(1): 1–3.
229. Lobmaier P, Kornor H, Kunoe N, Bjorndal A. Sustained-release naltrexone for opioid dependence. Cochrane Database Syst Rev 2008; (2): CD006140.
230. Cunningham N, Anisfeld E, Casper V, Nozyce M. Infant carrying, breast feeding, and mother–infant relations. Lancet 1987; 1: 379.
231. Hendershot GE. Trends in breast-feeding. Pediatrics 1984; 74(4 Pt 2): 591–602.
232. Kreek MJ, Schecter A, Gutjahr CL, et al. Analyses of methadone and other drugs in maternal and neonatal body fluids: use in evaluation of symptoms in a neonate of mother maintained on methadone. Am J Drug Alcohol Ab 1974; 1(3): 409–19.
233. Blinick G, Inturrisi CE, Jerez E, Wallach RC. Amniotic fluid methadone in women maintained on methadone. Mt Sinai J Med 1974; 41(2): 254–9.
234. Geraghty B, Graham EA, Logan B, Weiss EL. Methadone levels in breast milk. J Human Lactat 1997; 13(3): 227–30.
235. McCarthy JJ, Posey BL. Methadone levels in human milk. J Human Lactat 2000; 16(2): 115–20.
236. Wojnar-Horton RE, Kristensen JH, Yapp P, et al. Methadone distribution and excretion into breast milk of clients in a methadone maintenance programme. Brit J Clin Pharmacol 1997; 44(6): 543–7.
237. Jansson LM, Velez M, Harrow C, et al. Methadone maintenance and lactation: a review of the literature and current management guidelines [see comment]. J Human Lactat 2004; 20(1): 62–71.
238. Lesher GA, Beierschmitt WP. l-alpha-Acetylmethadol administration to lactating rat dams. Effect on hepatic aniline hydroxylase and ethylmorphine N-demethylase activities in rat pups. Drug Metab Dispos: The Biological Fate of Chemicals 1988; 16(1): 9–14.
239. Marquet P, Chevrel J, Lavignasse P, et al. Buprenorphine withdrawal syndrome in a newborn. Clin Pharmcol Ther 1997; 62(5): 569–71.
240. Jansson LM, Choo RE, Harrow C, et al. Concentrations of methadone in breast milk and plasma in the immediate perinatal period. J Human Lactat 2007; 23(2): 184–90.

241. Jansson LM, Choo R, Velez ML, et al. Methadone maintenance and long-term lactation. Breastfeeding Medicine: The Official Journal of the Academy of Breastfeeding Medicine 2008; 3(1): 34–7.
242. Kumar RM, Shahul S. Role of breast-feeding in transmission of hepatitis C virus to infants of HCV-infected mothers. J Hepatol 1998; 29(2): 191–7.
243. Lipsitz PJ. A proposed narcotic withdrawal score for use with newborn infants. A pragmatic evaluation of its efficacy. Clin Pediatr 1975; 14(6): 592–4.
244. Finnegan LP, Connaughton JFJ, Emich JP. Neonatal abstinance syndrome: assessment and management. Addict Dis 1975; 2: 141–155.
245. Zahorodny W, Rom C, Whitney W, et al. The neonatal withdrawal inventory: a simplified score of newborn withdrawal. J Dev Behav Pediatr 1998; 19(2): 89–93.
246. Green M, Suffet F. The Neonatal Narcotic Withdrawal Index: a device for the improvement of care in the abstinence syndrome. Am J Drug Alcohol Ab 1981; 8(2): 203–13.
247. Osborn DA, Jeffery HE, Cole M. Opiate treatment for opiate withdrawal in newborn infants [update of Cochrane Database Syst Rev 2002; (3): CD002059; PMID: 12137642]. Cochrane Database of Systematic Reviews 2005; (3): CD002059.
248. Osborn DA, Jeffery HE, Cole MJ, et al. Sedatives for opiate withdrawal in newborn infants [update of Cochrane Database Syst Rev. 2002; (3): CD002053; PMID: 12137641]. Cochrane Database Syst Rev 2005; (3): CD002053.
249. Jackson L, Ting A, McKay S, et al. A randomised controlled trial of morphine versus phenobarbitone for neonatal abstinence syndrome. Arch Dis Child Fetal Neonat Ed 2004; 89(4): F300–4.
250. Khoo K. The effectiveness of three treatment regimens used in the management of neonatal abstinence syndrome. PhD thesis, University of Melbourne, 1995.
251. Coyle MG, Ferguson A, Lagasse L, et al. Diluted tincture of opium (DTO) and phenobarbital versus DTO alone for neonatal opiate withdrawal in term infants. J Pediatr 2002; 140(5): 561–4.
252. Kraft WK, Gibson E, Dysart K, et al. Sublingual buprenorphine for treatment of neonatal abstinence syndrome: a randomized trial. Pediatrics 2008; 122(3): e601–7.
253. NSW Department of Health. National clinical guidelines for the management of drug use during pregnancy, birth and the early development years of the newborn. Commissioned by the Ministerial Council on Drug Strategy under the Cost Shared Funding Model. North Sydney: Commonwealth of Australia, 2006.

chapter 10

Politics, practice, and research into treatment of heroin addiction

James Bell

Introduction

The drug treatment industry in Australia was thrown into chaos in June 1997, when the banner headline for a popular women's magazine read 'I woke up cured of heroin addiction'. The accompanying story told of how a young heroin user, with the help of a media organization, had flown to Israel and undergone rapid detoxification under anesthesia.

The story precipitated a series of events, most notably a surge of demand for naltrexone treatment from consumers. Within months of that headline, rival groups of entrepreneurs from Israel had visited Australia to promote their competing programs, each of which was based on 'rapid detoxification' followed by naltrexone treatment. Media coverage was intense. The publicity spurred several Australian practitioners to establish clinics, and within a few months testimony from recovering individuals added to the excitement over the new 'cure' for heroin addiction. Practitioners with no prior interest nor training in treatment of addiction began running flourishing clinics, delivering treatment for which there was little or no evidence of either safety or efficacy.[1] Critics and protagonists of 'rapid detoxification' became embroiled in often bitter debates about the respective merits of naltrexone and methadone treatment. In one of several 'culture wars' which have occurred in Australia in the last decade, a political, academic, and media conflict was under way which would determine the direction of treatment services.

Culture wars have raged over the last two decades in many nations. While superficially about issues of scholarship or science, culture wars are primarily struggles within academic and public life between factions seeking to impose a particular paradigm or interpretation of history.[2] There is substantial booty to be won in such conflicts, in terms of funding and prestige, and Australia's naltrexone wars, like other culture wars, were not only grounded in philosophic differences, but driven by ambition and competition for a lucrative market. A newspaper report in 1998 claimed that investors were pouring money into rapid detoxification treatment, and estimated that in Sydney alone heroin users (and their families) had paid more than a million dollars for rapid detoxification in the preceding few months.[3]

Heroin addiction had become an important political issue in the mid-1990s, in part due to concerted pressure for research into prescribing heroin. In July 1997, after 6 years of concerted pressure to stage a 'heroin trial', the Ministerial Council on Drug Strategy (a council of Australian health and police ministers) voted in favor of commencing a trial of prescribed heroin. This remarkable vote, and the rapid veto of such a trial imposed by the Prime Minister, intensified public debate, which became increasingly polarized. Supporters of 'zero tolerance' policies argued that the government should be supporting rapid detoxification using naltrexone rather than supporting trials of heroin.[4] Several politicians, predominantly conservative representatives of rural electorates, called for the public health system to provide rapid detoxification. Most State Governments responded to this pressure by allocating funds to conduct clinical trials of rapid detoxification and naltrexone treatment. The Federal Government provided further funding to ensure that results of different State trials could be compared, and this was the origin of a multisite collaboration, the National Evaluation of Pharmacotherapies for Opioid Dependence (NEPOD).

This chapter describes the context in which NEPOD was conducted, and the impact of the NEPOD studies on policy, practice, and research. In particular, it analyzes the relative contributions of research and political actions in resolving the conflict within the community over how to respond to heroin addiction.

Philosophical divisions in addiction treatment

Ideologic divisions are an essential prerequisite for the development of culture wars, and the addiction treatment field has a long history of alternate paradigms of treatment. In both the treatment of alcohol dependence and opioid dependence, the focal point of difference between the competing paradigms has been over the importance of abstinence as the primary goal of treatment. In the field of treatment for alcohol problems, the first research claims that some alcohol-dependent people could achieve controlled drinking were met with quite disproportionate hostility, signaling that at issue was not merely an empirical issue, but an assault on a dominant paradigm.

In the treatment of heroin addiction, the primacy of abstinence as the objective of treatment has contributed to widespread questioning over whether methadone maintenance treatment (MMT) is a valid way to treat heroin addiction. It is counter-intuitive for a community to countenance provision of drugs as treatment of addiction, and there has been understandable community, professional, and consumer scepticism towards maintenance treatment.[5] Precisely because it is counter-intuitive and subject to widespread hostility, MMT has been extensively researched, and there is a substantial literature documenting what can be expected from it. Treatment of a heroin user in MMT reduces the risk of death, reduces the risk of transmission of blood-borne viruses, reduces heroin use, improves quality of life, and reduces involvement in crime.[6] However, entry to MMT probably does not increase the likelihood of an individual becoming long-term abstinent from all opioids; rather, it is a long-term intervention, in which most benefits of treatment are observed so long as the patient remains in treatment.[7] People who believe that abstinence from opioids should be the primary measure of treatment effectiveness ignore the documented benefits of MMT, and continue to call for curative treatment – despite evidence that such a cure remains elusive.[8]

Even among practitioners delivering MMT, the relative importance of abstinence as a goal of treatment also influenced the way in which treatment came to be given. The DARP (Drug Abuse Reporting Program) researchers identified two broad approaches to MMT: 'change-oriented' and 'adaptive.'[9] This distinction referred to the extent to which programs were prepared to tolerate a degree of continuing drug use (tolerant programs being 'adaptive'). There was a tendency for the adaptive programs to favor long-term treatment with high-dose methadone, and for the change-oriented programs to favor lower methadone doses and encourage patients to withdraw from treatment in time, with a view to long-term abstinence. A later study[10] refined the broad distinction between programs, identifying the key philosophic difference as the extent of 'orientation to abstinence'. 'Abstinence-oriented' programs tended to be less tolerant of continued drug use and less committed to indefinite maintenance, seeing abstinence from all drugs, including methadone, as the primary goal of treatment, and tended to prescribe lower doses of methadone. These differences between methadone clinics in the extent of orientation to abstinence are not mere matters of style, but have implications for treatment effectiveness. Clinics characterized by an orientation to abstinence appear to have poorer outcomes than those oriented to maintenance.[11–13] The extent to which philosophical and attitudinal issues were more influential than evidence in determining how treatment was delivered was illustrated in a survey conducted in the US, which reported that most methadone treatment was out of line with research evidence.[14]

Rosenbaum[15] has argued that, in America, the increasing orientation to abstinence seen in treatment programs was a product of a conservative shift in North American politics. She argued that moves to define deviance not as 'sickness' but as 'badness', for which moral rather than medical solutions were more appropriate, had altered the way MMT was approached in America, suggesting that the orientation to abstinence was part of the reframing of treatment into a moral paradigm, with moral objectives. Among many consequences, zero tolerance attitudes to drug use in the US have had a profound effect on methadone treatment in that country. Critics have characterized MMT as 'soft' on drug users, a weakening of the community's hard line against heroin use, and community suspicion of MMT is probably one factor which contributed to increasing bureaucratic regulation of treatment in the US.[15–17]

It seems plausible that underlying the polarization between orientation to abstinence and to maintenance are alternate paradigms of drug use and its treatment, which may be labeled 'morally grounded' and 'empirically grounded'. In a morally grounded paradigm, heroin use (perhaps, all drug use) is inherently wrong, individuals are held to be responsible for their actions, and punishment is the appropriate response to deviance. This view is intuitive, and appealingly simple, as summed up in the phrase 'Just say "no" to drugs' – the policy stance adopted by the Reagan administration. The moral paradigm is characterized by support for 'zero tolerance' policies, a hard and unwavering stance against drug use that permits no ambiguity or uncertainty. The empirically grounded paradigm makes no assumptions about whether drugs are inherently bad, but assumes that the objective of treatment is to minimize adverse consequences of personal choice. It takes as a starting point for treatment the failure of criminal sanctions and social stigma to deter dependent drug users, and the need for tolerance and support in fostering the social reintegration of marginalized drug users. The empirically grounded paradigm of treatment loosely corresponds to a 'harm minimization' policy position, and the morally grounded position to 'zero tolerance'.

For purposes of discussion, the two polarities will be referred to as 'zero tolerance' and 'harm minimization' views. However, as will be argued later, these labels do not adequately characterize the deep but ill-defined range of differences over drug policy, treatment practices, and attitudes to drug users which exist in the community.

Politics and drug policy

Prior to 1985, there was little availability of MMT in most jurisdictions, and most treatment agencies were primarily oriented towards treating alcohol problems. However, recognition that the spread of HIV infection among injecting drug users represented a serious public health issue changed attitudes sharply. The importance of reducing transmission of blood-borne viruses by needle-sharing became, for a time, a higher priority than maintaining a politically acceptable but potentially harmful policy of zero tolerance. Recognizing the political risks in introducing potentially unpopular, counter-intuitive policies, the Federal Government decided to stage a national 'Drug Summit' in 1985. The summit was an attempt to reach a consensus on a potentially divisive topic, without politicizing the issues – the antithesis of using drug policy as a campaign strategy. The most important outcome of the Summit was that, based on expert advice, governments around Australia made a commitment to policy based on 'harm minimization' – a stance which assumed that abstinence from all drugs was only one of a number of valuable objectives which could be achieved by treatment, but by no means the only valid or even most important goal.[18] The importance of research in informing policy was emphasized by the allocation of funding to establish two National Centres to undertake research into prevention and treatment. It was decided to fund needle and syringe programs, and to expand access to methadone treatment.

This outbreak of pragmatism was not restricted to Australia. In the late 1980s and early 1990s, the convergence of two factors – a global increase in heroin supply, and recognition of the need for effective ways to contain HIV transmission among injecting drug users – meant that, for a period, pragmatism prevailed in drug policy. There was a marked increase in substitution treatment, particularly MMT, worldwide. This expansion of treatment was based on some empirical evidence, namely the consensus that substitution treatment could reduce the harm associated with heroin addiction.[19]

Methadone treatment in Australia 1985–97

At the Drug Summit of 1985, the Federal Government provided funding to expand treatment, and several new, publicly funded clinics were established. These clinics were staffed to provide counseling and welfare services in addition to medical services and dispensing. However, demand for treatment rapidly outstripped allocated funding, and alternate ways of funding continued expansion of treatment had to be found. Continued growth was only possible because of Australia's then system of universal health insurance, under which office-based treatment by a general practitioner or psychiatrist could be provided at no cost to the patient. This funding source was the major factor defining the characteristics of treatment in Australia, in which medical practitioners became the key providers of methadone treatment, with relatively little emphasis on counseling or welfare services. There were about 1,000 in methadone treatment in 1985, and this rose progressively to about 25,000 in treatment in 1997. By the mid-1990s, Australia had one of the highest per capita rates of participation in methadone treatment in the world.[20]

In addition to the original, publicly funded 'free' clinics, two other modes of treatment were allowed: private clinics, in which consumers paid a dispensing fee, and had medical consultations funded through government rebates to doctors, and office-based treatment, involving a dispensing fee and medical consultations, again funded through universal health insurance. This came to be the major modality by which people accessed MMT in Australia, emphasizing that the dramatic expansion would not have been possible without Australia's public health infrastructure – universal health insurance, and subsidized medication.

The rise in office-based prescribing has not been unique to Australia, and in Europe and Canada, more than 50% of all methadone is prescribed in the office of a general practitioner. There is now some limited evidence suggesting that treatment in primary care settings is as effective as treatment in specialist clinics.[21,22]

As in other countries, expansion of office-based prescribing was hampered in all Australian jurisdictions by the reluctance of practitioners to become involved.[23] In most Australian jurisdictions moves were made to recruit and train doctors. The training programs 'medicalized' methadone maintenance, partly as a way of making it acceptable to practitioners and thus encouraging them to participate.[24] The training presented the management of opioid dependence as being mainstream health care. It was 'marketed' to practitioners with the argument that skills in treating opioid-dependent people were valuable clinical skills in many areas of behavioral medicine. The training program presented clinical skills – assessment, exploring motivation, explaining treatment options and obtaining informed consent, and regular monitoring and review. It presented treatment as based on an empathic, non-judgmental therapeutic relationship. It emphasized tolerance of continuing drug use, use of high doses of methadone, and an orientation to maintenance rather than abstinence, as being components of treatment supported by research evidence. Thus, out of a pragmatic decision to fund treatment by shifting it into office-based care, a distinct 'medical' approach to maintenance treatment was shaped. This approach influenced treatment in most public and private clinics, as well as office-based practice, so that throughout the treatment system there was little emphasis on counseling, ancillary services, or involvement with 12-step fellowships.[25]

Precipitants of change

By 1996 in Australia, the consensus that had supported harm minimization since the 1985 drug summit was fragmenting, and views were becoming increasingly polarized. There appear to have been two factors contributing to this polarization. Firstly, as noted in the introduction, there had been sustained and growing pressure to undertake research into prescribed heroin as a way to minimize harm associated with dependence on the drug. This contributed to a backlash from proponents of zero tolerance. Secondly, and more importantly, in 1996 there had been a change in the Federal Government.

The change of government marked a shift in the political and ideologic climate in Australia. This shift was away from technocratic and administrative approaches to policy towards populist politics based on conservative social values. For the previous decade, drug policy in Australia had embraced many counter-intuitive measures such as supplying needles and syringes to injecting drug users as a way of minimizing drug-related harm. On social issues, the new government was populist; the theme the Prime Minister often expressed was that people should be able to feel 'relaxed and comfortable' with their own assumptions and beliefs. If counter-intuitive policies, such as supplying clean needles and syringes to drug users, caused people difficulty, they were encouraged to trust their own instincts. A prominent aspect of the political shift was the distrust of experts, who were disparaged as 'elites', groups who were out of touch with community values (usually referred to as 'family values'). In relation to drug policy and treatment approaches, populist conservative politicians explicitly rejected 'harm minimization', arguing that it was more important to 'send the right message' than to risk displaying any tolerance of drug use.

When sensational claims for rapid detoxification began appearing in 1997, the changed political climate meant that people were much more receptive to a radical change in drug policy and treatment practices. There were also two reasons why the politicians, practitioners, and consumers were receptive to change. First, there was a marked increase in availability and use of heroin. Second, among consumers and the community, disillusion with methadone treatment was a key factor which contributed to the remarkable rise in demand for naltrexone treatment.

Availability of heroin

Between 1995 and 1999, heroin was plentiful and cheap in most Australian jurisdictions. There appears to have been a marked increase in the number of people using heroin, reflected in a dramatic increase in heroin overdose over the decade of the 1990s.[26] Moreover, where previously heroin use had seemingly been largely a problem of marginalized and disaffected young people, often with established criminal involvement, in the 1990s there appeared to a rise in 'middle-class' heroin use. Young people with reasonable education and opportunities were taking up heroin use, as illustrated by the observation from a research trial at the time that 37% of heroin-dependent people presenting for treatment had tertiary educational qualification.[22] A consequence of this was that the problem of heroin use became more visible, and a major focus of community concern. This was reflected in a dramatic increase in media attention devoted to heroin use.[27]

Disillusion with methadone treatment

There was a widespread perception, among consumers, health providers, and the public, that much MMT was of poor standard. There was considerable diversion of methadone[28] and there had been a number of methadone-related deaths.[29] These factors caused considerable concern among people delivering treatment, and provided scope for criticism from people philosophically opposed to MMT. Perhaps most importantly, the sharp rise in heroin overdoses made it clear that expanding access to methadone treatment had not stemmed an increasing prevalence of heroin addiction.

Many potential participants, and their families, were deterred from MMT by the institutionalized nature of treatment (daily attendance at clinic). Perhaps most importantly, there is profound stigma associated with MMT.[6] For all these reasons, there was considerable openness to alternative approaches to treatment. When media reports of a rapid cure for heroin addiction appeared, there was enthusiasm among consumers. For many prospective patients, naltrexone represented 'hope', where methadone represented defeat or despair – resignation to long-term treatment. Many thousands of Australian heroin users underwent 'rapid detoxification' and periods on a daily dose of naltrexone. While naltrexone was at times promoted with quite inappropriate claims of 'curing' heroin addiction, there is little doubt that, as with methadone treatment, the growth of naltrexone clinics was driven primarily by consumer demand – and this was driven, in part, by discontent with MMT.

Alternative models of treatment

The alignment of three factors – rising heroin use, disillusion with MMT, and an increasingly polarized political culture – meant that when naltrexone treatment began to feature in media stories, there were many people who welcomed the debate. Some were simply receptive to the idea that a cure for heroin addiction had been found, others were keen to join the ideologic struggle over the future shape of drug treatment in Australia.

Public debate came to be reduced to the question of whether methadone or naltrexone was 'better' treatment. This superficial and divisive topic replaced the similarly superficial and divisive topic of whether Australia should conduct a heroin trial, but for people involved in treatment – both consumers and practitioners – it was far from an academic issue. The debate intensified the stigma associated with MMT, and challenged the credibility of professionals involved in treatment. Practitioners who questioned the safety and efficacy of naltrexone treatment were dismissed as representing the 'methadone industry'.[27] The debate often became personal. At one point, a prominent conservative demanded that public servants involved in formulating drug policy should themselves undergo drug testing, and that 'those who returned positive tests should undergo compulsory rehabilitation'.[30]

What gave the polarization between methadone and naltrexone such life (and, indeed, gave the debate over 'heroin trials' such animus) was probably the underlying philosophic polarization between harm minimization and zero tolerance. The complexity and intensity of the assumptions and beliefs which can be grouped together under the rubric 'zero tolerance' can be illustrated by practices of some of the practitioners who began delivering naltrexone treatment. For example, the largest, most high-profile and influential naltrexone program in Australia during the late 1990s illustrated a re-emerging model of service delivery quite different to the 'medical' paradigm. This clinic had close links to an evangelical church group, and placed strong emphasis on recovery through faith. Its literature stated explicitly 'our outcomes depend totally on optimism. We must believe in our God....'[31] Prospective candidates for naltrexone treatment were encouraged to attend the clinic on particular days, where those who presented were inducted – up to 21 in one day – using 'rapid detoxification'. People undergoing induction were supported through the procedure by volunteers, many of whom were themselves on naltrexone. In another naltrexone clinic, the doctor performing rapid detoxification was reported to have used 'religion, exorcisms, calls to prayer' on patients during precipitated withdrawal.[32]

These naltrexone clinics were offering models of service delivery radically different from the neutral, non-judgmental frame of reference supported in the 'empirical' approach to treatment. Underlying arguments about the superiority of 'methadone' or 'naltrexone' were in reality a clash of different models of treatment, each with a long tradition behind them. One model is 'faith-based', incorporating religious affiliation, hope, and 'moral clarity' – an unambiguous rejection of heroin use. Its 'evidence base' is personal testimony from recovering people. The alternate model is based on clarification of the patients' problems and goals, voluntary treatment after informed consent, empathic and non-judgmental attitude, and tolerance of a degree of continued heroin use. The evidence base for such an approach is research findings and professional consensus.

Faith-based treatment, generally based on the self-help fellowship of Alcoholics Anonymous, had coexisted reasonably peacefully with empirical approaches to treatment for many years before the controversy over naltrexone emerged. Most workers in the field had been comfortable with this coexistence, recognizing that people with drug problems frequently moved between different approaches to treatment, finding help from different sources at different times. When conflict over naltrexone broke out in 1997, it was not primarily from within existing services. Rather, for the most part it was medical practitioners who had not previously been closely involved in treatment of heroin addiction who became enthusiastic proponents of naltrexone. Rather than suggesting naltrexone was a treatment alternative for some people (the position adopted by most practitioners within the field), several of the newcomers claimed that the availability of naltrexone treatment would make methadone treatment 'unnecessary'.

The NEPOD project

In response to public pressure in 1997, most State Governments decided to fund clinical trials of naltrexone treatment, as a way of making it available, while also placating critics who argued that the safety and effectiveness of the treatment had not been demonstrated. The State Government in Victoria had already committed to funding research into treatment of heroin addiction, under a project called the New Pharmacotherapies Project. This funding enabled researchers in that state to develop a program of research investigating a variety of pharmacologic treatments. However, in most states, funding was allocated for trials with very little preparation and no peer review of proposals.

In an attempt to ensure that the best value and results were obtained from these trials, the Federal Government provided substantial funding to coordinate these diverse state-funded trials. This funded the NEPOD. The National Drug and Alcohol Research Centre (NDARC) was asked to coordinate a project to bring together the investigators. The funding provided by the Commonwealth was used to establish standardized data collection, pooling of results, and undertaking of pre-planned analyses. Funding was provided for external monitoring of the trials, and for the provision of an external randomization service. These measures were designed to ensure that the trials would be high-quality, rigorous research. In addition, funding was used to provide health economic analyses on the different treatments.

A NEPOD investigators group was formed comprising staff from NDARC and the principal investigators of the trials and sites. All investigators in State Government trials of pharmacotherapies were invited to participate. The group met regularly, to agree on data collection, health economic evaluation, and planned analyses; and later, to report on recruitment and results.

The NEPOD project included 13 individual trials conducted over 3 years, investigating the costs and outcomes of different pharmacotherapies (methadone, buprenorphine, LAAM, and naltrexone) in the treatment of opioid dependence. Twelve of the trials were funded directly by governments, one was part funded by a pharmaceutical company, and one was a peer-reviewed trial funded by the National Health and Medical Research Council. In total, 1430 subjects entered the trials, 1075 heroin users and 355 people on methadone moving to an alternative treatment. More than 250 clinical and research staff were directly involved, mostly in delivering care.

The overall findings from the NEPOD pooled data set are reported elsewhere.[33-35] The important finding in relation to maintenance treatment was that 6 months after entry to treatment, outcomes of treatment with naltrexone, methadone, and buprenorphine were quite similar in terms of levels of heroin use. All subjects entering trials of naltrexone had chosen that form of treatment, and none of the trials randomized subjects to either naltrexone or a maintenance treatment; therefore, the similarity in outcomes does not suggest equal efficacy, nor can it be concluded that the treatments are equally able to attract heroin users into treatment. The NEPOD pooled data indicated that, adjusting for differences in observation periods, subjects treated with naltrexone had significantly higher risk of heroin overdose after leaving treatment than did patients from methadone or buprenorphine treatment.[34] Overall, the results were sufficient to indicate that contrary to community and consumer hopes, naltrexone was not a wonder drug; and contrary to prevailing negativity towards methadone, MMT was moderately effective, and the most cost-effective treatment. Neither of these were new findings, but in the context in which this research was conceived, these findings were an important contribution to continuing political support for methadone treatment.

The limitations of research and collaboration

For participating researchers, most of whom had not been involved in previous multisite collaboration, participating in the NEPOD process was challenging. One researcher who was conducting a State Government funded trial of naltrexone treatment declined to participate. Among participating researchers, there was difficulty agreeing on planned analyses. On one issue, that of cost-effectiveness of different treatments, despite agreement on how to collect and analyze the data, it was not possible to reach consensus on how to report the findings.

Difficulty in defining outcomes of 'detoxification'

There was particular difficulty within the group in reaching consensus on suitable outcomes against which to judge the effectiveness of 'detoxification'. 'Rapid detoxification' procedures led to very high rates of completing detoxification, and most subjects remained heroin-free for the first week. Those who continued to take naltrexone generally remained abstinent from heroin, but engagement in post-withdrawal treatment was poor, and attrition from treatment was rapid. The converse situation occurred in people undergoing detoxification using buprenorphine. A majority of people treated with buprenorphine used heroin occasionally during treatment, and numbers 'completing detoxification', defined either as one week without heroin, or reversal of neuroadaptation, were quite low.[33] However, many people who presented for detoxification often found that buprenorphine 'worked' for them, allowing them to function more stably, and chose to extend the period of treatment (such that at 3 months one third of people who had initially presented for 'detoxification' were still taking buprenorphine, in de facto maintenance treatment). Most subjects in maintenance treatment used heroin infrequently, and at 3 months after entry to treatment, the group that had entered buprenorphine treatment was doing much better than at entry.[22,36]

If the primary goal of detoxification were defined as abstinence from heroin for 1 week, or as achieving complete reversal of neuroadaptation to opioids, rapid detoxification procedures were clearly more effective than all other treatments. If engagement in ongoing treatment at 3 months is the key measure of efficacy, then buprenorphine was clearly more effective than either rapid detoxification or conventional inpatient detoxification. Depending on the criteria used to evaluate treatments, quite different findings could be reported.

Several researchers came to the conclusion that it was artificial to distinguish between 'detoxification' and 'maintenance', and that heroin use at 3 months or 6 months after entry to treatment was the most appropriate outcome measure for effectiveness of an episode of treatment.

The problem of how to interpret outcomes was intensified by the adversarial atmosphere in which the research was conceived and conducted. Reducing issues to whether naltrexone or buprenorphine was 'better' is a superficial interpretation of the research findings. Furthermore, what the research findings led to were not clearcut empirical answers, but raised ethical and value questions about the basis of treatment.

It appeared that people mostly sought treatment – either detoxification or maintenance – at a time when drug use had escalated out of control. At this time they were desperate, and wanted a complete change in lifestyle. Their motivation at entry was towards abstinence from all drugs. Many participants may well have been quite unclear, or at least ambivalent, as to whether they wanted short-, medium-, or long-term treatment; at the time of entry, the important issue was an urgent solution to a pressing problem. It was observable that once the acute crisis was resolved, motivation to abstinence and lifestyle change was poorly sustained. Retention in all forms of treatment, particular naltrexone, was very poor. However, this did not imply prompt relapse to dependent heroin use. After leaving treatment, some subjects did rapidly return to levels of use similar to pre-treatment, but many more returned to controlled, infrequent use of heroin. A few remained abstinent from heroin over the follow-up observation period. These observations suggest that, over time, many heroin users go in and out of phases of heavy, dependent use, sometimes with the assistance of episodes of treatment. Short- and medium-term episodes of treatment may be viewed as part of their adaptation to a drug-using lifestyle.

This pattern of involvement in treatment and heroin use raised a critical issue in treatment of addiction. Treatment effectiveness is limited by compliance, and consumers often make decisions which appear to be self-defeating – in particular, dropping out of treatment prematurely, with the high probability of returning to heroin use. Is a consumer able to make a rational decision to discontinue naltrexone treatment with the intention of having a 'taste' of heroin; or is the nature of 'addiction' such that consumers should be regarded as sick, and unable to make such a rational choice? In general, proponents of 'harm minimization' adopted the pragmatic position of accepting the autonomy of drug users, their choices to enter and leave treatment, and sought to make treatment more effective by finding ways of making it more attractive – by providing more flexibility and support. Proponents of zero tolerance tended to be more in favor of measures to enhance compliance, with involvement of family members or carers in supervising treatment, trying to enforce compliance by providing more structure to treatment.

Adverse consequences of involvement in research

The atmosphere generated by publicity over naltrexone generated unrealistic expectations among consumers and researchers, and this in turn had some adverse consequences. Methadone was stigmatized, and in low standing among participants. Despite extensive literature indicating high likelihood of relapse, investigators established trials to investigate ways of withdrawing from methadone in order to become drug-free. When trials were set up to explore using rapid detoxification to help long-term patients withdraw from methadone, consumer interest was overwhelming. Later, there was also a trial to see if transfer to buprenorphine could improve the outcomes in people seeking to withdraw from methadone.

These trials were responding to strong consumer demand – and to the hope that new treatments might change the outcome of withdrawal from MMT. There were relatively few potential subjects who met the criteria for entry to the trial – those who had been stably abstinent from heroin for a period, and appeared to have the best prospects for successfully withdrawing. Unfortunately, and predictably, most subjects who withdrew from MMT relapsed after withdrawing. In one study involving slow withdrawal using buprenorphine, 69% had relapsed to heroin use within one month of completing withdrawal.[37]

One result of enthusiasm to undertake research into new treatments may have been to destabilize a number of previously stable participants.

What NEPOD trials did not answer

Is the 'moral' or 'empirical' paradigm more effective?

It was suggested earlier in this chapter that underlying the intensity of the debate over naltrexone was a clash of paradigms, between a morally grounded, directive treatment oriented to abstinence, and a technical approach to treatment, oriented towards minimizing harm. However, these different paradigms were never compared in the research trials. All trials involved the medical paradigm of treatment.

In some ways, this is disappointing. Although it would be both ethically and logistically challenging to randomize people to either a faith-based program, with objectives of promoting abstinence and recovery, or to an empirically based program, with objectives of reducing heroin use, distress, and risks, it would presumably have been possible. The comparison would have been a fascinating one. However, it is also a potentially destructive and sterile comparison, which few people would want to happen. Faith-based treatment programs and empirically based programs have coexisted peacefully for many years prior to the naltrexone war, and since about 2002, this relatively peaceful and stable coexistence has returned. At best, to set the two paradigms of treatment in opposition to each other seems academic. If and when there are further attempts by individuals to launch careers or new treatment programs by exploiting philosophic differences within the community, then perhaps it would be an opportunity to conduct such research. Indeed, anyone making large claims for treating heroin addiction should be subject to the discipline of conducting monitored research, if for no other reason than to reign in the unrealistic expectations engendered by talk of cure. There will always be people wanting to believe such claims, and even instinctively feeling that claims for a cure are plausible.

What is the appropriate basis for drug policy?

The critical issue for the community which precipitated the NEPOD exercise was whether we should be promoting treatment that 'works' to reduce harm, while accepting ongoing heroin use; or whether drug use in the community responds better to the 'right' messages of zero tolerance and treatment based on abstinence. That policy question was never going to be answered in these trials. Whether it is better to maintain a hard line against tolerating drug use, and opposing maintenance by using naltrexone rather than agonists, is potentially amenable to empirical answers (and, indeed, many would argue we have ample evidence on this question already), but that issue was not addressed in the NEPOD clinical trials.

Impact of NEPOD studies

Less than might be expected

Several of these trials, particularly those involving 'rapid detoxification', were launched urgently and under intense media scrutiny. They were expected to provide answers that would determine the extent to which rapid detoxification came to be offered through the public health system, and would determine the extent to which naltrexone treatment would replace MMT in the treatment of heroin addiction. However, as is so often the case, events ran ahead of research. Three developments occurred before the pooled NEPOD trials were completed and reported.

Reduced demand for naltrexone

First, and perhaps most importantly, consumer demand for naltrexone waned over time. In July 1998, the *Sydney Morning Herald* had reported 'Investors are pouring money into the controversial naltrexone rapid detoxification treatment'.[1] A year later, at the time of the collapse of Sydney's first private naltrexone clinic, the newspaper reported that 'A turf war has erupted in Sydney's lucrative heroin treatment market'.[38] However, one year further on, the same paper was reporting, in a story headed 'City's naltrexone clinics go to the wall', that the largest private clinic had gone into receivership.[39] The decline in demand for naltrexone may have been partly influenced by published results of trials reporting poor outcomes, but was undoubtedly also influenced by the disappointment of many consumers who had hoped for a cure, only to experience failure.

The NSW Drug Summit

The second critical issue was the decision by the NSW State Government to hold a 'Drug Summit' in 1999. Leading up to the State election in 1999, there had been enormous criticism of the methadone program, and of needle and syringe programs. The State opposition campaigned on a policy of reviewing the state's methadone program, and devoting vastly increased resources to residential, drug-free treatment.[40] The decision to hold the summit was a strategy to defuse drugs as an electoral issue.

The summit was held over several days, and community representatives, experts, and consumers all had an opportunity to address the politicians. A wide range of views was presented, ranging from advocacy for ceasing methadone treatment to opening a medically supervised injecting center for street drug users. Debate over the future of methadone treatment was a key issue, and several expert delegates gave evidence as to the value of methadone treatment. The turning point in that debate, and in many ways the turning point of the whole summit, came when an articulate young woman rose to address the assembled delegates and declared 'methadone saved my life'. Against a background of research evidence and expert opinion, it was personal testimony which appeared to cause opinion to swing behind MMT. In the final analysis, the summit resolved to expand access to MMT, and to support improvements in the quality of treatment. It was a remarkable turnaround after the summit had commenced in an atmosphere so hostile to substitution treatment.

The drug summit – which occurred before results of the NEPOD studies were available – proved to be a very effective process for achieving community and political consensus on a controversial and potentially divisive issue. It gave voice to all perspectives, with expert and consumer input. The final outcome included an affirmation of harm minimization as the guiding principle of policy. The summit even endorsed the establishment of a medically supervised injecting center at the heart of one of Sydney's street drug markets.

Protagonists of 'zero tolerance' were appalled. Indeed, the following year, with the blessing of the Prime Minister, opponents of harm minimization announced they were staging a 'Zero Tolerance Drug Summit'.[41] Given that the notion of a 'summit' involved the expression of divergent viewpoints, staging a summit devoted to expressing a single viewpoint seemed slightly incongruous – or, perhaps, underlined the difficulty that organizers had in accepting the idea that there were alternate, valid viewpoints.

The heroin 'drought'

The third factor contributing to a cooling of the conflict over drug policy was that abruptly, at the end of 2000, the availability of heroin in Australia dropped sharply. For a brief period, as supplies of heroin dried up, there was a huge demand for treatment as people found they could no longer obtain heroin. This was followed by a sustained drop in people seeking treatment, and a profound drop in rates of heroin overdose. The 'heroin drought' has meant that heroin use rapidly dropped off the political agenda. By the time the NEPOD report was presented to Federal Cabinet, the intense community anxiety over heroin addiction was already dissipating.

More than might have been expected

Although the political climate had already changed at the time the NEPOD studies became available, the studies were nonetheless important. Most importantly, they were a restatement of how elusive is the cure of heroin addiction. Addiction has long been a source of intense frustration, as the solution – abstinence from drugs – seems tantalizingly simple, and available to all. The fact that people dependent on heroin usually cannot achieve stable abstinence has repeatedly been demonstrated in research, yet continually needs restatement. Perhaps it is in part a matter of 'corporate memory', that every decade or so a new generation of practitioners entering the field needs to rediscover for themselves the difficulty of achieving cure of heroin addiction.

The NEPOD studies also had a profound effect on participating staff. Prior to the NEPOD studies, there was virtually no clinical research culture within existing services and clinics. Undertaking research changed practices to meet research needs. Staff had to improve the documentation of treatment, as required by research protocols, and in several studies had to integrate structured intervention protocols into treatment. Conducting research was in itself a successful form of technology transfer. It both established a culture of research, and transformed treatment practices. It also, for the first time in most clinics, provided staff with systematic follow-up data about the outcomes of the treatment they were delivering.

Impact on directions of treatment in Australia

The NEPOD studies demonstrated that in voluntary treatment settings, naltrexone was of very limited efficacy, and actually increased the risk of overdose. However, even before these results were available, the conflict between zero tolerance and harm minimization had moved on from the question of the effectiveness of rapid detoxification. In the last 5 years, frustration with moral relativism, ambivalence, and poorly sustained motivation to abstinence has seen a swing towards government and community support for mandatory treatment, through Drug Courts and other diversion programs. Huge resources have been invested in an expansion of diversion programs in Australia, although it appears that a majority of offenders referred for treatment may be cannabis users rather than heroin users.

Attempts to enhance compliance with naltrexone treatment have also been made. One Australian group has been employing naltrexone implants in an attempt to overcome the tendency of people to drop out of treatment. This is a logical extension of the process of rapid detoxification. One motive for offering rapid detoxification is the sense that it minimizes the scope for ambivalence and for patients changing their mind, as once a dose of naltrexone has been administered, detoxification proceeds irrevocably. This is a key reason why rapid detoxification procedures achieve higher rates of short-term abstinence than other detoxification procedures. Removing the voluntary element of compliance with treatment by using naltrexone implants is an extension of the theme of committing people to treatment at the time when they are motivated. This is a critical area for research.

The opposite trend is towards offering greater autonomy and choice in treatment to heroin users. The French experience with buprenorphine has challenged the assumption that substitution treatment needs to involve the supervised administration of medication, and the development of new formulations of medication designed to minimize diversion has also contributed to a re-appraisal of the extent to which supervised administration is required.[42] In addition, there is ongoing discussion of trials of injectable opioids as a treatment alternative.

Conclusion

In a review of the impact of research on policy, Wayne Hall identified the key role of research centers, particularly the National Drug and Alcohol Research Centre, in providing governments with quality information and advice to inform policy.[27] However, while research is necessary, it is not sufficient to ensure support for unpopular and stigmatized programs, which are always vulnerable. The critical ingredient in Australia's efforts to minimize the harm from injecting drug use was political consensus informed by research; when political consensus broke down, and particularly when attempts were made to exploit the drug issue for political gain, research was easily ignored.

In the naltrexone wars, several individuals, probably with a range of different motivations, tapped into community anxiety over heroin addiction to promote naltrexone treatment. Their message of optimism and hope was far more appealing to consumers, and the community, than a complex message about what treatments can realistically be expected to deliver. Proponents of naltrexone offering optimism were able to attract consumers, and public support, and it took several years and some assistance from research for the enthusiasm for naltrexone to fade.

Presumably, if recruitment to heroin use again accelerates in the future in Australia, as it has done periodically over the last 4 decades, there will again be individuals offering dramatic cures, and politicians seeking to exploit community fear and frustration by promising to get 'tough on drugs'.

The unresolvable polarization between harm minimization and zero tolerance remains a tension within the community, and within treatment and research circles. To the extent to which it drives informed debate and quality research, it is a constructive tension. To the extent to which it degenerates into a culture war, exploited by individuals seeking advantage and advancement, it has the potential to diminish the effectiveness of treatment, the quality of research, and the professionalism of the field.

References

1. Doherty L, Sweet M. Clutching for the million-dollar cure. Sydney Morning Herald, 1998 Jul 9: Sydney, 1.
2. Moses A.D. Revisionism and denial. In: Whitewash R. Manne, ed. 2003, Black Inc. Agenda: Melbourne.
3. Sweet M. A Quick Fix. Sydney Morning Herald, 1998 Jul 9: Sydney, 11.
4. Parrett C. Good news on the drugs front. Canberra Times, 1997 Jan 17: Canberra, 10.
5. Bell J, et al. Substitution therapy for heroin addiction. Subst Use Misuse 2002; 37(8–10): 1145–74.
6. Bell J, Zador D. A risk-benefit analysis of methadone maintenance treatment. Drug Safety 2000; 22(3): 179–90.
7. Ward J, Hall W, Mattick RP. Methadone maintenance treatment and other opiate replacement therapies. Amsterdam: Harwood Academic, 1998.
8. Newman RG. The need to redefine 'addiction'. New Engl J Med 1983; 308: 1096–8.
9. Cole SG, James LR. A revised treatment typology based on the DARP. Am J Drug Alcohol Ab 1975; 2: 37–49.
10. Allison M, Hubbard RL, Drug abuse treatment process: a review of the literature. Int J Addict 1985; 20: 1321–45.
11. Ball JC, Ross A. The effectiveness of methadone maintenance treatment: patients, programs, services, and outcomes. 1991, New York: Springer-Verlag.
12. Bell J, Chan J, Kuk A. Investigating the effect of treatment philosophy on outcome of methadone maintenance. Addiction 1995; 90: 823–30.
13. Capelhorn J, Lumley TS, Irwig L. Staff attitudes and retention in methadone maintenance programs. Drug Alcohol Depen 1998; 52(1): 57–61.
14. D'Aunno T, Vaughan TE. Variation in methadone treatment practices: results from a national study. JAMA 1992; 267: 253–8.
15. Rosenbaum M. The demedicalization of methadone maintenance. J Psychoactive Drugs 1995; 27(2): 145–9.

16. Des Jarlais DC, Paone D, Friedman SR, et al. Regulating controversial programs for unpopular people: methadone maintenance and syringe exchange programs. Am J Public Health 1995; 85(11): 1577–84.
17. Dole VP, Nyswander M, Des Jarlais D, Joseph H. Performance-based ratings of methadone maintenance programs. New Engl J Med 1982; 306: 169–72.
18. Blewett N. Assumptions, arguments and aspirations. In: National Campaign Against Drug Abuse Monograph No 1; Australian Government Publishing Service: Canberra, 1987.
19. Stimpson JV. AIDS and injecting drug use in the UK 1987–1993: the policy response and the prevention of the epidemic. Soc Sci Med 1995; 41(5): 699–916.
20. Berbatis CG, et al. Trends in licit opioid use in Australia, 1984–1998: comparative analysis of international and jurisdictional data. Med J Australia 2000; 173: 524–7.
21. Gossop M, Marsden J, Stewart D, et al. Methadone treatment practices and outcome for opiate addicts treated in drug clinics and in general practice: results from the National Treatment Outcome Research Study. Brit J Gen Pract 1999; 49(438): 31–4.
22. Gibson AE, Doran CM, Bell JR, et al. A comparison of buprenorphine treatment in specialist and primary care settings: a randomised trial. Med J Australia 2003; 179: 38–42.
23. Roche A, Hotham ED, Richmond RL. The general practitioner's role in AOD issues; overcoming individual, professional and systemic barriers. Drug Alcohol Rev 2002; 21: 223–30.
24. Bell J. Lessons from a training programme for methadone prescribers. Med J Australia 1995; 162: 143–4.
25. Bell J, Ward J, Mattick RP, et al. An evaluation of private methadone clinics. In: National Drug Strategy Research Report No 4; Australian Government Publishing Service: Canberra, 1995.
26. Hall WD, Ross JE, Lynskey MT, et al. How many dependent heroin users are there in Australia? Med J Australia 2000; 173: 528–31.
27. Hall W. The contribution of research to Australian policy responses to heroin dependence 1990–2001: a personal retrospective. Addiction 2004; 99(5): 560–9.
28. Lintzeris N, Lenne M, Ritter A. Methadone injection in Australia: a tale of two cities. Addiction 1999; 94(8): 1175–8.
29. Sunjic S, Zador D. Methadone related deaths in New South Wales, July 1990–December 1995. Drug Alcohol Rev 1999; 18: 409–16.
30. Cornford P. Test Public Servants for Drugs: PM Adviser. Sydney Morning Herald 2000 Mar 20: Sydney, 3.
31. O'Neill G. How to care for patients with heroin addiction. 1997, Perth: Australian Medical Procedures Research Foundation.
32. Thomas H. Doctor accused in 31 deaths. Brisbane Courier Mail. 2002 Sep 11: Brisbane.
33. Digiusto E, Lintzeris N, Breen C, et al. Short-term outcomes of five heroin detoxification methods in the Australian NEPOD project. Addict Behav 2005; 30(3): 443–56.

34. Digiusto E, Shakeshaft A, Ritter A, et al. Serious adverse events in the Australian National Evaluation of Pharmacotherapies for Opioid Dependence (NEPOD). Addiction 2004; 99(4): 450–60.
35. Mattick RP, et al. National evaluation of pharmacotherapies for opioid dependence (NEPOD). In: NDS Monograph Series No.52; Australian Government Department of Health and Ageing: Canberra, 2001.
36. Lintzeris N, et al. A randomised, controlled trial of buprenorphine in the management of short-term ambulatory heroin withdrawal. Addiction 2002; 97: 1395–404.
37. Breen CL, et al. Cessation of methadone maintenance treatment using buprenorphine: transfer from methadone to buprenorphine and subsequent buprenorphine reductions. Drug Alcohol Depen 2003; 71: 49–55.
38. Totaro P. Heroin quick fix pioneer collapses in "a field of agony." Sydney Morning Herald. 1999: Sydney, 1.
39. Totaro P. City's naltrexone clinics go to the wall. Sydney Morning Herald. 2000: Sydney, 4.
40. Bernoth A. Libs pledge 4000 places for addicts. Sydney Morning Herald. 1999: Sydney, 8.
41. Totaro P. PM backs summit on drugs zero tolerance. Sydney Morning Herald. 2000: Sydney, 6.
42. Bell J, et al. A pilot study of buprenorphine-naloxone combination tablet (Suboxone) in treatment of opioid dependence. Drug Alcohol Rev 2004; 23(3): 311–17.

chapter 11

Clinical guidelines and procedures for the use of methadone in the maintenance treatment of opioid dependence

Sue Henry-Edwards, Linda Gowing, Jason White, Robert Ali, James Bell, Rodger Brough, Nicholas Lintzeris, Alison Ritter, and Allan Quigley

Introduction

Methadone was first used as a treatment for heroin dependence in Vancouver in 1959 and was subsequently introduced into Australia in 1969 for the same purpose. Methadone maintenance treatment (MMT) was endorsed by State, Territory, and Commonwealth Governments as an appropriate and useful treatment for heroin dependence at the launch of the National Campaign Against Drug Abuse in 1985. Since that time there has been substantial growth in the number of individuals receiving methadone treatment in most jurisdictions of Australia.

The aims of MMT are to: reduce or eliminate illicit heroin and other drug use by those in treatment; improve the health, well-being, and social rehabilitation of those in treatment; reduce the spread of blood-borne diseases associated with injecting opioid use; reduce the risk of death associated with opioid use; and reduce the level of involvement in crime associated with opioid use.

These clinical guidelines have been prepared to aid authorized medical practitioners in the selection and management of patients seeking methadone maintenance treatment for opioid dependence. The content has been designed to complement the National Policy on Methadone Treatment and local jurisdictional policies and requirements for methadone prescribing.

These guidelines were prepared under the auspices of the National Expert Advisory Committee on Illicit Drugs (NEACID) in collaboration with the National Evaluation of Pharmacotherapies for Opioid Dependence (NEPOD) project, the Royal Australian College of General Practitioners (RACGP), and the Australian Professional Society on Alcohol and Other Drugs (APSAD) and are funded by the Commonwealth Department of Health and Ageing.

The clinical guidelines are based on national and international research literature, previously published guidelines, and clinical experience with the use of methadone in Australia. They have undergone a rigorous process of review and have been formally endorsed by the RACGP and APSAD.

The authors gratefully acknowledge the contribution of a number of individuals and organizations in the drafting and review of these guidelines. Mr Andrew Preston generously gave permission for material from his book *The New Zealand Methadone Briefing* to be included in the guidelines. Dr Tony Gill and the Drug Programs Bureau, NSW Health Department gave valuable feedback and allowed us to reproduce sections of the *NSW Methadone Maintenance Treatment Clinical Practice Guidelines* in the appendices. Dr Hendree Jones, Director of Research at the Centre for Addiction and Pregnancy in the USA, provided valuable comments on the sections on Pregnancy and Lactation. We are indebted to Dr Michael Farrell and the UK Department of Health. To all those who patiently reviewed and commented on successive drafts of the document – our grateful thanks.

Clinical pharmacology

General information

What is methadone?

Methadone is a potent synthetic opioid agonist which is well absorbed orally and has a long, although variable plasma half-life. The effects of methadone are qualitatively similar to morphine and other opioids.

Clinical pharmacology

Effects of methadone

The actions of methadone include analgesia, sedation, respiratory depression, and euphoria. The degree of euphoria is less with oral methadone than intravenous heroin.

Other actions include decreased blood pressure, constriction of the pupils (miosis), cough suppression, and histamine release causing itchy skin. Gastrointestinal tract actions include: reduced gastric emptying, reduced motility, elevated pyloric sphincter tone, and elevated tone of sphincter of Oddi, which can result in biliary spasm. Endocrine actions include reduced follicle stimulating hormone, reduced luteinizing hormone, elevated prolactin, reduced adrenocorticotrophic hormone, reduced testosterone, and elevated antidiuretic hormone. Endocrine function may return to normal after 2 to 10 months on methadone.

Side-effects from methadone administration include sleep disturbances, nausea and vomiting, constipation, dry mouth, increased sweating, vasodilation and itching, menstrual irregularities in women, gynecomastia and sexual dysfunction including impotence in males, fluid retention, and weight gain.

Most people who have used heroin will experience few side-effects from methadone. Once on a stable dose, tolerance develops until cognitive skills and attention are not impaired. Symptoms of constipation, sexual dysfunction, and occasionally increased sweating can continue to be troubling for the duration of MMT.

Methadone is fat soluble and binds to a range of body tissues including the lungs, kidneys, liver, and spleen such that the concentration of methadone in these organs is much higher than in blood. There is then a fairly slow transfer of methadone between these stores and the blood. Because of its good oral bioavailability and long half-life, methadone is taken in an oral daily dose.

Methadone is primarily broken down in the liver via the cytochrome P450 enzyme system. Approximately 10% of methadone administered orally is eliminated unchanged. The rest is metabolized and the (mainly inactive) metabolites are eliminated in the urine and feces. Methadone is also secreted in sweat and saliva.

Pharmacokinetics

There is wide individual variability in the pharmacokinetics of methadone but, in general, blood levels rise for about 3–4 hours following ingestion of oral methadone and then begin to fall. Onset of effects occurs approximately 30 minutes after ingestion. The apparent half-life of a single first dose is 12–18 hours, with a mean of 15 hours. With ongoing dosing, the half-life of methadone is extended to between 13 and 47 hours with a mean of 24 hours. This prolonged half-life contributes to the fact that methadone blood levels continue to rise during the first week of daily dosing and fall relatively slowly between doses.

Methadone reaches steady state in the body (where drug elimination equals the rate of drug administration) after a period equivalent to 4 to 5 half-lives or approximately 3 to 10 days. Once stabilization has been achieved, variations in blood concentration levels are relatively small and good suppression of withdrawal is achieved. For some, however, fluctuations in methadone concentrations may lead to withdrawal in the latter part of the interdosing interval. If dose increases or multiple dosing within a 24-hour period do not prevent this, other agonist replacement treatment approaches such as buprenorphine should be considered.

Withdrawal syndrome

The signs and symptoms of the opioid withdrawal syndrome include irritability, anxiety, restlessness, apprehension, muscular and abdominal pains, chills, nausea, diarrhea, yawning, lacrimation, piloerection, sweating, sniffing, sneezing, rhinorrhea, general weakness, and insomnia. Signs and symptoms usually begin two to three half-lives after the last opioid dose, i.e. 36 to 48 hours for long half-life opioids such as methadone, and 6 to 12 hours for short half-life opioids such as heroin and morphine.

Following cessation of heroin, symptoms reach peak intensity within 2 to 4 days, with most of the obvious physical withdrawal signs no longer observable after 7 days. The duration of methadone withdrawal is longer and may last between 5 and 21 days. This first, or acute, phase of withdrawal may then be followed by a period of protracted withdrawal syndrome. The protracted syndrome is characterized by a general feeling of reduced well-being. During this period, strong cravings for opioids may be experienced periodically.

The opioid withdrawal syndrome is rarely life-threatening. However, completion of withdrawal is difficult for most people. Untreated methadone withdrawal symptoms may be perceived as more unpleasant than heroin withdrawal, reflecting the more prolonged nature of methadone withdrawal.

Factors that have been identified as having the potential to influence the severity of withdrawal include the duration of opioid use, general physical health, and psychological factors, such as the reasons for undertaking withdrawal and fear of withdrawal. Buprenorphine appears to have a milder withdrawal than other opioids.

Drug interactions

Toxicity and death have resulted from interactions between methadone and other drugs. Some psychotropic drugs may increase the actions of methadone because they have overlapping, additive effects, For example, benzodiazepines and alcohol add to the respiratory depressant effects of methadone. Other drugs interact with methadone by increasing or decreasing metabolism. Drugs which induce the metabolism of methadone can cause a withdrawal syndrome if administered to patients maintained on methadone. These drugs should be avoided in methadone patients if possible. If a cytochrome P450 inducing drug is clinically indicated for the treatment of another condition seek specialist advice. Cytochrome P450-3A inhibitors can decrease the metabolism of methadone and cause overdose.

Safety

The long-term side-effects of methadone taken orally in controlled doses are few. Methadone does not cause damage to any of the major organs or systems of the body and those side-effects which do occur are considerably less harmful than the risks of alcohol, tobacco, and illicit opiate use. The major hazard associated with methadone is the risk of overdose. This risk is particularly high at the time of induction to MMT and when methadone is used in combination with other sedative drugs. The relatively slow onset of action and long half-life mean that methadone overdose can be highly deceptive and toxic effects may become life-threatening many hours after ingestion. As methadone levels rise progressively with successive doses during induction into treatment, most deaths in this period have occurred on the third or fourth day of treatment.

Formulations

Two preparations are available for methadone maintenance treatment in Australia:

- Methadone Syrup® from Glaxo Smith Kline. This formulation contains 5 mg/ml methadone hydrochloride, sorbitol, glycerol, ethanol (4.75%), caramel, flavoring, and sodium benzoate.
- Biodone Forte® from McGaw Biomed. This formulation contains 5 mg/ml methadone hydrochloride and permicol-red coloring.

Entry into methadone maintenance treatment

Note: Jurisdictional requirements stipulating eligibility for entry to MMT may vary from state to state and change over time. These guidelines are an attempt to present the clinical basis for MMT. If in doubt consult your jurisdictional policy.

Indications

Methadone maintenance treatment is indicated for those who are dependent on opioids and who have had an extended period of regular opioid use.

The diagnosis of opioid dependence should be made by eliciting the features of opioid dependence in a clinical interview. The definitional criteria of the *Diagnostic and Statistical Manual of Mental Disorders*, 4th edn (DSM-IV),[1] are useful to diagnose dependence.

Dependence is defined as 'A maladaptive pattern of substance use leading to clinically significant impairment or distress as manifested by three or more of the following occurring at any time in the same 12 month period.'

- Tolerance as defined by either a need for markedly increased amounts of opioids to achieve intoxication or desired effect, or a markedly diminished effect with continued use of the same amount of opioids.

- Withdrawal as manifested by either the characteristic withdrawal syndrome for opioids, or opioids, or a closely related substance, being taken to relieve or avoid withdrawal symptoms.
- Opioids often taken in larger amounts or over longer periods than intended.
- A persistent desire or unsuccessful attempts to cut down or control opioid use.
- A great deal of time regularly spent in activities necessary to obtain opioids, use opioids, or recover from their effects.
- Important social, occupational, or recreational activities given up or reduced because of opioid use.
- The opioid use continued, despite knowledge of having a persistent or recurrent physical or psychological problem that is likely to have been caused or exacerbated by opioids.

Note: A person diagnosed as opioid dependent may or may not be physically dependent on opioids at the time of presentation. If there is no current physical dependence MMT will not usually be appropriate. For those not physically dependent at the time of presentation, the prescribing practitioner must clearly document that the potential benefits to the individual's health and social functioning outweigh the disadvantages of MMT.

The patient will usually be at least 18 years of age. The prescribing doctor should seek a second or specialist opinion before treating anyone under 18 years of age. However, methadone treatment should not be precluded on the grounds of age alone. The patient must be able to provide proof of identity – a requirement for treatment with any S8 medication.

The patient must be able to give informed consent to treatment with methadone.

Contraindications

Some categories of patients are not suitable for treatment with methadone. These include patients with severe hepatic impairment or decompensated liver disease as methadone may precipitate hepatic encephalopathy. Generally, treatment other than methadone should be considered for a person under the age of 18 years, however methadone treatment should not be precluded solely on the grounds of age. The prescribing doctor should check jurisdictional requirements regarding age limits for MMT. Where patients are unable to give informed consent due to the presence of a major psychiatric illness or being underage, the prescribing doctor should consider relevant secondary consultation and check jurisdictional requirements regarding obtaining legal consent. Patients who are hypersensitive to methadone or other ingredients in the formulation are not suitable for treatment with methadone.

Other contraindications identified by the manufacturers of methadone include severe respiratory depression, acute asthma, acute alcoholism, head injury and raised intracranial pressure, ulcerative colitis, biliary and renal tract spasm, and patients receiving monoamine oxidase inhibitors or within 14 days of stopping such treatment. It is recommended that specialist advice be sought in these cases.

Precautions

Particular caution should be exercised by prescribers when assessing individuals with the following clinical conditions as to their suitability and safety for treatment with methadone. Concomitant medical and psychiatric problems and other drug use increase the complexity of management of patients on MMT and may also increase the risk of overdose and death. The prescribing doctor should seek specialist advice or assistance in such cases.

All opioid substitution treatments should be approached with caution in individuals using other drugs, particularly those likely to cause sedation such as alcohol, as well as benzodiazepines and antidepressants in doses outside the normal therapeutic range. Particular attention should be given to assessing the level of physical dependence on opioids, codependence on other drugs, and overdose risk.

Due to the significant management problems presented by people with concomitant alcohol dependence, consideration should be given to concurrent disulfiram or acamprosate therapy. If disulfiram or acamprosate are used, a methadone liquid formulation that does not contain alcohol should be considered to reduce the risk of reactions.

After a period of treatment with naltrexone, or having recently completed a period in prison or an opioid withdrawal program, the patient can be expected to have reduced tolerance to opioids and is at significant risk of overdose if they use opioids. Caution is advised if methadone is prescribed after a recent history of reduced opioid tolerance.

People whose mental state impairs their capacity to provide informed consent, such as those with an acute psychotic illness, cognitive impairment, or a severe adjustment disorder, should receive adequate treatment for the psychiatric condition so that informed consent can be obtained before initiation of MMT. At entry to MMT most patients exhibit some degree of depression which usually resolves quickly with methadone, and the majority of these patients do not require antidepressant treatment before commencement of methadone. Individuals at moderate or high risk of suicide should not be commenced on methadone in an unsupervised environment and specialist consultation should be sought.

A significant proportion of methadone-related deaths involves individuals who were in poor health and had other diseases, particularly hepatitis, HIV, and other infections which may have contributed to their death. This emphasizes the importance of giving consideration to concomitant medical problems.

Refer patients with chronic pain for specialist assessment first. Caution is advised in patients with head injury and increased intracranial pressure, although generally such cases are only seen in the hospital emergency setting. Aggravated hypertension has been reported in patients with pheochromocytoma in association with heroin use. In patients with asthma and other respiratory conditions even usual therapeutic doses of opioids may decrease the respiratory drive associated with increased airways resistance. Methadone should be used with caution in the presence of hypothyroidism, adrenocortical insufficiency, hypopituitarism, prostatic hypertrophy, urethral stricture, shock, and diabetes mellitus. Patients who exhibit poor compliance with treatment for major coexisting illnesses such as asthma or diabetes pose a particular challenge in MMT.

Assessment for treatment with methadone

Initial assessment procedures are similar for all opioid users seeking treatment. A comprehensive assessment of the patient's drug use, medical, psychological, and social conditions, previous treatment history, and current treatment goals should be conducted and documented. Specific attention should be given to assessment of dependence and tolerance, and the indications, contraindications, and precautions for methadone treatment. Obtain evidence of identity and aspects of the history relating to drug use and medical and psychiatric conditions to clarify any inconsistencies between physical examination findings and reported history. Accuracy of clinical assessment may be improved by using corroborating evidence such as urine tests and examination of veins for evidence of injecting drug use.

Evidence of dependence should also be obtained. The best evidence is observed signs of opioid withdrawal, either spontaneous or precipitated by naloxone challenge, or a verifiable history of previous treatment for opioid dependence with detoxification or maintenance. The initial assessment will result in an initial management plan which can be implemented directly. However, extra information will also need to be gathered at subsequent reviews so that more comprehensive treatment plans can be developed.

Key features of the assessment

Assessment includes the following key features:

- Opioid use: opioids used, quantity, frequency, route of administration, duration of current episode of use, time of last use, and use in the last 3 days; severity of dependence; age of commencement, age of regular use, age of dependence, timing and duration of periods of abstinence; episodes of overdose.
- Other drug use: alcohol, illegal and prescribed drugs, current medications.
- Health status: diseases from drug use, blood-borne viruses or infection, coexisting general or psychiatric health conditions.
- Psychosocial status: legal; social – employment, education, vocational skills, housing, financial, family; psychological – mood, affect, cognition.
- Past treatment for opioid dependency and other drug use: where and when, periods of abstinence, and degrees of success and acceptance of treatment.
- Selection of treatment: motivation for treatment, trigger for seeking treatment, patient goals for treatment episode, stage of change.

- Physical examination: observation of clinical signs related to drug use, evidence of medical problems such as liver disease, jaundice, ascites, and encephalopathy.
- Investigations: urine drug screening tests if there are concerns about the accuracy of the drug history and diagnosis; hepatitis B and C and HIV testing may also be indicated.

Informed consent and patient information

Obtain informed consent to methadone treatment in writing from the patient before commencing treatment. For patients to make a fully informed decision, they should be provided with written information addressing the nature of methadone treatment, other treatment options, program policies and expectations, consequences of breaches of program rules, recommended duration of treatment, side-effects and risks associated with taking methadone, risks of other drug use, the potential impact of methadone on their capacity to drive or operate machinery, and access to further information about treatment.

Methadone may affect the capacity of patients to drive or operate machinery during the early stages of treatment, after an increase in dose, or when patients are also taking other drugs. Warn patients about this effect before entry into treatment, and again when the dose of methadone is increased, or when the use of other drugs is suspected.

Meeting legislative requirements

Methadone is a registered Schedule 8 medication that is approved for the purpose of treating opioid dependence and withdrawal. Each jurisdiction is responsible for a system for authorizing medical practitioners to prescribe methadone for the purpose of treating addiction. Prescribers must obtain authority for each patient. Check your jurisdictional policy for details of authorization procedures. Patient identity must be verified at the time of assessment.

Patients must not begin MMT until approval has been obtained from the jurisdictional authority. Once authorization has been obtained, commencement of methadone should not be delayed. Successful commencement and continuation of treatment is enhanced by prompt program access.

Coordinated care

The relationship between the prescriber and dispenser of methadone requires ongoing communication to ensure consistency in the overall treatment program. This communication can be facilitated by the development of coordinated care plans.

The prescriber and dispenser and other members of the therapeutic team have a duty of care to the patient that may necessitate sharing of information despite professional obligations to maintain patient confidentiality. The dispenser is legally required to assess whether a dose of methadone is appropriate for the patient, and can withhold treatment if deemed necessary.

There are jurisdictional requirements regarding child protection and notification of at-risk children. Occasionally staff may experience a conflict between their duty of care to the patient and their jurisdictional responsibilities.

Induction to methadone treatment

Commencing methadone from heroin use

Objectives during induction to methadone are to retain individuals in treatment by reducing the signs and symptoms of withdrawal and to ensure their safety. This can be achieved by careful explanation regarding intoxicating effects and withdrawal during the induction and maintenance phases of methadone treatment, establishment of a therapeutic relationship, safe dosing, and repeated observation of patients.

It is particularly important to clearly explain that it takes time to complete induction onto methadone and that patients will experience increasing effects from methadone over the first few days of treatment even if the dose is not increased.

There is a need to achieve a balance between adequate relief of withdrawal symptoms and the avoidance of toxicity and death during the induction phase of MMT. The aim is to minimize the symptoms and signs of withdrawal while simultaneously minimizing the risks of sedation and toxicity.

While doses of methadone which are too high can result in toxicity and death, inadequate commencement doses may cause a patient experiencing withdrawal symptoms to 'top up' the prescribed dose of methadone with heroin, benzodiazepines, or illicit methadone. This can have potentially lethal consequences. For most patients, withdrawal symptoms will be alleviated but not entirely eliminated by doses less than 30 mg of methadone.

Deaths during the induction phase of methadone treatment have been related to: concomitant use of other drugs, particularly sedatives such as alcohol and benzodiazepines; inadequate assessment of tolerance; commencement on doses that are too high for the level of tolerance; a lack of understanding of the cumulative effect of methadone; inadequate observation and supervision of dosing; and individual patient variation in metabolism of methadone.

Size of the first dose

The first dose of methadone should be determined for each patient based on the severity of dependence and level of tolerance to opioids. The history of quantity, frequency, and route of administration of opioids, findings on examination, corroborative history, and urine testing together provide an indication of the level of tolerance a patient has to opioids, but do not predict it with certainty.

A defined period of observation for signs and symptoms of opioid toxicity and withdrawal is a more accurate method of assessing opioid tolerance than history alone. In circumstances where there is doubt about the degree of tolerance, a review of the patient at a time when withdrawal symptoms are being experienced may help to resolve uncertainty about a safe starting dose.

Prescribers should make every effort to communicate with other medical practitioners who may have seen the patient previously in order to corroborate significant elements of the patient's history and to assist in decision-making about commencing treatment.

New patients should be dosed with caution. Deaths in the first 2 weeks of MMT have been associated with doses in the range of 25 to 100 mg/day, with most occurring at doses of 40 to 60 mg/day. If at all possible, patients should be observed 3 to 4 hours after the first dose for signs of toxicity or withdrawal during this time of peak effect. If the patient is experiencing persistent withdrawal symptoms at 4 hours, a supplementary dose of 5 mg of methadone can be considered.

When deciding on the commencing dose also consider: where dosing is to occur, whether staff and facilities are available for observation and assessment of the patient before and after dosing, and who will assess withdrawal/intoxication prior to dosing.

The risk of overdose increases most markedly when other central nervous system (CNS) depressants are also used. If the patient shows signs of intoxication with benzodiazepines or alcohol, the dose should be withheld or reduced. Induct morphine, codeine, and oxycodone users as if they were heroin users.

A dose of less than or equal to 20 mg for a 70 kg patient can be presumed to be safe, even in opioid-naïve users, as this is the lowest dose at which toxicity has been observed. Caution should be exercised for starting doses of 30 mg or more. Exercise extreme caution if an initial dose of methadone exceeding 40 mg is considered necessary. Specialist consultation may be advisable.

Stabilization

During the first 2 weeks of MMT the aim is to stabilize the patient so that they are not oscillating between intoxication and withdrawal. This does not necessarily mean that the patient will reach an optimum maintenance dose in that time, and further dose adjustments may be required after the patient has been initially stabilized.

Monitoring during the first 2 weeks

Patients should be observed daily prior to dosing and an assessment made of intoxication. If there is any concern the patient should be assessed by a doctor before the dose is administered.

To ensure safety, it is desirable that patients are reviewed at least once, and preferably twice, by an experienced clinician in the first week with a view to assessing intoxication from methadone. Dose increases should only be considered subject to assessment by the prescriber.

Assessment should include withdrawal severity, intoxication, other drug use, side-effects, and patient perception of dose adequacy and adherence to dosing regimen.

Dose titration

Stabilization is about titrating the dose of methadone against the needs of the individual patient. Do not increase the methadone dose for at least the first 3 days of treatment unless there are clear signs of withdrawal at the time of peak effect (i.e. 3 to 4 hours after dose) as the patient will experience increasing effects from the methadone each day. Consider dose increments of 5 to 10 mg every 3 days subject to assessment. Total weekly increase should not exceed 20 mg of methadone. The maximum dose at the end of the first week should typically be no more than 40 mg. Patients should be warned not to drive or operate machinery during periods of dose adjustments.

Transfer from other pharmacotherapies

Prescribers may need to seek specialist advice when prescribing for patients who are transferring from other pharmacotherapies with which they are unfamiliar.

Buprenorphine

Consideration should be given to transferring a patient from buprenorphine to methadone under the following circumstances: the patient is experiencing intolerable side-effects to buprenorphine; there is an inadequate response with buprenorphine treatment; the patient is transferring to a program where buprenorphine is not available.

Patients should be stabilized on daily doses of buprenorphine and their buprenorphine dose reduced to 16 mg or less for several days prior to transfer. Methadone can be commenced 24 hours after the last dose of buprenorphine. The initial methadone dose should not exceed 40 mg. Patients transferring from lower doses of buprenorphine of 4 mg or less should be commenced on lower doses of methadone. Care should be taken not to increase the dose of methadone too quickly.

Naltrexone

Transfer will generally be considered because of relapse to opioid use following cessation of naltrexone. After a short period, possibly only a few days, on naltrexone the patient loses tolerance to opioids. Consequently, patients transferring from naltrexone should be treated as if they were naïve to opioids and non-tolerant to their effects unless the clinical circumstances clearly indicate a return to regular, heavy heroin use. Do not administer methadone until at least 72 hours after the last dose of naltrexone. Extreme caution should be exercised with commencing doses of methadone, which should be no greater than 20 mg.

Maintenance dosing

Dose levels

Doses should be determined for individual patients but generally a higher dose is required for maintenance than is required for initial stabilization. Typically effective maintenance doses are greater than 60 mg/day.

There is a dose–response relationship between maintenance doses of methadone, retention in treatment, and continued use of heroin. Methadone doses in excess of 60 mg/day are associated with higher retention rates and less heroin use. This has been demonstrated in both randomized controlled trials (RCTs) and cohort studies. Cross-tolerance to heroin increases as a function of increasing methadone dose and results in blockade of the euphoric effect of concurrent heroin use. A daily methadone dose of 60 mg or greater should be sufficient to ensure a substantial level of tolerance to effects of heroin in the majority of individuals. Maintenance doses for effective MMT are typically 60 to 100 mg/day.

Doses in excess of 100 mg/day may be necessary to achieve successful maintenance with patients who have a fast methadone metabolism, but there is no evidence from treatment outcome studies to suggest that routine dosing at levels in excess of 100 mg/day results in any additional benefit for the majority of patients.

Changing dose level

Patient input to treatment decisions, including determination of dosing levels, promotes a good therapeutic relationship by enhancing patient trust and responsibility. When making decisions about changes in dosage the following should be taken into consideration: concurrent use of illicit opioids and continued injecting use may indicate the need for a higher dose; individual variation in methadone metabolism; use of other medications; pregnancy; and polydrug use.

Compliance

Daily administration of methadone is recommended to ensure that plasma methadone levels are maintained and to avoid withdrawal symptoms. If plasma levels are not maintained, cross-tolerance to heroin will be lessened, reducing the capacity of MMT to moderate the euphoric effect of heroin. Reduced compliance is therefore associated with an increased risk of relapse to heroin use.

Monitoring drug use

Assessment of drug use enables monitoring of progress in treatment and can give useful information for making decisions on clinical management. Monitoring can also be used to support contingency management approaches. Concurrent use of other drugs with methadone by patients may threaten their safety. Monitoring drug use can also provide a basis for program evaluation. There is little evidence to support the use of drug monitoring as a deterrent against unsanctioned drug use.

Options for the monitoring of drug use include: self-report, urine testing, and clinical observation. Analysis of hair, saliva, and sweat may be an option in the future.

Self-report can be a reliable guide to drug use in settings where no negative consequences result from disclosure. However, in the clinical situation there are always contingencies which patients may perceive as punitive. Consequently, caution should be exercised when making clinical decisions based solely on self-reported drug use. The best information is usually obtained from a combination of self-report and urinalysis.

Urinalysis is an objective measure of drug use, however it may not be a reliable indication of drug use if patient urine collection is not observed. Observed urines are demeaning to both patients and staff. Reliability of unobserved urine samples may be increased by checking the temperature of the urine sample. Urinalysis will only detect recent drug use. The actual time frame varies depending on the drug being measured and will also depend on the threshold level set by the testing laboratory.

In urinalysis, it should be noted that false positives and false negatives do occur and research literature suggests that urine testing does not reliably reduce drug use. Methadone programs should not be punitive. Urinalysis is most useful where patients are in the early stages of treatment, and where clarity of drug use is required for diagnostic purposes.

Australian Medicare allows for a maximum of 21 urinalysis tests per patient per year. It is expected that the average number of tests will be significantly lower than this maximum and will decrease the longer a patient has been in treatment.

Adjunct treatment

There is compelling evidence that treatment factors other than an adequate dose of methadone contribute to improved outcomes. In particular, the quality of the therapeutic relationship between treatment providers and client is important. Where clients are treated respectfully with regard to their dignity, autonomy, and privacy, the outcomes of treatment are likely to be improved.

Social services

Multiple social problems are common among opioid-dependent people and a history of physical, sexual, and emotional abuse is prevalent among opioid-dependent people, particularly for female clients. These factors may have a negative impact on treatment outcome. Providing reinforcement and referral to vocational, financial, housing, and family assistance contributes positively to the progress of treatment.

Counseling

Counseling should not be mandatory within methadone programs, however there is evidence that access to counseling as an adjunct to MMT improves the effectiveness of MMT and is associated with greater retention in treatment and reduced use of illicit opioids. Therapeutic tools such as motivational interviewing, relapse prevention, and social skills training have been associated with improved outcomes. All ancillary services should be provided on the basis that the patient freely consents to be involved. For further information on counseling strategies see the report by Jarvis et al.[2]

Take-away doses

The take-away policy for methadone is determined for each jurisdiction in line with the National Policy on Methadone Treatment, which underpins all methadone management programs in Australia.

The benefits of take-away doses include: enhancement of integration into the community through reduction of time and associated travel costs for the patient; promotion of patient responsibility for treatment; reduced inconvenience and cost of daily dispensing for the pharmacist or clinic; and reduced inconvenience of regular attendance for the patient, thereby enhancing retention. Studies have indicated that programs which have take-away policies have better retention rates than programs which restrict take-aways.

Concerns regarding take-away doses of opioid medications include the risk of deliberate or accidental overdose by the patient or others, particularly through the use of a take-away dose by children and other non-tolerant individuals, and/or use in combination with other sedative drugs. Injection of take-away medication can also result in overdose, damage to veins, or other health consequences. All patients in receipt of take-away doses should have an inspection of their veins at regular clinical review. People with evidence of continued injection should have take-away doses suspended until they show evidence that injecting has ceased. Diversion of take-away doses can result in poor outcomes for the patient due to poor compliance with the treatment regimen and abuse by other individuals.

Uncontrolled access to take-away doses is associated with greater diversion and adverse consequences, including bringing the program into disrepute. The safety of take-away doses of methadone is increased by careful selection of suitable patients, close patient monitoring by the prescriber and dispenser, and patient education.

Take-away doses for interstate or overseas travel must be organized by the prescriber through the jurisdictional authorities responsible for controlling methadone. The Coordinating and Information Resource Center for International Travel by Patients Receiving Methadone and other Substitution Treatments for Opiate Addiction ('The Travel Resource Center') provides information and advice on importation regulations for methadone and on the possibilities of maintaining treatment abroad in over 190 countries as well as a range of other topics related to international travel by methadone patients. The information is aimed at both patients and doctors and is available at http://www.indro-online.de/nia.htm.

Missed doses and reintroduction

When patients miss methadone doses they may use other drugs including other CNS depressants such as alcohol or benzodiazepines. When methadone doses are missed for 3 or more days, tolerance to opioids may be reduced, thus placing patients at increased risk of overdose when methadone is reintroduced.

Reintroduction

Patients should be assessed for signs of intoxication and withdrawal before dosing is recommenced after missed doses. If the dose has not been collected for 3 or more consecutive days the dose should be withheld or reduced until the patient has been assessed by the prescriber.

In general, the following schedule can be presumed to be safe and effective. If the patient has missed:

- 1 day – there should be no change in dose
- 2 days – the normal dose can be administered if there is no evidence of intoxication
- 3.days – administer half a dose in discussion with the prescriber
- 4 days – the patient must be reviewed by their prescriber. Recommence dosing at 40 mg or half dose, whichever is the lower
- 5 days or more – regard the patient as a new induction to methadone.

Cessation of methadone maintenance treatment

Voluntary withdrawal

Factors that motivate patients to consider detoxification include lifestyle issues, tangible and intangible personal rewards, and perceptions and attitudes directed towards methadone.

Length of time in treatment

Studies have found the length of time in treatment is predictive of an improved treatment outcome. This relationship was evident for durations between 3 months and 2 years and was linear. A significant reduction in heroin use after treatment was only observed for those who spent more than 1 year in MMT. Significant reductions in criminality were observed only while patients remained in treatment. The findings of multiple observational studies indicate that it is a combination of treatment duration and behavior change including ceasing heroin use, a stable relationship, and maintaining employment during treatment which predicts positive post-treatment outcomes. It is recommended that patients be encouraged to remain in treatment for at least 12 months to achieve enduring lifestyle changes.

Management of withdrawal from MMT

Dose reductions should be made in consultation with the patient. Continued reduction in the face of distress is usually counterproductive. It may be appropriate to maintain a patient at a reduced dose for a prolonged period until the patient feels comfortable recommencing the reduction regimen. During this phase the aim of any intervention is to ensure that the withdrawal process is completed with safety and comfort.

When a regimen of reducing doses of methadone is used to manage withdrawal from heroin or methadone, typically signs and symptoms of withdrawal will begin to rise as the methadone dose falls below 20 mg/day, with peak symptoms occurring 2 to 3 days after cessation of methadone. Subsidence of the symptoms is slow, with studies reporting withdrawal scores not falling below baseline until 10 to 20 days after the cessation of methadone, depending on the duration of the methadone taper.

Clonidine offers no benefit as an adjunct to a regimen of reducing doses of methadone, primarily because of a high incidence of hypotensive side-effects when clonidine is used in this way. Clonidine can be given after cessation of methadone to manage withdrawal symptoms.

Voluntary withdrawal schedule

Recommend reducing the dose by 10 mg/week to a level of 40 mg/day, then 5 mg/week. Rates of reduction should be negotiated with patients, and dose changes should occur no more frequently than once a week.

Abrupt cessation of methadone could be considered from 40 mg/day in conjunction with clonidine and symptomatic medications to manage withdrawal signs and symptoms. Other approaches to the management of opioid withdrawal that have been the subject of research in recent years include the use of buprenorphine to ameliorate the signs of symptoms of withdrawal, and the use of opioid antagonists to induce withdrawal. The efficacy of these approaches to manage withdrawal from MMT remains uncertain.

Risk of relapse

Longer duration and greater intensity of pretreatment opioid use is associated with an increased probability of relapse to opioid use after leaving treatment. The likelihood of a patient maintaining abstinence after leaving treatment is increased in people who have established drug-free social supports, are in stable family situations, employed, and have good psychological strengths.

Supportive care and after care

There is evidence from RCTs that structured after care reduced the risk of relapse and self-reported crime, and facilitated unemployed patients finding employment. Supportive care should be offered for at least 6 months following cessation of methadone. For recently discharged patients an automatic fast track for readmission to MMT should be available if needed.

Involuntary withdrawal

It is sometimes necessary to discharge a patient from treatment for the safety or well-being of the patient, other patients, or staff. This may be the result of violence or threat of violence against staff or other patients, property damage or theft from the methadone program, drug dealing on or near program premises, or repeated diversion of methadone.

Interruption to treatment may also occur as the result of a change in the patient's situation such that they are no longer able to access methadone.

Management of involuntary discharge from MMT

In some instances problems may be resolved by transferring the patient to another program rather than discharging them from methadone. Abrupt cessation of methadone or rapid dose reduction may occasionally be warranted in cases of violence, assault, or threatened assault against staff or patients.

Where treatment is interrupted for less severe breaches of clinic rules or for other reasons, patients should, where possible, be withdrawn to 40 mg/day according to the above voluntary withdrawal schedule. Patients being discharged must be warned about the risks of illicit drug use and informed of other treatment options.

Transfer to naltrexone

Administration of naltrexone to a patient who is physically dependent on opioids will precipitate a severe withdrawal syndrome. MMT patients being transferred to naltrexone should undergo methadone detoxification followed by a 14-day drug-free period to allow methadone to be eliminated from the body. Seek specialist advice if it is not possible to follow this regimen.

Transfer to buprenorphine

Buprenorphine has a higher affinity for μ opioid receptors than methadone, but has a weaker action at these receptors. Consequently, when methadone patients take a dose of buprenorphine, methadone is displaced from the μ opioid receptors.

Patients on low doses of methadone of less than 30 mg per day generally tolerate this transfer with minimal discomfort. Patients on higher doses of methadone may find that replacement of methadone with buprenorphine precipitates transient opioid withdrawal.

Very low doses of buprenorphine of 2 mg are generally not adequate to substitute for methadone, while higher doses of 8 mg or more are more likely to precipitate withdrawal.

Buprenorphine should not be dispensed within 24 hours of the last methadone dose. The first dose of buprenorphine should be delayed as long as possible and ideally until there are signs of withdrawal such as lacrimation, rhinorrhea, and piloerection. Increasing the interval between the last dose of methadone and the first dose of buprenorphine reduces the incidence and severity of precipitated withdrawal. It is important that the patient is aware of the reason for the delay in dosing, and does not supplement the buprenorphine dose with other opioids (especially heroin) as this will further exacerbate withdrawal.

Common management issues

Side-effects

A number of resources are available for patients experiencing sleep problems which include guidance regarding sleep hygiene and simple relaxation techniques. Patients on methadone appear to be at increased risk of sleep apnea and the use of hypnotic drugs may therefore paradoxically worsen sleep by exacerbating sleep apnea.

All opioids including methadone reduce the production of saliva, while illicit use is associated with poor nutrition and poor dental hygiene. Consequently, dental problems are common for clients at entry to MMT. However, it is common for patients to blame methadone for their dental problems. Salivary flow can be increased by chewing. Encourage patients to improve dental hygiene.

Changes in libido and sexual function may be helped with a reduction in methadone dose, however this must be balanced against the risk of return to heroin use.

Elucidate the cause of excessive lethargy as the methadone dose may need to be reduced.

Excessive sweating may be reduced in line with a reduced dose of methadone. Sweating can also be a prominent symptom in withdrawal, so careful history-taking and observation of the patient prior to dosing may be necessary to assist in determining the cause of the sweating.

People rarely develop tolerance to the constipating effects of opioids and so many patients may experience chronic constipation. Encourage patients to consume plenty of fruits and vegetables and non-alcoholic fluids each day.

Overdose

In Australia, more than 90% of deaths during stabilization on methadone involved other drugs, in particular alcohol, benzodiazepines, and antidepressants. Patients should be warned of the risks associated with using other drugs with methadone.

Death following methadone induction often occurs at home during sleep, many hours after peak blood methadone concentrations have occurred. Typically, overdose occurs around the third or fourth day of methadone induction.

Given that many deaths occur during sleep, administration of methadone in the morning will ensure that peak methadone concentrations occur when patients are normally awake and there is an increased likelihood of other people being available for support if overdose should occur.

Naloxone, which promptly reverses opioid-induced coma, should be given as a prolonged infusion when treating methadone overdose. A single dose of naloxone will wear off within one hour, leaving the patient at risk of relapse into coma due to the long-lasting effects of methadone. Patients who are thought to have taken a methadone overdose require prolonged observation.

Family members should be warned that deep snoring during induction to treatment could be a sign of dangerous respiratory depression and should be reported to the prescriber. Heavy snoring during maintenance treatment may be associated with sleep apnea and should also be reported.

Signs and symptoms of methadone overdose include: pinpoint pupils, nausea, dizziness, feeling intoxicated, sedated, nodding off, unsteady gait, slurred speech, snoring, hypotension, slow pulse, shallow breathing, frothing at the mouth as an indicator of pulmonary edema, and coma. Symptoms may last for 24 hours or more. Death generally occurs from respiratory depression.

Intoxicated presentations

Patient safety is the key consideration in responding to those who present for methadone administration while intoxicated due to opioids, alcohol, or other drugs. Patients should always be assessed by the person responsible for dispensing the methadone before the dose is given. The assessment should ensure that the patient is not showing evidence of intoxication due to opioids, alcohol, or other drugs.

Patients who appear intoxicated with CNS depressant drugs should not be given their usual methadone dose or a take-away dose at that time. The patient can be asked to attend later when they are no longer intoxicated.

If intoxication is evident but appears mild the patient may be given a reduced dose, but only after being reviewed by the prescriber.

Incorrect dose administered

A patient who receives a methadone dose in excess of that prescribed is at risk of overdose. To prevent accidental methadone overdose establish procedures for easy and accurate identification of patients to minimize the risk of inappropriate dosing, and ensure that patients are informed of the risks and signs and symptoms of overdose.

In the case of an accidental overdose, the critical issues which determine how clinicians should respond are the patient's level of tolerance and the amount of methadone given in error. Patients in the first 2 weeks of methadone treatment who receive an overdose of any magnitude require observation for at least 4 hours after dosing. If signs of intoxication continue, more prolonged observation is required which may require sending the patient to an Emergency Department. Patients who have been on a dose >40 mg/day consistently for 2 months will generally tolerate an increased dose which is double that of their usual dose, without significant symptoms. For an overdose with greater than double the usual daily dose, the patient will require observation for at least 4 hours. If signs of intoxication are observed, more prolonged observation must be maintained.

If patients are receiving regular take-away doses, or if they do not attend daily, it cannot safely be assumed that they have been taking their daily dose and have a known level of tolerance. Therefore, such patients require observation in the event of overdose of >50% of their usual dose. Patients in whom the level of tolerance is uncertain with a methadone dose less than 40 mg/day, or who have been in treatment for less than 2 months, require observation for at least 4 hours if they are given a dose at least 50% higher than their usual dose.

In all cases of dosing error the following procedures should be followed:

- Overdose up to 50% of the normal dose: advise the patient of the mistake and carefully explain the possible consequences. Inform the patient about signs and symptoms of overdose and advise him/her to go to a hospital Emergency Department if any symptoms develop. The dispenser must advise the prescribing doctor of the dosing error and record the event.

- Overdose greater than 50% of the normal dose: advise the patient of the mistake and carefully explain the possible seriousness of the consequences. The dispenser must contact the prescribing doctor immediately. If the prescriber is unable to be contacted consult a drug and alcohol medical specialist. If it is decided by the prescriber or drug and alcohol specialist that the patient requires hospitalization, the reasons should be explained to the patient and they should be accompanied to the hospital to ensure admitting staff receive clear information on the circumstances. If the patient has left before the mistake is realized, every attempt must be made to contact the patient.

Inducing vomiting may be dangerous and is contraindicated if the patient has any signs of CNS depression. Emesis after the first 10 minutes is an unsatisfactory means of dealing with methadone overdose as it is impossible to determine if all of the dose has been eliminated. In circumstances where medical help is not readily available, or the patient refuses medical care, induction of vomiting (by mechanical stimulation of the pharynx) within 5 to 10 minutes of ingesting the dose may be appropriate as a first aid measure only. Ipecac syrup is contraindicated as its action may be delayed.

Continued high-risk drug use

Continued high-risk drug use is evidenced by: frequent presentations when intoxicated; overdoses; chaotic drug-using behavior; and deteriorating medical or mental states due to drug use.

Continued drug use can affect patient stability and treatment progress and place the patient at risk of relationship, social, and employment problems, contracting infectious diseases, and involvement in crime.

Attempts to stabilize such patients should include review of psychosocial interventions and supports, precipitants to continued drug use, and the risks of combining methadone with other drug use against the benefits of continued treatment.

If the patient's safety is not at risk from ongoing drug use it will generally be in the patient's interest to persist with treatment. If the risks of combining methadone with other drug use outweigh the benefits to the patient of MMT, arrange the patient's gradual withdrawal from methadone.

Increases in methadone dose may be helpful if this is considered safe by the prescriber.

Analgesia and anesthesia

Analgesic requirements for patients on methadone

Consider non-opioid analgesics such as NSAIDs or paracetamol. Where parenteral analgesics are required, consider ketorolac or tramadol.

Management of acute pain in hospital for patients on MMT

Patients on methadone who are experiencing acute pain in hospital often receive inadequate doses of opiates for serious pain. Analgesia should be provided to patients in MMT in the same way as for other patients. This includes the use of injectable and patient-controlled analgesia. Because of their tolerance of opioids, patients taking methadone frequently require larger doses of opioid analgesia for adequate pain relief. Partial agonists such as buprenorphine should be avoided as they may precipitate withdrawal symptoms. There is evidence of cross-tolerance between methadone and anesthetic agents and so patients on methadone may require higher doses of anesthetic agents in the event of dental or surgical procedures.

Management of patients with chronic pain

Patients needing methadone for ongoing management of chronic pain need a comprehensive management plan. It is recommended that specialist advice be sought regarding such patients.

Diversion of methadone

Diversion of methadone to illicit use can result in opioid overdose and undermines the therapeutic rationale and effectiveness of MMT. Injection of methadone carries significant additional risks including sorbitol toxicity, bacterial infection, and transmission of blood-borne viruses.

Research into methadone-related deaths has consistently shown that between one third and two thirds of all methadone-related deaths occurred in persons not prescribed methadone treatment. The major source of diverted methadone is take-away doses prescribed for patients in MMT.

The risk of diversion of prescribed methadone can be reduced by: ensuring that, in general, methadone is consumed under supervision; careful selection and monitoring of patients eligible to receive take-away doses taking into account the patient's stability, reliability, and progress in treatment; and by limiting the number of consecutive take-away doses.

Pregnancy and lactation

Pregnant women who are dependent on opioids are at high risk of experiencing complications, generally as a result of: inadequate antenatal care; lifestyle factors including smoking, poor nutrition, high levels of stress, and deprivation; and repeated cycles of intoxication and withdrawal which can harm the fetus or precipitate premature labor or miscarriage.

In most Australian jurisdictions, pregnant opioid-dependent women have high priority for access to methadone maintenance programs in order to minimize the risk of complications.

Methadone maintenance treatment enables stabilization of drug use and lifestyle, reduces or eliminates illicit opioid drug use and can help stabilize the in utero environment, facilitates access to comprehensive antenatal and postnatal care, and does not increase the risk of congenital abnormalities in the fetus.

Methadone is classed as a Pregnancy Category C drug in Australia because of the potential risk of respiratory depression in the neonate and the likelihood of neonatal withdrawal syndrome. Respiratory depression is not a significant problem in babies born to opioid-dependent mothers receiving methadone maintenance treatment. Babies born to mothers on MMT may experience a withdrawal syndrome. Available evidence gives little support to the existence of a relationship between the severity of the neonatal withdrawal syndrome and maternal methadone dose at delivery, and its occurrence is unpredictable. The benefits of methadone maintenance treatment for both the mother and the baby outweigh any risks from the neonatal withdrawal syndrome.

Management in pregnancy

Opioid-using pregnant women not already in treatment should be given high priority for assessment. Naloxone challenge should not be used in pregnant women because this may precipitate miscarriage or premature labor. Pregnant women should be maintained on an adequate dose of methadone, to achieve stability and prevent relapse or continued illicit opioid drug use. Women already in methadone treatment who become pregnant can safely be maintained on their current dose.

The bioavailability of methadone is decreased in the later stages of pregnancy due to increased plasma volume, an increase in plasma proteins which bind methadone, and placental metabolism of methadone. It may be necessary to divide the daily dose and possibly to increase the dose in the third trimester of pregnancy to avoid withdrawal symptoms and minimize additional drug use.

Antenatal and postnatal care should be managed in collaboration with a specialist obstetric service experienced in the management of drug dependency during pregnancy.

Dose reductions or detoxification during pregnancy

Opioid withdrawal in the first trimester of pregnancy is thought to be associated with an increased risk of miscarriage. Opioid withdrawal in the third trimester of pregnancy may be associated with fetal distress and death. Therefore, it is important that pregnant women are not exposed to withdrawal during the first and third trimesters.

If dose reductions or detoxification are to be undertaken during pregnancy these should be implemented in the second trimester and only if the pregnancy is stable. The magnitude and rate of reduction needs to be flexible and responsive to the symptoms experienced by the woman concerned. Careful monitoring of the pregnancy and fetus should be undertaken during dose reduction. In most instances, dose reductions of 2.5 mg to 5 mg per week are considered safe and withdrawal is avoided.

Breastfeeding

Breast milk contains only small amounts of methadone and mothers can be encouraged to breastfeed regardless of methadone dose provided that they are not using other drugs. Breastfeeding may reduce the severity of the neonatal withdrawal syndrome. Women receiving high doses of methadone should be advised to wean their babies slowly to avoid withdrawal in the infant.

Neonatal withdrawal syndrome

The occurrence and severity of neonatal withdrawal is very unpredictable. Severity of withdrawal is probably ameliorated if neonates can be kept with their mothers rather than in the neonatal intensive care nursery, which may be stressful and overstimulating. However, this is not always possible.

All babies born to opioid-dependent mothers should be observed by experienced staff for the development of withdrawal signs. It is recommended that a validated scale be used to assess the presence and severity of the neonatal withdrawal syndrome.

Common signs include: irritability and sleep disturbances, sneezing, fist sucking, a shrill cry, watery stools, general hyperactivity, ineffectual sucking, poor weight gain, dislike of bright lights, tremors, and increased respiration rate. Less common signs include: yawning, vomiting, increased mucus production, increased response to sound, and convulsions (rare).

Withdrawal symptoms usually start within 48 hours of delivery, but may be delayed for 7–14 days in a small number of cases. Experience in the US suggests that in cases where withdrawal is delayed it may be because methadone was being used in conjunction with illicit benzodiazepines and the infant is actually withdrawing from the benzodiazepines.

Supportive treatment of neonatal withdrawal syndrome involves minimizing environmental stimuli and enhancing the baby's comfort and may include: soothing by holding close to the body or swaddling, keeping nostrils and mouth clear of secretions, use of a dummy to relieve increased sucking urge, and frequent small feeds.

Treatment with opioids should be considered for infants who exhibit severe withdrawal symptoms. Indications for treatment include: seizure, weight loss due to poor feeding, diarrhea, vomiting and dehydration, poor sleep, and fever.

Treatment should be based on the severity of the withdrawal signs. Use of the Finnegan Screening Instrument is recommended. Treatment should be commenced when the score is 9 or more on two consecutive observations. Improvement should be monitored using scores on the screening tool. Specialist advice should be sought. Treatment with opioids may depress respiration and should be used with extreme caution. Options to be considered include:

- morphine oral preparation – 2 mg/ml morphine dilution which can be further diluted if necessary
- tincture of opium – 0.4 mg/ml dilution
- paregoric (camphorated tincture of opium)
- methadone.

Treatment with opioids should be used with extreme caution. It is recommended that neonatal care be managed in collaboration with a specialist obstetric or pediatric service which is experienced in the management of babies born to drug-dependent mothers.

Polydrug use

Polydrug use is prevalent among opioid users. One in 5 patients seeking MMT are likely also to be dependent on benzodiazepines, 1 in 20 are likely to be alcohol dependent, and high percentages of patients are likely to be using benzodiazepines or alcohol at hazardous or harmful levels.

Patients at high risk from polydrug use frequently present intoxicated or with signs of benzodiazepine or alcohol withdrawal, and regularly use other drugs at levels above normal therapeutic doses. It is recommended that specialist advice be sought when treating patients at high risk from polydrug use, especially where sedatives are involved.

Benzodiazepine users exhibit overall patterns of increased risk and poorer psychological functioning than other patients. Benzodiazepine injection is associated with vascular damage as well as mortality. Over the years, injection of the gel capsule formulation of temazepam has been reported to lead to limb amputations. This formulation was withdrawn in Australia in March 2004 due to increased abuse and intentional misuse. Advise patients about the interactions of benzodiazepines and methadone. Caution should be exercised in prescribing benzodiazepines for patients in MMT. The clinical supervision of patients receiving maintenance benzodiazepines must be of the same standard as that provided for MMT.

HIV

Methadone treatment programs should ensure that HIV-positive patients have access to specialist HIV medical care so that the patient's overall health may be monitored and appropriate treatment provided as required.

In general, patients who are HIV positive are able to comply with the requirements and conditions of the program, however the medical, psychological, and social implications of HIV infection may necessitate the provision of additional services. Methadone doses must be monitored due to the potential for interactions between methadone and HIV medications and the effects of related illnesses. Higher methadone doses may be necessary if HIV medications increase methadone metabolism.

Flexibility in dosing arrangements may be needed if patients are unable to attend for daily dosing due to illness. This may need to be negotiated with the responsible jurisdictional authority. Options include collection of daily methadone dose by a responsible adult, home deliveries, and take-away doses.

In the terminal stages of HIV/AIDS, methadone service providers may need to work with hospice services in managing methadone treatment and AIDS-linked conditions.

Hepatitis B and C

Hepatitis B

Hepatitis B vaccinations are recommended to all patients on the methadone program who are found to have no immunity to the hepatitis B virus. Patients who are acutely infected or who are chronic carriers of hepatitis B should be referred to a gastroenterologist for specialist assessment and follow-up.

Hepatitis C

A high percentage of patients entering methadone programs will be hepatitis C antibody positive. Patients should be managed in accordance with the RACGP supplement *Hepatitis C. A management guide for general practitioners*[3] and the RACGP Australian Family Physician *Hepatitis C update.*[4]

Patients who are hepatitis C antibody positive but who have three normal serum alanine aminotransferase (ALT) and aspartate aminotransferase (AST) results over 6 months should have liver function tests repeated at 6-monthly intervals and a hepatitis C polymerase chain reaction test at 12 months. If the patient has three abnormal serum aminotransferase results over 6 months, a referral to a gastroenterologist or liver clinic for specialist assessment and shared care is indicated.

Impaired liver function

Patients with chronic liver disease on long-term methadone maintenance generally do not need dose alterations but abrupt changes in liver function might necessitate substantial dose adjustments.

Psychiatric comorbidity

Many opioid users exhibit symptoms of anxiety and depression at the time of presentation for treatment. Most, but not all studies link psychiatric distress to poorer treatment outcome. Multiple studies have indicated that MMT can reduce levels of psychiatric distress, with improvement apparent within weeks of commencement of treatment. After stabilization on methadone, all patients need to be rescreened for psychiatric disorders. A careful and detailed mental state examination will usually suffice.

Psychotherapy as an adjunct to MMT may benefit patients with medium and high levels of psychiatric problems, but for those with low-severity psychiatric problems the addition of psychotherapy offers no advantage. Depression has been found to predict poor psycho-social functioning and to increase the risk of relapse to heroin use in the event of life crises. Evidence of the effectiveness of antidepressants as adjuncts to MMT is equivocal, with only a few studies demonstrating favorable effects on mood. One Australian cohort study found antidepressant use was associated with higher levels of polydrug use, poorer health and higher levels of psychiatric distress, and a greater risk of heroin overdose. The excess risk of overdose was specifically associated with tricyclic antidepressants.

References

1. American Psychiatric Association. Diagnostic and statistical manual of mental disorders. 4th ed. Washington, DC: American Psychiatric Association; 1994.
2. Jarvis T, Shand F, Tebbutt J, Mattick R. Treatment approaches for alcohol and drug dependence: an introductory guide. 2nd ed. Chichester, UK: Wiley, 2005.
3. Royal Australian College of General Practitioners. Hepatitis C. A management guide for general practitioners. Australian Family Physician 1999; 28(Special Issue).
4. Royal Australian College of General Practitioners. Hepatitis C update. Australian Family Physician 2003; 32(10).

Further reading

Avants SK, Margolin A, Sindelar JL, et al. Day treatment versus enhanced standard methadone services for opioid dependent patients: a comparison of clinical efficacy and cost. Am J Psychiat 1999; 156(1): 27–33.

Department of Health, The Scottish Office Department of Health, Welsh Office, Department of Health and Social Services Northern Ireland. Drug Misuse and Dependence – Guidelines on Clinical Management. Norwich, UK: Her Majesty's Stationery Office: 1999.

Dilppoliti D, Davoli M, Perrucci CA, Pasqualini F, Bargagli AM. Retention in treatment of heroin users in Italy: the role of treatment type and methadone maintenance dosage. Drug Alcohol Depen 1998; 52: 167–71.

Drug and Alcohol Services Council 1994 Private Methadone Program. Policies and Procedures. Adelaide: Drug and Alcohol Seniors Council.

Gowing, LR, Ali, RL, White J. The management of opioid withdrawal: an overview of research literature. DASC Monograph No 9, Research Series. Drug & Alcohol Services Council, 2000.

Griffith JD, Rowan-Szal GA, Roark RR, Simpson DD. Contingency management in outpatient methadone treatment: a meta-analysis. Drug Alcohol Depen 2000; 58(1): 55–66.

Humeniuk R, Ali R, White J, Hall W, Farrell M, eds. Proceedings of expert workshop on the induction and stabilisation of patients onto methadone. National Drug Strategy Monograph 39. Commonwealth Department of Health and Aged Care, Canberra: 2000.

Jarvis T, Tebbutt J, Mattick R, Shand F. Treatment Approaches for Alcohol and Drug Dependence. 2nd edn. Sussex, UK: Wiley, 2005.

Latowsky M. Improving detoxification outcomes from methadone maintenance treatment: the interrelationship of affective states and protracted withdrawal. J Psychoactive Drugs 1996; 28(3): 251–7.

Mental Health and Drug and Alcohol Office, NSW Department of Health. Opioid Treatment Program: Clinical Guidelines for Methadone and Buprenorphine Treatment. Sydney: NSW Department of Health, 2006.

Nunes EV, Quitkin FM, Donovan SJ, et al. Imipramine treatment of opiate dependent patients with depressive disorders. Arch Gen Psychiat 1998; 55: 153–60.

Petry NM. A comprehensive guide to the application of contingency management procedures in clinical settings. Drug Alcohol Depend 2000; 58(1): 9–25.

Preston A. The New Zealand Methadone Briefing 1999. Drugs and Health Development Project. Wellington New Zealand: 1999.

Prochaska JO, DiClemente CC, Norcross JC. In search of how people change: applications to addictive behaviours. In: Addictive Behaviours: Readings on etiology, prevention and treatment. Marlatt GA, VandenBos GF, eds. Washington DC: American Psychological Association, 1997; 671–96.

Strain EC, Bigelow GE, Liebson IA, Stitzer ML. Moderate versus high dose methadone in the treatment of opioid dependence: a randomised controlled trial. JAMA 1999: 281(11): 1000–5.

Ward J, Mattick R, Hall W, eds. Methadone maintenance treatment and other opioid replacement therapies. Harwood Academic Publishers, Amsterdam: 1998.

chapter 12

National clinical guidelines and procedures for the use of buprenorphine in the treatment of heroin dependence

Nicholas Lintzeris, Nicholas Clark, Peter Muhleisen, Alison Ritter, Robert Ali, James Bell, Linda Gowing, Lynn Hawkin, Sue Henry-Edwards, Richard P Mattick, Benny Monheit, Irvin Newton, Allan Quigley, Sue Whicker, and Jason White

Introduction

Buprenorphine in sublingual tablet form (Subutex®) is registered in Australia for the management of opioid dependence including maintenance and detoxification, within a framework of medical, social, and psychological treatment. This preparation is effective both in the long term, as a maintenance treatment program, and in the short term as part of a heroin withdrawal program. To assist in the safe and effective implementation of buprenorphine treatment in Australia, the following national guidelines were commissioned by the Commonwealth Department of Health and Aged Care under the auspices of the National Expert Advisory Committee on Illicit Drugs (NEACID).

These guidelines cover both the maintenance and withdrawal programs using buprenorphine. Section 1 explains the clinical pharmacology of buprenorphine; Section 2 covers the commencement of treatment with buprenorphine; Section 5, complications and adverse events; and Section 6 prescribing and dispensing issues. In each of these sections, both maintenance and withdrawal programs are covered. In Sections 3 and 4, however, guidelines and procedures are set out separately for each program with maintenance treatment addressed in Section 3, and withdrawal programs in Section 4.

This set of guidelines has been developed through a consensus process by a working party of senior Australian clinicians and researchers with experience in the use of buprenorphine in a variety of jurisdictions. The original draft of the maintenance guidelines for this project was developed as part of the Buprenorphine Implementation Trial by the Turning Point Alcohol and Drug Centre. The *Clinical Guidelines for the Buprenorphine Implementation Trial* were piloted by over 20 medical practitioners, both specialists and general practitioners, and 30 pharmacies involved in delivering buprenorphine maintenance treatment. In addition to the patients, doctors, pharmacists, and researchers participants of the Buprenorphine Implementation Trial, the following individuals have contributed to the development of these clinical guidelines: In the USA: Paul Fudala, Alice Huber, Ed Johnson, Surita Lao, Walter Ling, Laura McNicholas, Boris Meandzija, Charles O'Brien, Richard Rawson, Richard Schottenfeld, and George Woody. In France: Marc Auricombe. In the UK: Fergus Law, Judith Myles, David Nutt, Chris Chapleo, and Don Walter. And in Australia: Louise Rushworth, Reckitt Benkizer; Gabriele Bammer, National Centre for Population Health and Epidemiology; Adrian Dunlop, Nadine Ezard, Alan Gisbjers, Sandra Hocking, Jozica Kutin, Paul Murray, and Greg Whelan.

The guidelines have been endorsed by the Royal Australian College of General Practitioners, the Royal Australian College of Physicians, and the Australian Professional Society on Alcohol and other Drugs.

The contribution of Ms Elizabeth Vorrath, Medical Editor, in ensuring that the guidelines are clear and easy to read is gratefully acknowledged.

Clinical pharmacology

General information

What is buprenorphine?

Buprenorphine is a derivative of the morphine alkaloid thebaine, and is a partial opioid agonist at the μ opioid receptors in the nervous system. It is also an opioid receptor antagonist at the κ opioid receptors. It has low intrinsic agonist activity, only partially activating μ opioid receptors, thus producing a milder, less euphoric, and less sedating effect than full opioid agonists such as heroin, morphine, and methadone. Nevertheless, its activity is usually sufficient to diminish cravings for heroin, and prevent or alleviate opioid withdrawal in dependent heroin users. Buprenorphine also has a high affinity for μ opioid receptors, binding more tightly to these receptors than full opioid agonists. It therefore reduces the impact of additional heroin or other opioid use, by preventing the opioid from occupying these receptors. By its dual effects of producing opioid responses while blocking the effects of additional heroin use, buprenorphine reduces the self-administration of heroin.

What form does it come in?

The buprenorphine product registered in Australia for treating opioid dependence is Subutex®, a sublingual tablet preparation of buprenorphine hydrochloride in 0.4, 2, and 8 mg strengths. Buprenorphine is also registered in Australia for the management of short-term relief of moderate to severe pain, including post-operative and terminal and chronic pain, as Temgesic® sublingual tablets and ampoules for intramuscular or subcutaneous injection. Sublingual buprenorphine tablets have approximately 30–35% of the bioavailability of intravenous buprenorphine preparations. Buprenorphine undergoes extensive first-pass metabolism when taken orally.

How is it metabolized?

Peak plasma concentrations are achieved 1–2 hours after sublingual administration. Buprenorphine has a distribution half-life of 2–5 hours. It is principally metabolized by two hepatic pathways: conjugation with glucuronic acid and *N*-dealkylation. The metabolites are excreted in the biliary system, with enterohepatic cycling of buprenorphine and its metabolites. Most of the drug is excreted in the feces and urine.

Buprenorphine has an elimination half-life of 24–37 hours. It is long acting, relative to the dose administered. Peak clinical effects occur 1–4 hours after sublingual administration, with continued effects for up to 12 hours at low doses (2 mg), but as long as 48–72 hours at higher doses (16 or 32 mg). The extended duration of action of buprenorphine is thought to relate to three factors: a very high affinity for opioid μ receptors (once bound to these receptors it is dislodged only slowly); a high lipophilicity (low levels of buprenorphine are released slowly from fat stores, particularly with chronic dosing); and reabsorption of buprenorphine after intestinal hydrolysis of the conjugated metabolite.

The prolonged duration of effect at high doses enables alternate-day, and even 3 days a week dispensing regimens.

The majority of early studies with sublingual buprenorphine used a liquid solution of buprenorphine in 30% aqueous ethanol, with a bioavailability of approximately 40% of subcutaneous preparations. The commercial sublingual tablet preparation of buprenorphine (Subutex®) is reported as having 50–80% of the bioavailability of the ethanol solution.[1] In practice, sublingual tablet doses should be approximately 50% greater than sublingual solution doses referred to in earlier research studies; for example, an 8 mg sublingual solution corresponds approximately to a 12 mg sublingual tablet.

Buprenorphine also exhibits antagonist effects at the κ opioid receptor. The role of these receptors in humans is still poorly understood, but excess endogenous κ agonist activity appears to be implicated in both affective and psychotic conditions. Buprenorphine's antagonist effects at the κ receptor are thought to produce antidepressant and antipsychotic effects in some people. However, as further research is needed into these effects, buprenorphine is not currently indicated for these conditions.

Withdrawal syndrome from buprenorphine

Its partial agonist properties, along with its slow dissociation from opioid receptors, are thought to explain why opioid withdrawal syndrome is milder with the cessation of buprenorphine treatment, than with heroin, morphine, or methadone.

Typically, the withdrawal syndrome following the abrupt cessation of long-term buprenorphine treatment emerges within 3 to 5 days of the last dose, and mild withdrawal features continue for up to several weeks. Treatment with opioid antagonists such as naltrexone can be commenced within days of the cessation of low-dose buprenorphine treatment without precipitating severe opioid withdrawal. This enables patients to transfer promptly to naltrexone treatment, and avoid relapse and treatment drop-out. By contrast, naltrexone is not usually started until 10 to 14 days after the cessation of methadone.

Safety and side-effects

Dose–response studies show that, because of its ceiling effects, high doses of 16 mg daily or more do not result in substantially greater peak opioid effects than lower doses of 8 or 12 mg. Doses many times greater than normal therapeutic doses appear to be well tolerated, and rarely result in clinically significant respiratory depression, even in non-opioid-tolerant individuals.

The safety of buprenorphine mixed with high doses of other sedative drugs, such as alcohol or benzodiazepines, is still unclear with several deaths having been reported. Naloxone is of limited use in resuscitating individuals who have overdosed on high doses of buprenorphine.

Precaution should be exercised when buprenorphine is administered concomitantly with CYP3A4 inhibitors such as protease inhibitors, some drugs in the class of azole antimycotics such as ketoconazole, or calcium channel antagonists such as nifedipine and macrolide antibiotics as this may lead to increased plasma concentrations of buprenorphine.

The side-effects of buprenorphine are similar to those of other opioids, the most common being constipation, disturbed sleep, drowsiness, sweating, headaches, and nausea.

Many patients report less sedation on buprenorphine than on methadone. Like all opioid medications, buprenorphine may affect the capacity of patients to drive or operate machinery during the early stages of treatment or following dose increases. It appears to have minimal impact on hepatic function, although its effects in very high doses remain unclear.

Under certain circumstances, buprenorphine may precipitate opioid withdrawal symptoms 1–4 hours after the first dose. It has a higher affinity and lower intrinsic activity than agonists such as methadone, morphine, or heroin. Consequently, buprenorphine displaces agonists from opioid receptors and in the short term may not produce sufficient agonist effects to compensate for the displaced methadone or heroin, producing opioid withdrawal as the buprenorphine reaches its peak effects about 1 to 4 hours after initial administration. The phenomenon of precipitated withdrawal has particular clinical relevance during the induction of heroin users and methadone patients.

Drug interactions

The principal drug interactions of buprenorphine relate to its opioid activity. Buprenorphine exerts additive sedative effects when used in conjunction with other sedating medications. These include other opioids, benzodiazepines, alcohol, tricyclic antidepressants, sedating antihistamines, and major tranquilizers. A number of deaths have been reported involving the combination of buprenorphine with benzodiazepines and other sedatives.

Buprenorphine has higher affinity for μ opioid receptors than the opioid antagonists. In the event of overdose with buprenorphine, very high doses of naloxone of between 10 and 35 mg are required to reverse its effects. Naltrexone can precipitate a delayed withdrawal reaction in patients on buprenorphine.

Buprenorphine exerts a degree of blockade to the effects of full agonist opioids, which may complicate the use of additional opioids for analgesia. The initial dose of buprenorphine can precipitate opioid withdrawal in patients with high levels of neuroadaptation to full opioid agonists.

Buprenorphine is metabolized by the hepatic microsomal CYP3A4 enzyme system. While current evidence is inconclusive, it is thought that the concurrent use of medications which induce or inhibit microsomal enzyme activity will have minimal clinical impact on buprenorphine dosing requirements.

Entry into buprenorphine treatment

Suitability for treatment with buprenorphine

The following guidelines should be taken into account when considering a person's suitability for treatment with buprenorphine in either the maintenance or the withdrawal program.

Buprenorphine treatment is only indicated for those who are opioid dependent.

Diagnostic definition of opioid dependence (DSM-IV)

'A maladaptive pattern of substance use leading to clinically significant impairment or distress as manifested by three or more of the following, occurring at any time in the same 12 month period.'

- Tolerance as defined by either a need for markedly increased amounts of opioids to achieve intoxication or desired effect, or a markedly diminished effect with continued use of the same amount of opioids.
- Withdrawal as manifested by either the characteristic withdrawal syndrome for opioids, or opioids, or a closely related substance, being taken to relieve or avoid withdrawal symptoms.
- Opioids often taken in larger amounts or over longer period than intended.
- A persistent desire or unsuccessful attempts to cut down or control opioid use.
- A great deal of time regularly spent in activities necessary to obtain opioids, use opioids, or recover from their effects.
- Important social, occupational, or recreational activities given up or reduced because of opioid use.
- The opioid use continued, despite knowledge of having a persistent or recurrent physical or psychological problem that is likely to have been caused or exacerbated by opioids.

Neuroadaptation to opioids

Evidence of neuroadaptation or physical dependence includes tolerance of the opioid and onset of withdrawal syndrome on stopping or decreasing use.

Neuroadaptation is not a prerequisite for the diagnosis of drug dependence. However, in the absence of neuroadaptation, the prescribing medical practitioner must clearly demonstrate potential benefits to the individual's health and well-being that outweigh the potential disadvantages of buprenorphine treatment, and alternative treatment options should be carefully considered.

The patient must be at least 18 years of age. The prescribing doctor should seek a second or specialist opinion before treating anyone under 18 years of age. While buprenorphine has been registered for administration to people aged 16 and over, caution should be exercised in prescribing a drug of dependence for anyone in the 16–17 age group.

The patient must be able to provide proof of identity – a requirement for treatment with any S8 medication.

The patient must also be capable of giving informed consent to treatment with buprenorphine.

Contraindications

Anyone with known hypersensitivity and/or severe side-effects from previous exposure to buprenorphine is ineligible for buprenorphine treatment.

Pregnant women and nursing mothers are also ineligible at this stage, as there is insufficient evidence that buprenorphine is safe for either the developing fetus or the breastfed neonate, and there is evidence of harm in other species. Developmental toxicity studies of buprenorphine in pregnant rats and rabbits have shown fetotoxicity, including post-implantation loss, and decreased post-natal survival with no evidence of teratogenicity. The described effects occurred at systemic exposures similar to the maximum anticipated human dose of 32 mg/day. In addition, maternal oral administration at high doses of 80 mg/kg/day during gestation and lactation resulted in a slight delay in the development of some neurologic functions in neonatal rats. In humans there is currently not sufficient data to evaluate potential teratogenic or fetotoxic effects of buprenorphine in pregnancy. However, high doses even for short durations may induce respiratory depression in neonates. During the last 3 months of pregnancy, chronic use of buprenorphine may be responsible for a withdrawal syndrome in neonates.

Animal studies indicate buprenorphine has the potential to inhibit lactation. Buprenorphine passes into the mother's milk, therefore breastfeeding while using buprenorphine is contraindicated until its safety has been fully established.

Severe respiratory or hepatic insufficiency is also a contraindication for buprenorphine treatment.

Precautions

Particular caution should be exercised when assessing the suitability of buprenorphine treatment for anyone with any of the following clinical conditions.

All opioid substitution treatments should be approached with caution in individuals using other drugs, particularly sedative drugs such as alcohol, benzodiazepines, or antidepressants. Particular emphasis should be given to assessing the level of neuroadaptation to opioids, the likelihood of continued use of other sedative drugs, and overdose risk.

Buprenorphine is an opioid medication and caution should be exercised in using it in patients with recent head injury, increased intracranial pressure, or acute abdominal conditions.

Buprenorphine, like other opioids, should be used with caution in patients with chronic obstructive airways disease or cor pulmonale, and in individuals with a substantially decreased respiratory reserve, pre-existing respiratory depression, hypoxia, or hypercapnea. In such patients, even normally safe therapeutic doses of opioids may decrease respiratory drive whilst simultaneously increasing airways resistance to the point of apnea.

Caution needs to be taken in considering buprenorphine treatment for people with clinically significant hepatic failure. Severe hepatic disease may alter the hepatic metabolism of the medication. However, the presence of elevated enzyme levels on liver function testing, in the absence of clinical evidence of liver failure, does not exclude someone from treatment with buprenorphine.

Opioids should only be given with caution, and at a reduced initial dose, to patients with any of the following conditions: advanced age or debilitation; prostatic hypertrophy or urethral stricture; pre-existing diabetes mellitus or a predisposition to it, with the possibility of increases in serum glucose on buprenorphine; and severe renal disease.

Opioid substitution treatment should not be initiated in anyone with acute psychosis, severe depression, or other psychiatric conditions which severely compromise the capacity to give informed consent. The first priority should be an attempt to manage and stabilize the psychiatric condition. People at moderate or high risk of suicide should not be commenced on buprenorphine without adequate supervision, and specialist advice should be sought.

Buprenorphine may be used as an analgesic in the management of acute and chronic pain conditions, but at much lower doses than for heroin dependence. Ideally, chronic pain is best managed under the supervision of a specialist multidisciplinary team, and appropriate referral or consultation should be considered.

Buprenorphine may cause difficulties in transferring from methadone by precipitating withdrawal. This is most likely to occur in patients on high doses of methadone, and attempts to reduce the methadone dose to below 60 mg, and preferably below 40 mg, should be made before initiating buprenorphine. Methadone patients who relapse into regular heroin use following the reduction of their methadone dose are likely to find transition to buprenorphine difficult, if not unachievable.

Assessment procedures

A careful assessment should be conducted at the outset of buprenorphine treatment. It is recommended that the patient history include: heroin and other opioid use including quantity and frequency, duration, route of administration, when last used, and features and severity of dependence; use of other drugs including benzodiazepines, alcohol, cannabis, and psychostimulants; participation in high-risk drug behaviors; history of prior attempts at treatment; social circumstance including home environment, social supports, employment, and barriers to change; medical and psychiatric history, with particular attention to unstable or active conditions which might potentially complicate treatment; pregnancy and contraception; motivations and goals for treatment.

The examination should include: vital signs – blood pressure, pulse, and respiratory rate; evidence of intoxication or withdrawal from heroin or other drugs; and evidence of complications of injecting drug use, including injection site problems, hepatic disease, lymphadenopathy, and systemic infections.

Urinary drug screens can be helpful in clarifying or confirming an unclear drug use history. However, delays in getting the results of routine urine tests often limit their usefulness at initial assessment.

Liver function tests and viral serology (HIV, hepatitis B and C) should be considered at some stage with appropriate pre- and post-test counseling. This is advisable after stabilization, when the patient is better able to understand the significance and consequences of testing.

A comprehensive assessment for buprenorphine treatment can rarely be completed at the initial appointment, and generally needs to be conducted over several sessions. Initially, clinicians should target key issues important in the selection and initiation of treatment, and assess indications, contraindications, and precautions. Referral or consultation with a specialist is recommended for patients with complex presentations.

Informed consent and patient literature

The participation of an informed patient in the clinical decision-making process is important in the treatment of all opioid dependence. It is particularly important when incorporating opioid medications – such as buprenorphine or methadone – as part of the treatment plan. In considering the commencement of buprenorphine for maintenance or withdrawal treatment, the service provider should also explore alternative treatment options with the patient, including alternative approaches to withdrawal or substitution maintenance treatment, self-help, residential rehabilitation programs, counseling, and naltrexone.

All patients commencing treatment with buprenorphine must give their informed consent to treatment. This process requires fully informed patients and their opportunity to discuss with the service provider the following topics: what is buprenorphine and how does it work; duration of treatment; cost and associated 'routines' including urine testing, take-aways, and transfers; known side-effects; pregnancy and contraception issues; dangers of additional drug use and overdose; potential impact on driving and employment; and the conditions of involuntary discharge.

Specific patient literature should be provided prior to the commencement of treatment. It is recommended that consent be documented and that patients be given their own copies of the documents they have signed.

Permits and registration of patients

Buprenorphine is registered as a Schedule 8 medication in Australia. Each jurisdiction is responsible for a system of authorizing medical practitioners to prescribe buprenorphine to a particular patient.

Guidelines for maintenance treatment

Selecting maintenance pharmacotherapies

Current evidence suggests that key treatment outcomes for maintenance buprenorphine and methadone treatment are comparable under optimal treatment conditions. Whilst there is no evidence of the greater efficacy of one treatment over the other, patients or clinicians may develop personal preferences.

Ultimately, the continued use of a medication should depend on its ability to meet the aims and objectives of treatment. This requires the identification of treatment goals by the patient and the individual service provider, and decisions about how the treatment outcomes will be assessed.

Where these goals are not being met, a review of treatment strategies should occur, including: the role of psychosocial interventions; levels of supervision, monitoring, and review; dose of a substitution opioid; the role of adjuvant interventions; and a review of alternative opioid pharmacotherapies. For example, patients who cannot stabilize their continued use of heroin, even on high doses of buprenorphine, may be better suited to high doses of an agonist treatment such as methadone.

There may be considerable pharmacokinetic and pharmacodynamic differences between individuals in their response to different opioid substitution pharmacotherapies.

Individuals experiencing significant side-effects from one opioid medication may benefit from treatment with an alternative medication. In particular, buprenorphine may be preferred by individuals complaining of continued sedation under methadone.

Logistics of participating in treatment may be an important consideration, including issues such as ease of access for participants, frequency of dispensing, convenient location of treatment services and the costs to patients, service providers, and funding bodies. Once stabilized on a daily dosing regimen, the majority of patients on buprenorphine will be able to switch to an alternate-day, or three times a week dosing regimen. This should be more convenient for patients and reduce the need for regular take-away doses. Not all patients will be comfortable on alternate-day buprenorphine dosing, and may require daily doses.

A limiting factor for many patients considering maintenance treatment is the problem of dependence on the maintenance opioid. As it is only a partial agonist and dissociates slowly from receptors, buprenorphine appears to have a milder withdrawal syndrome than methadone. Nevertheless, current research indicates that relapse rates to heroin use are comparable for patients discontinuing maintenance treatment from either opioid.

Expectations of any medication may impact seriously on its perceived outcomes. The introduction of new pharmacotherapies for heroin dependence may give rise to unrealistic expectations in patients, their families, and even service providers.

Some patients require high doses of methadone to stabilize their heroin use, and a marked reduction can cause a relapse to regular heroin use. For patients who cannot reduce below high doses of 60 mg of methadone without becoming destabilized, transfer to buprenorphine should not be recommended unless it is part of a broader plan of gradual withdrawal from maintenance substitution treatment.

Induction to buprenorphine treatment

Commencing buprenorphine from heroin use

There are a number of factors which must be taken into consideration when considering the initial dose of buprenorphine. Patients with a low degree of neuroadaptation or tolerance to opioids should be commenced on a dose of 2 or 4 mg. In instances where the medical practitioner is uncertain of the degree of neuroadaptation, the patient should be commenced on a dose of 4 mg. Patients with high levels of neuroadaptation should commence on 6 or 8 mg.

Patients experiencing considerable opioid withdrawal at the time of the first dose require higher doses of buprenorphine to alleviate withdrawal symptoms. Patients with little or no indication of opioid withdrawal at the time of the first dose should be prescribed a lower dose, or be asked to return for treatment at a later time.

If there is a high perceived likelihood of concurrent drug abuse, including alcohol consumption, unauthorized use of prescription sedative drugs, particularly benzodiazepines, or illicit drug use, lower doses of buprenorphine should be prescribed, with frequent reviews.

Concurrent medical conditions, particularly impaired hepatic function, and interactions with other medications warrant the use of lower initial doses of buprenorphine with regular monitoring.

Care should be taken by prescribing clinicians, pharmacists, and nursing staff not to administer the first dose to a patient within 6 hours of heroin use, or intoxicated on opioids, as the patient may experience opioid withdrawal as the buprenorphine displaces the opioid from the opioid receptors. Buprenorphine precipitated withdrawal typically begins 1 to 4 hours after the first buprenorphine dose, is generally mild to moderate in severity, and lasts for up to 12 hours. If this happens, patients may require symptomatic withdrawal medication, and should be directed to see their doctor.

Subsequent doses of buprenorphine commencing the following day should result in light or minimal withdrawal discomfort if the patient has not used heroin during the intervening period. Patients who continue to use heroin between their first and second doses of buprenorphine may have difficulty stabilizing on the treatment, with ongoing features of opioid withdrawal. If so, patients should be advised to cease heroin use at least 6 hours prior to the next dose of buprenorphine.

Transferring from methadone maintenance treatment

Buprenorphine has a higher affinity for μ opioid receptors than methadone, but is a weaker agonist at these receptors. When methadone patients take a dose of buprenorphine, the methadone is displaced from the μ opioid receptors by buprenorphine. Patients on low doses of methadone, that is, less than 30 mg, generally tolerate this transition with minimal discomfort. However, patients on higher doses of methadone may find the replacement of methadone with buprenorphine precipitates transient opioid withdrawal.

This has a number of clinical implications. Wherever possible, patients in methadone treatment should have their methadone dose reduced and stabilized on this low dose prior to transferring to buprenorphine, in order to minimize any opioid withdrawal features. Table 12.1 describes key factors in the development of precipitated withdrawal.

Transferring to buprenorphine from doses of methadone of 40 mg or less

Wherever possible, patients should be on a methadone dose of less than 40 mg, and preferably 30 mg or less, for at least one week prior to receiving their first dose of buprenorphine. Indeed, it is preferable for patients to be experiencing a mild degree of methadone withdrawal prior to converting to buprenorphine. For many patients, the optimal methadone dose prior to transferring to buprenorphine may be below 30 mg of methadone.

Table 12.2 lists the conversion rates that should be used when converting from low-dose methadone to sublingual buprenorphine.

The likelihood of precipitating withdrawal on commencing buprenorphine is reduced as the time interval between the last methadone dose and the first buprenorphine dose increases. A precipitated withdrawal may be avoided by ensuring the last dose of methadone is taken early in the morning, and the first dose of buprenorphine is taken late the following day.

Features of a precipitated withdrawal following the first dose of buprenorphine are typically mild to moderate in severity, which can distress the unprepared patient. Symptoms commence 1 to 4 hours after the first buprenorphine dose and last for up to 12 hours before subsiding. Patients experiencing discomfort may attend the prescribing doctor later in the day and require symptomatic withdrawal medication such as clonidine 100 µg 3 to 4 hourly. Subsequent doses of buprenorphine on the following day are less likely to precipitate withdrawal symptoms.

Transferring to buprenorphine from doses of methadone greater than 40 mg

Most patients in methadone treatment require maintenance doses of greater than 40 mg of methadone to achieve abstinence from heroin, and

Table 12.1

Factor	*Discussion*	*Recommended strategy*
Dose of methadone	Doses greater than 30 mg of methadone are more often associated with precipitated withdrawal. In general, the higher the methadone dose, the more severe the withdrawal experienced	Attempt transfer from low dose of methadone (<40 mg where possible). Patients on >60 mg methadone should not attempt transfer
Time between last methadone dose and first buprenorphine dose	Buprenorphine should not be taken within 24 hours of last methadone dose. Increasing the interval between last dose of methadone and first dose of buprenorphine reduces the incidence and severity of precipitated withdrawal	Cease methadone and delay first dose of buprenorphine until patient is experiencing features of methadone withdrawal
Dose of buprenorphine	Very low doses of buprenorphine (e.g. 2 mg) are generally inadequate to substitute for methadone (unless the methadone dose is very low). High first doses of buprenorphine (e.g. 8 mg or more) are more likely to precipitate withdrawal, as there is greater displacement of methadone from the receptors. This is a common mistake by inexperienced practitioners	First dose of buprenorphine should generally be 4 mg, with review of the patient 2 to 4 hours later (or early the following day)
Patient expectancy	Patients who are not prepared for the possibility of precipitated withdrawal are more likely to be distressed and confused by its onset, with potential negative consequences such as treatment drop-out or abuse of other medications	Inform patients and carers fully. Provide written information. Prepare a contingency management plan for severe symptoms
Use of other medications	Symptomatic medication like clonidine can be useful in relieving any precipitated withdrawal	Prescribe and dispense in accordance with a management plan

Table 12.2

Last oral methadone dose (mg)	*Initial buprenorphine dose (mg)*	*Day 2 buprenorphine dose (mg)*
20–40	4	6–8
10–20	4	4–8
1–10	2	2–4

are unable to reduce their dose of methadone to 40 mg or less without considerable withdrawal discomfort or relapse to heroin use. As it may be difficult to get these patients' doses of methadone below 40 mg, transfer to buprenorphine may need to be considered at higher methadone doses, with the inherent risks associated with such a procedure explained fully to the patient. It is possible to transfer to buprenorphine from methadone doses of 40–60 mg for those patients who choose to do so.

The general principle is to cease methadone dosing, and delay the initiation of buprenorphine treatment until the patient experiences significant, observable features of opioid withdrawal. This generally means that buprenorphine is not commenced until 48 to 96 hours after the last dose of methadone. Patients should be warned that the use of heroin or other opioids at this stage increases the likelihood of a difficult initiation to buprenorphine. Symptomatic withdrawal medication may be prescribed to ease the discomfort of methadone withdrawal, although the quantities of medications, such as benzodiazepines or clonidine, should be limited. Medications containing codeine or d-propoxyphene should be avoided.

Patients should have the possibility of precipitated withdrawal explained, as well as the relevant strategies for dealing with its symptoms. Transfer should be organized for a time when the patient has no significant work or other commitments, and the doctor is available for review.

Patients should be reviewed by their prescriber immediately prior to commencing buprenorphine, to ensure they are indeed in opioid withdrawal.

After the first dose of buprenorphine, the patient should be reviewed by a medical practitioner within 3 to 4 hours. If the patient is experiencing no increase in withdrawal severity, either subjectively or objectively, a further 2 or 4 mg of buprenorphine can be given. If the patient is experiencing a worsening of withdrawal, do not give any further doses of buprenorphine that day. Symptomatic withdrawal medication may be required for the rest of the day, such as clonidine 100 µg 3 to 4 hourly. Peak withdrawal discomfort is generally experienced during the first day of buprenorphine treatment.

The patients should also be reviewed by their prescriber prior to buprenorphine dosing on the second day. Buprenorphine can generally be increased to 6 or 8 mg. Subject to the outcomes of review of the patient by their prescriber, further increases in buprenorphine dose are possible on subsequent days. Patients may feel uncomfortable during their first week on buprenorphine.

Summary of proposed procedures for medium-dose methadone (40–60 mg) to buprenorphine transfer

- Prepare the patient for the transition to buprenorphine with information and organization of support, and communicate proposed changes with the pharmacist and/or other relevant staff.
- Cease methadone and delay administration of the first buprenorphine dose until the patient experiences significant withdrawal discomfort, which is generally 48 to 96 hours after last methadone dose. Symptomatic medication may be required.
- Administer the first dose of 4 mg buprenorphine in the morning or early afternoon.
- Review the patient 2 to 4 hours after their first buprenorphine dose. If withdrawal worsens following this first dose, provide symptomatic medication to manage opioid withdrawal for the remainder of the day. If there is no change in withdrawal, or an improvement following the first dose of buprenorphine, a further 2 to 4 mg dose can be dispensed that afternoon or evening.
- Review the patient prior to dosing on the following day. Titrate the dose of buprenorphine to 6 to 10 mg, according to the responses of the previous day.
- Review frequently and titrate the dose of buprenorphine until stable. Mild withdrawal and/or dysphoria may continue for 1 to 2 weeks after transfer.

Stabilization

The optimal maintenance dose should be individualized according to the patient's response to buprenorphine. Responses vary considerably and are influenced by the following factors: rates of absorption or metabolism of buprenorphine; levels of opioid neuroadaptation and dependence; experience of side-effects; and continued use of other drugs.

These variations require the clinician to titrate the buprenorphine dose to optimize treatment objectives.

Initial doses of buprenorphine can serve as 'test doses' to enable both the patient and the clinician to monitor responses to buprenorphine. For some individuals initial doses of buprenorphine may not be adequate to prevent withdrawal over the initial 24-hour period, while others may feel sedated or 'drugged' possibly due to additional drug use, or too high a dose of buprenorphine.

A steady state with buprenorphine can be achieved quickly, and the effects of a dose change should become apparent within 2 to 3 days. Consequently, dose levels of buprenorphine can be more rapidly titrated according to patient response than with methadone.

Regular patient review

Frequent reviews by the prescriber are required in the first few weeks to titrate the optimal doses of buprenorphine for the individual, to ensure a comprehensive assessment of the patient, and to discuss further treatment plans.

The prescribing doctor should review the patient two or three times a week until the patient is stabilized to ensure adequacy of dose, inquire about withdrawal symptoms or side-effects, and to monitor any additional drug use.

Maintenance buprenorphine doses should be achieved within the first 1 or 2 weeks of treatment, subject to the patient's additional use of heroin or other drugs.

The following minimal schedule of reviews is recommended for prescribing doctors or nominated health care professionals involved in management:

- The day after the first dose of buprenorphine which enables the prescriber to identify the onset of any precipitated withdrawal and the general adequacy of the first dose.

- Every 2 to 4 days until the patient is stabilized.
- Every week for the following 4 to 6 weeks.
- Every 2 weeks during the next 6 to 8 weeks.
- Monthly reviews thereafter, although the prescriber may extend reviews to up to 3 months for stable patients.

Individuals with continuing high-risk patterns of drug use, or concomitant medical, psychiatric, or social problems, may require more frequent review. Increases in dose should be made only after review of the patient by the prescribing doctor.

Changes in buprenorphine dose

The dose–response curve of buprenorphine indicates that small increments have a greater impact at low doses, whereas at higher doses, larger increments in dose are required for a substantial change of effect. The following increments are proposed: below 16 mg buprenorphine, dose changes of 2 to 4 mg; and above 16 mg buprenorphine, dose changes of 4 to 8 mg.

Titrating the dose of buprenorphine

At each review, the buprenorphine dose should be titrated according to: features of intoxication or withdrawal over the preceding 24-hour period; cravings for heroin; additional drug use, and reasons for additional drug use; side-effects or other adverse events including intoxicated presentations or overdoses; adherence with dosing regimen; and patient satisfaction with buprenorphine dose and treatment.

Regular and high-risk use of heroin

Stabilization with prescribed opioids is hard to achieve if the patient is in the habit of using additional opioids, as such use complicates the interpretation of withdrawal or intoxication effects. In particular, patients who continue to use heroin during the first few doses of buprenorphine may experience difficulties in stabilizing on the new medication. The patient should be encouraged to make every effort to avoid heroin and any other opioid in the period prior to dosing to support their transition to buprenorphine treatment.

Alternative regimen for rapid induction onto buprenorphine

Evidence from overseas trials indicates that a faster rate of induction may be safely undertaken and may reduce the risk of early drop-out from the maintenance program. The alternative regimen achieves maintenance doses within 2 to 3 days using the following dose increments:

- day 1: 8 mg
- day 2: 16 mg
- day 3: 24 mg.

Prescribers who undertake this regimen should review patients daily, looking particularly for signs and symptoms of toxicity such as nausea and dizziness. If there is evidence of toxicity, increases in dose should be slowed.

Maintenance dosing

Dose levels

Buprenorphine doses need to be individually titrated according to the patient's response to treatment. Effective maintenance doses, resulting in reduced heroin use and improved treatment retention, are achieved with high buprenorphine doses in the range of 12 to 24 mg per day. Some patients may be satisfactorily maintained on daily doses of 8 to 12 mg, while doses of 4 mg or less will be less effective in retaining patients in treatment or reducing heroin use. There is little evidence to suggest that daily doses higher than 24 mg will result in improved outcomes or effects, and little is known regarding the nature of adverse events at maintenance daily doses greater than 32 mg. The maximum daily dose of buprenorphine routinely recommended is 32 mg.

People wishing to reduce their use of heroin, or other opioids, can do so with increases in the substitution dose of buprenorphine, as higher doses of this substance produce more effective antagonist reactions, blocking the effects of additional heroin use. However, this only succeeds up to a point. Continued heroin use despite adequate daily doses of buprenorphine may indicate that the patient needs more intensive psychosocial interventions, and/or an alternative opioid substitution with methadone.

Frequency of dosing: alternate-day and three times a week dosing regimens

Buprenorphine dosing begins on a daily basis. Most clinical studies with this therapy have examined daily dosing regimens, however recent work indicates that many patients stabilized on buprenorphine can be maintained on alternate-day dosing, some even on three times a week dosing, without experiencing features of intoxication or withdrawal. The convenience of reduced-frequency dosing should be considered for all patients found suitable for a trial of alternate-day dosing if they meet the following conditions: they have been on a stable dose of buprenorphine for at least 2 weeks; there is no high-risk drug use with frequent abuse of other sedatives including alcohol, benzodiazepines, heroin, or other opioids; there have been no intoxicated presentations to the pharmacy or medical practitioner; there is no recent history of overdose.

However, not all patients will be suited to an alternate-day, or three times a week, dispensing regimen, as some will experience increased cravings or features of withdrawal on the non-dosing days. Estimates suggest that about 15% of patients are more comfortable and more effectively maintained on daily, rather than alternate-day, dosing regimens. It is recommended that suitable patients be trialled for 2 weeks on an alternate-day dosing regimen of buprenorphine. If successful, the patient can then be trialled on a three times a week regimen. If a patient cannot be stabilized on such dosing regimens due to the onset of withdrawal, cravings, side-effects, or features of intoxication, they should be returned to a more frequent dosing regimen.

The alternate-day or four times a week regimen involves attending the pharmacy for dosing on alternate days, that is a dose every 48 hours, or attending four times a week for 3 × 48-hour doses and 1 × 24-hour dose, for example Monday, Tuesday, Thursday, and Saturday. The advantage of the four times a week dosing schedule is that the patient is on a regular attendance each week, with less likelihood of attendance errors on the patient's part and dosing errors by the pharmacist.

The dose dispensed for a 48-hour period is initially double that of the normal daily buprenorphine dose to a maximum of 32 mg dosed at a time. The patient should be reviewed following the first or second 48-hour dose, and the dose titrated according to the response. If the patient reports features of intoxication from the buprenorphine within the first 24 hours, the 48-hour dose should be reduced. If the patient reports that the dose does not prevent the onset of opioid withdrawal or cravings over a 48-hour period, then the 48-hour buprenorphine dose should be increased.

Some patients may tolerate three times a week dosing with buprenorphine, reducing the inconvenience and costs of treatment further. This should be attempted after a 2-week trial of 4 days a week dosing has been shown to be successful.

The recommended regimen for a 3-day dose is:

- 3-day dose = 3 times the normal 24-hour dose if the 24-hour buprenorphine dose <12 mg;
- 3-day dose = 32 mg when the 24 hour buprenorphine dose ≥ 12 mg.

The patient should be reviewed in the week following the first 72-hour dose, and the dose titrated accordingly. If a patient cannot be stabilized on a three times a week dosing regimen, the four times a week dosing regimen should be considered.

The recommended regimen for a 2-day dose is:

- 2-day dose = 2 times the normal 24-hour dose if the 24-hour buprenorphine dose <16 mg
- 2-day dose = 32 mg when the 24-hour buprenorphine dose ≥ 16 mg.

Some patients attempting alternate-day dosing may benefit from doses greater than 32 mg. However, there is limited evidence regarding the safety of higher doses, and buprenorphine is registered in Australia with a maximum recommended dose of 32 mg. Practitioners should be aware of the medicolegal implications of off-label prescribing before they prescribe doses of buprenorphine greater than 32 mg. Frequent clinical and hepatic monitoring is recommended under such circumstances.

Take-away doses

The take-away policy for buprenorphine will be determined by each jurisdiction. Take-away medication is not administered by the dispensing clinician, but given to the patient for administration at a later time.

The benefits of take-away opioid doses include reinforcement of patient responsibility for their own treatment; enhancement of patient integration into the community by cutting time and travel costs associated with the treatment; support for patient retention by minimizing the inconvenience of regular attendance for doses; and a reduction in the inconvenience and cost of daily dispensing to the pharmacist.

Concerns regarding take-away doses of opioid medications include:

- Possible overdose or accidental dose: take-aways increase the risk of deliberate or accidental overdose by the patient or others, particularly children and other non-tolerant individuals.
- Injection of take-aways, resulting in overdose, damage to veins, or other health consequences.
- Doubtful or poor compliance: diversion to others, resulting in poor outcomes for the patient.
- Diversion of buprenorphine to heroin-dependent individuals or methadone maintenance patients and precipitation of withdrawal.
- Negative 'publicity' over the treatment regimen.

The main issues regarding the safety of take-aways include the following:

- Close monitoring by the provider is vital to discern which patients are suitable for take-aways. This level of monitoring is not always achievable in community programs.
- Education of the patient is important regarding safe and responsible handling of the take-away doses.

Absence from pharmacy in patients ineligible for take-away doses

In circumstances where a patient is ineligible for buprenorphine take-aways, having recently commenced treatment or persisting with high-risk drug use, and is unable to attend for dosing for 1 or 2 days, it is possible to organize a one-off supervised multiple dose of buprenorphine. In this way, the dose of buprenorphine can be doubled in circumstances where the patient is away from the pharmacy for 1 day, or increased by three times the daily dose to maximum of 32 mg where the patient cannot attend the pharmacy for 2 consecutive days.

Ancillary interventions

People with a background of heroin dependence often have a range of social problems including financial, employment, parenting, legal, accommodation, and psychological difficulties such as anxiety and depression. The stability afforded by long-term substitution treatment provides an opportunity for these issues to be addressed. It is one of the key roles of treating clinicians to assist in this process, either as direct service providers, or as case managers referring the patient on to appropriate services for other areas of their lives.

There has been considerable debate over the role of counseling in maintenance substitution programs. The evidence from methadone treatment studies suggests that counseling should be available to all patients, and that patients should be positively encouraged to avail themselves of counseling services. However, there is no real place for mandatory attendance at counseling sessions, and all ancillary services should be offered on the basis of the patient freely consenting to be involved.

Counseling approaches, such as motivational interviewing, relapse prevention, and social skills training, which are all based on cognitive behavioral therapies, are frequently used and found to be effective. More intensive psychotherapy can be beneficial to people with concomitant affective disorders including anxiety and depression.

Continued high-risk drug use

People are said to be in continued high-risk drug use when there are frequent intoxicated presentations or overdoses of heroin or other substances, chaotic drug-related behaviors, or deteriorating medical or mental states due to drug use.

Attempts should be made to stabilize such patients. A review is required of their psychosocial interventions and supports, precipitants to continued drug use, and medication regimens. An adequate dose of buprenorphine should be prescribed, and the clinician must ensure that the patient is taking the buprenorphine as prescribed, which may require ceasing take-away doses, ensuring supervised consumption, and daily dosing regimens. Increases in the dose of buprenorphine may assist patients to reduce their heroin use.

Transfer to another pharmacotherapy such as methadone may be indicated if: there is little or no response to an increase in medication; the patient is already on a high dose of medication; or an increase in dose is considered 'unsafe' by the prescriber.

Alternatively, non-pharmacotherapeutic treatment options should be considered, such as therapeutic communities, counseling and support, and the patient withdrawn from prescribed opioid medication.

Missed doses

Single dose missed

Sometimes a patient who is on an alternate-day or three times a week regimen misses a 'dosing day', attending on the following 'non-dosing' day. When this happens, a lower dose of buprenorphine should be prescribed and dispensed in order to hold the patient over until the next scheduled dose.

The following procedures are recommended:

- The pharmacist should contact the prescriber. The buprenorphine dose prescribed should be sufficient to last until the next scheduled dose, so if this is 24 hours, then a 24-hour dose should be prescribed; if it is 48 hours, then a 48-hour dose should be prescribed.
- In circumstances where the pharmacist cannot contact the prescribing doctor, additional buprenorphine dosages cannot be dispensed as there is no valid prescription. However, this increases the risk that the patient will drop out of treatment. To prevent this happening, the prescriber can issue a prescription of buprenorphine to be administered by the pharmacist as a one-off dose for use if the patient on a three or four times a week regimen misses the scheduled dosing day and presents on a non-scheduled day.
- This prescription must not be greater than the usual 24-hour dose. The prescriber may wish to limit the maximum level of such an 'emergency dose' to a lower than usual dose in order to discourage such occurrences.
- Patients who repeatedly miss doses under these circumstances should be reviewed by their prescribing doctor to find out why, and whether these issues can be addressed. Alternatively, consideration might be given to a more feasible dosing regimen.

Multiple doses missed

Patients with erratic attendance for dosing are unlikely to achieve optimal outcomes. Patients who have missed more than 5 consecutive days of buprenorphine must be reviewed by their prescribing doctor prior to receiving a further dose, to ensure their safety.

The recommended recommencement doses of buprenorphine are given in Table 12.3.

Patients can be brought up to their usual maintenance doses over subsequent days using dosing increments if the prescribing clinician and patient think this is appropriate.

Cessation of buprenorphine maintenance treatment

Withdrawal from buprenorphine maintenance treatment

There is some clinical and anecdotal evidence that withdrawal from buprenorphine is less prolonged and less severe than methadone withdrawal, but the research on this is not conclusive. Withdrawal does appear to be milder during buprenorphine dose reductions, and the rate of buprenorphine dose reduction is normally more rapid than with methadone. The symptoms and signs of withdrawal from buprenorphine are qualitatively similar to withdrawal from other opioids.

The onset of symptoms is usually around 24 to 72 hours after the last 24-hour dose. Symptoms peak around days 3 to 5 following short maintenance courses of buprenorphine treatment, or days 5 to 14 for longer-term treatment. Duration of withdrawal from buprenorphine maintenance treatment has not been established, although mild to moderate

Table 12.3

Usual 24-hour buprenorphine dose	*Recommencement dose*
>8 mg	8 mg if <7 days with no dose 4 mg if >7 days with no dose
6–8 mg	4 mg
2–4 mg	2–4 mg

withdrawal symptoms, particularly cravings, and sleep and mood disturbances associated with protracted withdrawal, are likely to persist for weeks. One study described mild but ongoing withdrawal features 30 days after the last buprenorphine dose. Longer-term follow-up has not been reported.

Evidence from methadone research suggests that long-term outcomes are enhanced by longer treatment episodes, for example more than 12 months. The longer treatment episode allows the opportunity for the patient to establish a lifestyle away from heroin and other drug use prior to withdrawing from methadone treatment. Premature withdrawal from methadone before the patient has achieved a degree of stability in social circumstances and drug use is more likely to be associated with a relapse into dependent heroin use.

A patient may wish to withdraw from maintenance treatment for a range of reasons, such as the need for interstate travel, or concerns about side-effects or about remaining in treatment 'too long'. The prescribing clinician should address issues regarding the duration of treatment and withdrawal early in the treatment program, and provide information regarding the process of withdrawal. Patient literature is now available regarding withdrawal from methadone treatment[2] and parallels can be made with withdrawal from buprenorphine. Despite withdrawal from buprenorphine being frequently described as milder than from other opioids, patients should be informed of the likely withdrawal profile.

Except in the case of involuntary withdrawal, withdrawal from buprenorphine should occur only with the consent of the patient. Graduated reduction over weeks results in better outcomes, with less relapse to heroin use than reported for rapid reduction. The proposed rates of dose reduction are shown in Table 12.4, although reductions can occur both more rapidly and/or more slowly.

Table 12.4

Dose of buprenorphine	*Reduction rate*
Above 16 mg	4 mg per week or fortnight
8–16 mg	2–4 mg per week or fortnight
Below 8 mg	2 mg per week or fortnight

An increase in heroin or other drug use, or a worsening of the patient's physical, psychological, or social well-being, may warrant a temporary cessation or slowing down of the reduction rate.

Patients should be aware of their dose, except where an agreement has been reached between patient and service provider to the administration of a 'blind dose'. Increased supportive counseling, as well as information and education, should be available for patients withdrawing from buprenorphine. There may be a role for other medications for symptomatic relief. These include clonidine, NSAIDs, antiemetics, antidiarrheal agents, hypnotics, and smooth muscle relaxants such as hyoscine for patients experiencing severe withdrawal. However, caution should be applied regarding the use of potential drugs of abuse such as benzodiazepines.

Involuntary termination of treatment

The conditions for involuntary termination with patient consent or against the patient's wishes usually concern behavior which the service provider finds intolerable. This generally varies from program to program and conditions include: threatened or actual abuse of other patients or staff; illegal activities, such as theft, property damage, or drug dealing, in or near the service; or diversion of medications.

The rate of reduction under circumstances of involuntary treatment cessation can be up to a 4 to 8 mg reduction every 3 to 4 days. Patients who pose a considerable risk to the safety of other patients or staff may be abruptly terminated without a graduated dose reduction. Transfer to other service providers should always be considered as an alternative to rapid involuntary discharge.

The use of buprenorphine to assist withdrawal from methadone maintenance programs

Many patients on long-term methadone maintenance programs experience considerable difficulties in conventional approaches to withdrawing from methadone, including a prolonged period of withdrawal discomfort and/or relapse to heroin use. Consequently, there is considerable interest in finding alternative methods of withdrawing from methadone maintenance programs.

Two approaches have been recently proposed: either the use of opioid antagonists for rapid opioid withdrawal, or transfer to buprenorphine.

The transfer to buprenorphine requires a reduction in the dose of methadone, transfer to buprenorphine, and subsequent withdrawal from buprenorphine. However, as there is limited experience or evidence to support these approaches, they cannot be generally recommended at this time.

Commencing naltrexone following buprenorphine maintenance treatment

There is limited experience in commencing naltrexone following the cessation of maintenance buprenorphine treatment. The initiation of naltrexone must be delayed until several days after the last dose of a full opioid agonist, generally 7 days after heroin use and 10 to 14 days after methadone use. However, naltrexone can generally be initiated within days of the last dose of buprenorphine. The following procedures are recommended.

In circumstances where the last dose of buprenorphine was 2 mg or less for at least one week, naltrexone can be initiated 4 to 5 days after the last dose of buprenorphine providing there has been no heroin use in the previous 7 days.

Where the last dose of buprenorphine was greater than 2 mg, and to reduce the likelihood of precipitating withdrawal symptoms, the first dose of naltrexone can be delayed until more than 7 days after the last buprenorphine dose.

The initial 12.5 mg dose of oral naltrexone should be administered in the morning. The patient should be monitored for up to 3 hours after the first dose of naltrexone for features of opioid withdrawal.

Symptomatic withdrawal medication should be available for the patient to use in the 12 hours after the first dose of naltrexone, including clonidine (up to 150 µg 3 to 4 hourly), diazepam (up to 5 to 10 mg every 3 to 4 hours as needed), metoclopramide, hyoscine butylbromide, and NSAIDs.

Subsequent doses of naltrexone can be 25 mg for a further 2 to 3 days and then 50 mg per day as usually recommended. Clinical guidelines regarding the use of naltrexone should be consulted.[3]

The high receptor affinity of buprenorphine complicates the interpretation of a naloxone challenge test prior to commencing naltrexone in patients transferring from buprenorphine: a negative naloxone challenge test does not preclude the onset of withdrawal on commencing naltrexone; a positive naloxone challenge test is likely to reflect recent use of other opioids, and indicates that naltrexone induction should be delayed.

Given the potential for patients to use heroin or other opioids following the cessation of buprenorphine and prior to the commencement of naltrexone, some objective test should be conducted prior to commencing naltrexone in order to exclude recent opioid use. The naloxone challenge test or appropriate urine drug screening is recommended.

Transferring to methadone

Consideration should be given to transferring a patient from buprenorphine to methadone under the following circumstances:

- Intolerable side-effects to buprenorphine.
- Inadequate response with buprenorphine treatment. Treatment with buprenorphine should be considered unsuccessful if it has not resulted in marked improvements in the patient's drug use, injecting risk practices, or other outcomes identified by the patient and clinician as treatment goals. In such instances, treatment with an alternative substitution pharmacotherapy should be considered.
- Where buprenorphine is not available. As buprenorphine is a relatively new drug, it may not be available in certain jurisdictions, when the patient is overseas, during periods of incarceration, and in some hospitals. Patients should be transferred to methadone in such circumstances. To facilitate a planned return to buprenorphine treatment, the lowest effective methadone dose should be used.
- Complications with antagonists and analgesics. In patients who have frequent overdoses, the use of buprenorphine may complicate resuscitation efforts with naloxone. Such patients should be taken off substitution pharmacotherapies or transferred to methadone. Patients requiring frequent additional analgesia for recurrent acute or chronic pain conditions may be better stabilized on full agonists, such as methadone.

Transferring from buprenorphine to methadone treatment is less complicated than from methadone to buprenorphine. Patients transferring from 4 mg or lower doses of buprenorphine should be commenced on lower doses of methadone, such as 20 mg or less. The methadone dose can then be titrated accordingly. Care should be taken not to increase the dose of methadone too quickly, as buprenorphine can diminish or block the effects of methadone for several days, and there should be adequate time to allow 'wash out' of buprenorphine prior to marked increases in methadone dose.

Guidelines for the management of heroin withdrawal

Heroin withdrawal in context

Heroin withdrawal defined

Drug withdrawal is a substance-specific syndrome due to the cessation or reduction of heavy and prolonged drug use. This syndrome causes clinically significant distress and impairment in social, occupational, or other important areas of functioning.[4] The characteristic features of heroin withdrawal include: increased sweating, lacrimation, rhinorrhea, urinary frequency; diarrhea, abdominal cramps, nausea, vomiting; muscle spasm leading to headaches, back aches, leg cramps, twitching, arthralgia; piloerection, pupillary dilatation, elevated blood pressure, tachycardia; anxiety, irritability, dysphoria, disturbed sleep, and increased cravings for opioids.

Physical symptoms generally commence 6 to 24 hours after last use, peak in severity during days 2 to 4, and generally subside by day 7, while the psychological features of dysphoria, anxiety, sleep disturbances, and increased cravings may continue for weeks or even months. Heroin withdrawal is unpleasant, though rarely, if ever, life-threatening. It can, however, significantly complicate concomitant medical or psychiatric conditions.

Objectives of withdrawal services

Heroin users present for withdrawal services for a range of reasons and motivations, and the goals of individual patients may vary considerably. Withdrawal services should not be seen as a standalone treatment resulting in prolonged periods of abstinence. Indeed, research suggests that withdrawal treatment alone has little, if any, long-term impact on levels of drug use.[5–8] Unfortunately, many patients, families, friends, and health and welfare professionals hold unrealistic expectations regarding the outcomes of withdrawal services. Many are disappointed when people in these programs either cannot give up their heroin use in the first place, or recommence regular heroin use soon after a withdrawal attempt.

Palliation of the discomfort of heroin withdrawal symptoms is an important reason for patients presenting for treatment, and one of the primary aims of withdrawal services.

Although heroin withdrawal on its own is almost never life-threatening, withdrawal can present various serious problems, which services aim to prevent. These include the complication of concomitant medical or psychiatric conditions such as the precipitation of an acute psychotic episode in a patient with schizophrenia in remission, or dehydration in an individual with poor baseline nutritional status; and the increased risk of overdose following withdrawal. This can occur with resumption of heroin use following the reduction in opioid tolerance that accompanies withdrawal, and due to the combined sedative effects of heroin use and medications used for the management of heroin withdrawal, particularly benzodiazepines.

Many patients want treatment to end their heroin use completely during the withdrawal episode, intending to stay off it for a set period of time afterwards. However, giving up entirely is not the goal of every patient. Many see withdrawal as a means of reducing levels of heroin use, the severity of their dependence, and some of its associated harms. So, although the cessation of heroin use is an optimal outcome, a reduction in heroin use during a withdrawal attempt may still represent a very positive outcome for patients.

Withdrawal services are essentially acute services with short-term outcomes, whereas heroin dependence is a chronic relapsing condition, and positive long-term outcomes are more often associated with longer participation in treatment. Consequently, an important role of withdrawal services is to provide links with post-withdrawal services for those with other physical problems, or psychological or social needs.

Optimally, they should have automatic access to drug treatment services, such as 'drug-free' counseling, naltrexone treatment, residential therapeutic communities, self-help programs, or substitution maintenance programs with methadone or buprenorphine. But while some people will be unwilling or unable to continue in ongoing drug treatment programs, they may need – and be grateful for – contacts with welfare services; general support and case management services; or primary or specialist health services.

Non-pharmacologic aspects in managing heroin withdrawal

As well as the use of medications or pharmacotherapy, the delivery of withdrawal services requires assessment, treatment matching, planning for withdrawal, and supportive care.

Treatment selection is a synthesis of: assessment of the patient; examination of the available treatment options and likely outcomes; and negotiation with the patient around a suitable treatment pathway.

In considering possible modalities, it is important to remember that many people come for treatment with misconceptions and/or inadequate information about the two major options available.

In general, withdrawal treatment such as naltrexone, residential rehabilitation programs, counseling, or 12-step programs is appropriate for those who are considering abstinence-oriented, post-withdrawal treatment, or for those who are not interested in longer-term treatment, and merely want a 'break' from dependent heroin use.

However, maintenance substitution treatment with methadone or buprenorphine may be more appropriate for those with significant heroin dependence who will not accept residential rehabilitation or naltrexone treatment, but nevertheless want to stop or permanently reduce their heroin use and all the damage it is causing them. Clinical decision-making should have an evidentiary basis, and patients should be presented with the relative evidence addressing the merits and the limitations of treatment outcomes associated with each approach. Within such a framework, there is widespread evidence suggesting that maintenance substitution remains the 'gold standard' treatment for most people with chronic heroin dependence, by virtue of its success in keeping patients in treatment, and reducing drug-related harms.

Once it is established that withdrawal is to be attempted, consideration must be given to the services needed to achieve the best outcome. An optimal setting and adequate supports should be found for each patient, and monitoring arranged for their personal requirements and medication needs.

Withdrawal can occur in a continuum of settings, ranging from intensive residential services such as inpatient withdrawal unit or hospital to outpatient ambulatory or home-based withdrawal services. Most heroin withdrawal attempts can occur in outpatient settings, usually with the assistance of a general practitioner, alcohol and drug worker, or other health professional.

Some patients may wish to persevere with an outpatient withdrawal, despite unsuitable home environments or having repeatedly 'failed' as outpatients before. Such attempts at outpatient withdrawal may still be the way to go, if it is what the patient really wants. However, clinicians should first negotiate with their patient some mutually agreed criterion of failure, such as lack of significant progress within a week, at which point a switch will be made to an alternative treatment pathway.

Criteria for intensive residential settings include: unstable medical/psychiatric condition; polydrug dependence and withdrawal from multiple drugs; and unclear medical, psychiatric, or drug-use histories requiring close monitoring in a supervised environment.

Criteria for supported residential setting include: unsupportive home environment, such as living with other drug users, or without anyone reliable to supervise and support the patient; and repeated failure at outpatient withdrawal.

Getting organized for withdrawal

Residential withdrawal settings generally provide the full range of services needed for a withdrawal episode. Such settings are developed to be drug-free, with support available from staff and fellow patients, and the capacity for continuous monitoring, and usually have access to medical staff and medications. Unfortunately, such inpatient services often have waiting lists of days or weeks, and the patient may need short-term support in the interim.

Commencing an outpatient withdrawal requires planning, and the mobilization of the necessary supports and services. Patients should prepare themselves and their environment in advance, to maximize their chance of 'success'. For example, it is very hard to get through withdrawal in the company of others still using heroin.

A 'safe' place is one where drugs will not be easily accessible, and patients will not be confronted by other drug users. It is important to have caring people to support a patient during withdrawal, and these support people themselves need guidance and information about the process, and suggestions as to what they can reasonably do to help.

Supportive care

Patients need information regarding: the nature and duration of withdrawal symptoms; strategies for coping with symptoms and cravings; strategies to remove high-risk situations; and the role of medication.

Patients often have limited concentration during withdrawal, and information may have to be repeated, perhaps even rephrased, to be fully understood and absorbed. Written information is valuable in these circumstances, and is also recommended for support people. Local drug and alcohol authorities should be able to provide the relevant literature.

Counseling during the withdrawal episode should be aimed specifically at supporting the patient through problems associated with withdrawal and in facilitating post-withdrawal links.

Many patients will want to deal with a range of personal, emotional, or relationship problems during the withdrawal episode, but they should be persuaded to defer all this until later. Attempting to work through such issues will almost certainly be emotionally painful and anxiety provoking, which may intensify cravings and thus place the withdrawal program in jeopardy. Furthermore, patients in withdrawal tend to be irritable, agitated, tired, and run down; they can suffer from mood swings and poor sleep patterns, as well as difficulty in concentrating. This is definitely not the optimal frame of mind in which to try to solve significant, long-standing life problems. Assure your patients that you understand that they have many important issues to work through to get their lives together again, but it is best to take one step at a time. There will be opportunities for these wider problems to be addressed as part of their ongoing rehabilitation after they get through withdrawal. On the other hand, crisis intervention may be required during a withdrawal episode to ensure adequate accommodation, food, or other urgent welfare issues.

In addition to supportive counseling from health professionals and the support of family, friends, and peer workers, heroin users may also benefit from 24-hour telephone counseling services for help when others are unavailable.

Monitoring

An important part of the withdrawal service is regular and frequent monitoring, to check: general progress; drug use; response to the medication(s); severity of withdrawal symptoms which can be facilitated by the use of withdrawal scales; complications or difficulties; and ongoing motivation levels.

Doses of medication can then be adjusted according to the patient's progress. It is recommended that patients undergoing outpatient withdrawal be reviewed by a health professional – alcohol and drug worker, general practitioner, or experienced pharmacist – at least daily during the first few days of treatment.

Objective and subjective withdrawal scales

There are various opioid withdrawal scales available to refer to. Subjective scales are far more sensitive to changes in withdrawal severity, and are better predictors of patient outcomes. Objective scales are not only less sensitive, but usually need to be administered by a health professional. Nevertheless, such scales may be useful in corroborating subjective ratings, particularly in individuals who are thought to be over- or underrating their withdrawal severity.

Overview of buprenorphine in the management of heroin withdrawal

Efficacy of buprenorphine compared to other withdrawal medication regimens

The efficacy of buprenorphine in the management of heroin withdrawal has been compared to other withdrawal approaches in several randomized controlled trials conducted in inpatient[9–11] and outpatient settings.[12,13]

In general, these studies have demonstrated buprenorphine to be: more effective than symptomatic medications in reducing withdrawal symptoms;[9–11,13] more effective in retaining patients through the withdrawal episode and in post-withdrawal treatment;[13] and more effective in reducing heroin use in outpatient settings.[13]

Readers are referred to the Cochrane Review on buprenorphine for opiate withdrawal.[14]

Controlled trials comparing buprenorphine with other withdrawal medications for the management of heroin withdrawal in medically ill patients have not been conducted. Nevertheless, uncontrolled studies have reported favorably on the use of buprenorphine in these circumstances. Furthermore, the sublingual preparation is well suited to individuals who cannot tolerate oral medications. Caution should be used when employing buprenorphine or other opioids in individuals with certain medical conditions.

The role of buprenorphine in withdrawal

The aim of medication in withdrawal is the reduction of withdrawal symptoms and cravings; it is not the complete removal of all symptoms or the intoxication of the patient.

The clinician should discuss patient expectations of the medication with them, and address any misconceptions. In particular, the following principles regarding doses should be understood by the patient:

- Buprenorphine doses that are too high can result in increased rebound withdrawal, prolonged duration of symptoms, increased side-effects, and increased cost of the medication.
- Alternatively, use of doses that are too low can result in unnecessary withdrawal discomfort, continued heroin use, and treatment drop-out.
- Continued heroin use or cravings may not be due to inadequate doses of medication. For example, patients who continue to associate with other heroin users, and are present when others are acquiring or using heroin, can expect to have cravings regardless of their dose of buprenorphine.

Preventing precipitated withdrawal on commencing buprenorphine

Buprenorphine can precipitate opioid withdrawal in someone who has used heroin or methadone within the past 6 hours. Buprenorphine precipitated withdrawal typically commences 1 to 4 hours after the first buprenorphine dose, is generally mild to moderate in severity, and lasts for up to 12 hours. Patients experiencing severe discomfort may benefit from symptomatic withdrawal medication with clonidine 100 μg 3 to 4 hourly as required, and should be directed to see their prescribing doctor.

Patients should not receive the first dose of buprenorphine if they are experiencing heroin effects. In practice, it is recommended that patients wait at least 6 hours after their last use of heroin prior to receiving their first buprenorphine dose. It is preferable to withhold the first dose until the patient is beginning to experience the early features of withdrawal. If there are doubts or concerns, the patient should be asked to come back for dosing later in the day, or alternatively, a lower initial dose of 2 or 4 mg can be dispensed as it is less likely to precipitate withdrawal than a high initial dose.

Use of ancillary medications in conjunction with buprenorphine

Buprenorphine provides general relief of withdrawal symptoms, so that other symptomatic medications for opioid withdrawal are not routinely required. An exception to this rule is when patients experience difficulty sleeping during withdrawal, and may benefit from the limited use of benzodiazepines as a hypnotic. However, benzodiazepines should not be used routinely from the outset of the withdrawal episode, but rather should be added, as required, following clinical review of the patient. Low doses of a hypnotic agent such as temazepam 10 to 20 mg nocté, oxazepam 15 to 30 mg nocté, or nitrazepam 5 to 10 mg nocté are recommended, with daily dispensing from the pharmacy or supervision by a responsible adult. Under normal circumstances, benzodiazepines should not be continued beyond several days, with non-pharmacologic sleep hygiene strategies being encouraged.

Continued use of heroin and other drugs

Patients who keep on using heroin during buprenorphine treatment may have difficulty stabilizing on the medication, and may continue to experience features of precipitated withdrawal after each dose. Persistent features of precipitated withdrawal discomfort may be grounds for transfer to methadone, or other withdrawal medications.

All patients should be informed verbally and in writing of these risks. Intoxicated patients should not be dosed with buprenorphine or sedative medications.

Gateway model of treatment with buprenorphine

Buprenorphine is particularly useful in managing heroin withdrawal, in that it is not only effective during the withdrawal period, but also facilitates links to post-withdrawal treatment. Many patients entering withdrawal treatment do so without necessarily having considered all their treatment options, simply 'hoping' that an attempt at withdrawal will be sufficient to stop heroin use.

The use of buprenorphine for several days generally alleviates withdrawal symptoms without significant sedation, thereby allowing patients and clinicians to examine post-withdrawal issues relatively early on in the withdrawal episode. If patients require other withdrawal medications, such as benzodiazepines or clonidine, they may be psychologically distressed or sedated to levels which do not make this possible. A formal review of treatment plans should be structured several days into the withdrawal episode, at which time treatment can be tailored accordingly. For those patients who have successfully refrained from heroin use during withdrawal, and who are considering longer-term naltrexone treatment, naltrexone can be initiated either during buprenorphine administration or after a short course is ceased. Patients who are not interested in ongoing pharmacotherapy treatment can cease a short course of buprenorphine with minimal rebound discomfort. Alternatively, those patients who want to extend the duration of their withdrawal program, or have reconsidered the role of a maintenance treatment program, can continue buprenorphine treatment over a longer period of time. Care should be exercised in transferring patients with short histories of heroin dependence from short-term withdrawal programs on to long-term substitution maintenance programs.

Buprenorphine regimens in outpatient withdrawal settings

Buprenorphine is long acting, and so is well suited to outpatient withdrawal settings, allowing for once a day supervised dosing. Patients unable to attend an authorized pharmacy daily for supervised dispensing should consider alternative withdrawal medications.

The recommended duration of treatment with buprenorphine for the management of heroin withdrawal is 4 to 8 days. This short regimen ensures that the treatment covers the time when heroin withdrawal symptoms are most severe, typically up to the first 4 or 5 days, and then is promptly discontinued, thereby minimizing rebound withdrawal phenomena and limiting the duration of withdrawal discomfort.

There is no conclusive evidence of an optimal buprenorphine dosing regimen for heroin withdrawal. In general, daily buprenorphine doses of 4 to 16 mg appear to be most effective in reducing withdrawal severity and heroin use. The reader is referred to the Cochrane Review on buprenorphine withdrawal[14] for an analysis of relevant studies. The short-term outpatient withdrawal regimen shown in Table 12.5 is recommended.

Table 12.5

Proposed withdrawal regimen	*Recommended dose (mg)*	*Recommended lower and upper limits (mg)*
Day 1	6	4–8
Day 2	10	4–16
Day 3	10	4–16
Day 4	8	2–12
Day 5	4	0–8
Day 6		0–4
Day 7		0–2
Day 8		0–1
Total dose	36	

Some flexibility is allowable in doses to accommodate a range of factors, such as amount of heroin use and psychological condition, impacting on each patient's individual dosing requirements and withdrawal severity.

Review by a trained health professional is recommended on a daily basis during the first few days of the withdrawal regimen. This is important so that doses can be adjusted, if necessary, and any difficulties being experienced on the medication can be addressed. It is also needed to ensure provision of appropriate support care and monitoring.

Doctors may choose to prescribe a fixed daily dose, for example day 1: 6 mg, day 2: 8 mg, day 3: 10 mg, etc. Alternatively, they may prescribe a flexible regimen with upper and lower limits on any particular day and instructions for the pharmacist or nominated health care professional regarding dose titration, for example day 1: 6 mg, day 2: 6–10 mg; day 3: 8–12 mg, etc.

It is a good idea to attempt a short-term regimen, and schedule a formal review of progress within a few days. At this review, the clinician and patient can together consider the available post-withdrawal treatment options.

Those patients who remain ambivalent about long-term post-withdrawal treatment, and have not been able to cease their heroin use, may need referral to an inpatient supervised withdrawal program. Alternatively, an extension of the withdrawal regimen over several weeks may be warranted.

However, there are good reasons for not prolonging buprenorphine treatment. Intake for more than several days commonly produces rebound withdrawal when ceased, typically starting 1 to 3 days after the last dose of buprenorphine, peaking 2 to 5 days after the last dose, and with some symptoms persisting several weeks.

Prolonged, probably unsuccessful, attempts at withdrawal can be demoralizing for the patient, resulting in lowered capability, self-esteem, and/or confidence in the treatment provider. For this reason, a limit on the time spent on a gradual reduction regimen should be discussed with the patient early in the program. Longer-term maintenance substitution treatment with buprenorphine or methadone should be recommended to patients who: cannot stop, or markedly reduce, their heroin use during the withdrawal episode; relapse into regular heroin use as the dose of buprenorphine is reduced or ceased; or do not feel confident about maintaining abstinence, but do not want to relapse to dependent heroin use and the associated harms.

It is recommended that such patients stabilize on a maintenance substitution medication for a longer period of time before coming off their maintenance treatment, to give them the opportunity to first distance themselves from heroin use and possibly to address any problematic psychological and social issues which may be distressing them.

Buprenorphine for heroin withdrawal in residential settings

Buprenorphine is well suited to use in inpatient withdrawal settings, given its ability to alleviate the discomfort of withdrawal symptoms without significantly prolonging their duration.

It is recommended that an interval of at least 2 to 3 days be available from the time of the last buprenorphine dose to the time of planned discharge. Duration of dosing will be determined by the length of admission available, such as in a 7-day-admission treatment it will be limited to the first 4 to 5 days.

Approaches to dispensing in inpatient settings will depend on the level of supervision and staffing available. Titration regimens generally require nursing staff who can administer withdrawal scales and S8 (restricted access) medications, so places with limited access to nursing staff may be better suited to fixed regimens with the option of additional 'rescue' doses as required.

The additional rescue doses should only be administered at least 4 hours after the earlier dose, and if the patient is experiencing moderate or severe withdrawal discomfort.

Buprenorphine doses in inpatient settings can generally be lower as outpatient regimens must accommodate higher cravings and exert blockade effects, and outpatient regimens are generally limited to once a day dosing.

An evening dose between 1700 hours and 2200 hours is recommended to allow relief of withdrawal symptoms until the morning. Buprenorphine should not be administered if there are any features of intoxication or sedation.

Table 12.6 shows the regimen recommended for 7-day admission, and can be tailored accordingly.

Table 12.6

Day	*Buprenorphine sublingual tablet regimen*	*Total daily dose*
Day 1	4 mg at onset of withdrawal and additional 2–4 mg evening dose prn	4–8 mg
Day 2	4 mg mane with additional 2–4 mg evening dose prn	4–8 mg
Day 3	4 mg mane with additional 2 mg evening dose prn	4–6 mg
Day 4	2 mg mane prn, 2mg evening prn	0–4 mg
Day 5	2 mg prn	0–2 mg
Day 6	No dose	
Day 7	No dose	
Total dose	12–28 mg	

This regimen serves as a guide only, and considerable individual variation in withdrawal severity and medication requirements should be expected.

Post-withdrawal options should be explored prior to discharge. Patients commencing naltrexone treatment should do so during their admission. Patients wishing to commence buprenorphine maintenance treatment should continue their buprenorphine as inpatients until transfer to a community-based provider can be organized.

Transition to post-withdrawal treatment

Transition to maintenance treatment

Transition to a buprenorphine maintenance treatment program simply requires the continuation of treatment, often with upward titration of the dose to achieve optimal maintenance dose levels of 12–24 mg per day.

The transition to methadone maintenance treatment requires the cessation of buprenorphine, with the first dose of methadone given at least 24 hours later.

Commencing naltrexone treatment after short-duration buprenorphine withdrawal

One of the difficulties for many heroin users in commencing naltrexone treatment is staying off heroin for a whole week before the first dose, to avoid the precipitation of withdrawal. The recommended 7-day opioid-free period[3] also limits the use of opioids such as methadone, codeine, or d-propoxyphene as withdrawal medications, as they delay even further the initiation of naltrexone treatment. The pharmacology of buprenorphine allows the commencement of naltrexone without major delays. This is thought to be because buprenorphine has a higher affinity for opioid receptors than naltrexone, so the naltrexone does not significantly displace buprenorphine or cause the precipitation of severe opioid withdrawal.

Researchers are yet to determine the optimal method of inducting on to naltrexone from buprenorphine treatment, but two general procedures have been used: commencing low doses of naltrexone whilst continuing buprenorphine, or ceasing buprenorphine and commencing naltrexone several days later. Sample dosing regimens for the two approaches are shown in Table 12.7.

Which procedure is best?

Both procedures result in an increased severity of opioid withdrawal following the first dose of naltrexone. This typically commences 90 minutes to 4 hours after the first naltrexone dose, peaks around 3 to 6 hours after the naltrexone dose, and generally subsides in severity within 12 to 24 hours. The withdrawal is frequently experienced as moderate to severe at its peak. Subsequent doses of naltrexone produce considerably less severe withdrawal discomfort.

Most patients undergoing this procedure request symptomatic medication, and clonidine 100 to 150 µg every 3 to 4 hours as required, and a benzodiazepine such as diazepam 5 mg 3 to 4 hourly, as required should be prescribed.

Most patients find either procedure tolerable. All patients need supervision and access to the prescribing doctor. Table 12.8 illustrates the differences between the two procedures.

Table 12.7 Naltrexone induction regimens following buprenorphine treatment

Day	*Possible buprenorphine regimen (sublingual tablets, mg)*	*Early naltrexone induction regimen (oral, mg)*	*Delayed naltrexone induction regimen (oral, mg)*
1	6	0	0
2	10	0	0
3	8	12.5	0
4	6	12.5	0
5	4	25	0
6		50	0
7		50	0
8		50	12.5
9		50	12.5
10		50	25
11		50	50

An outpatient setting is appropriate only when there is a suitable and responsible person to support and supervise medications for the patient in the home, and if the prescribing doctor is available to manage any potential complications.

Complications or adverse events with buprenorphine treatment

Side-effects

The reported side-effects of buprenorphine are qualitatively similar to those of other opioids used in maintenance treatments. A side-effect is any undesired or unintended effect of drug treatment. Side-effects may be predictable on the basis of the drug's known actions, or unpredictable, such as allergic drug responses and idiosyncratic drug reactions.

Table 12.8 Comparison between early and delayed naltrexone induction

	Early naltrexone induction regimen	*Delayed naltexone induction regimen*
Potential advantages	Only 36 to 48 hours of abstinence from heroin use is required prior to first dose of naltrexone; hence more patients will get a first naltrexone dose	Allows more time for consideration and selection of optimal post-withdrawal treatment options
	More rapid resolution of withdrawal discomfort: naltrexone precipitated withdrawal peaks early in withdrawal episode, following naltrexone dose, with resolution of most withdrawal symptoms within days	Initial withdrawal episode is less severe for the patient and less intensive for service providers
Potential disadvantages	Greater drop-out reported after first naltrexone dose than in delayed induction regimen	Some patients will drop out or resume heroin use prior to day 8 or 9 of withdrawal episode, and therefore not commence naltrexone
	May 'rush' some patients into naltrexone treatment, whereas other post-withdrawal treatment such as maintenance substitution treatment may be preferred	Naltrexone precipitated withdrawal occurs later in the withdrawal episode on the day of first naltrexone dose

In large multicenter trials of buprenorphine maintenance treatment, opioid withdrawal symptoms were the most common side-effects reported by over 30% of patients, and these reports were most common in patients on a 1 mg daily dose of buprenorphine. Other commonly reported side-effects reported are shown in Table 12.9.

In general, most side-effects to buprenorphine are mild, well tolerated, and typically occur early in treatment, with symptoms subsiding over time.

Table 12.9 Commonly reported side-effects to buprenorphine

Side-effect	*Proportion of patients reporting side-effect (%)*	*Relation to dose*
Headache	8.7	Appears unrelated to dose
Constipation	7.5	More common on higher doses
Insomnia	7.3	Appears unrelated to dose
Asthenia	6.1	Appears unrelated to dose
Somnolence	4.3	Appears unrelated to dose
Nausea	3.5	More common on doses > 8 mg
Dizziness	2.7	More common on higher doses
Sweating	2.7	Appears unrelated to dose

Management of the side-effects, which will depend on their nature and severity, should be negotiated between patient and clinician. Conventional strategies should be adopted to manage opioid-related side-effects.

Overdose

The risk of lethal overdose on buprenorphine in an opioid-tolerant individual is less than that associated with the use of other opioid medications, such as methadone. This is due to the ceiling dose–response effects of buprenorphine.

As an opioid-naïve individual may overdose with a high dose of buprenorphine, all patients should be commenced on low 2 to 8 mg doses, and even lower doses (2 or 4 mg) should be considered where there is some doubt regarding the degree of neuroadaptation prior to commencing treatment.

The poor bioavailability of buprenorphine when taken orally reduces the risk of accidental overdose by children.

While overdose on buprenorphine is relatively uncommon, there is a greater risk when it is combined with other sedative drugs, such as alcohol, benzodiazepines, barbiturates, tricyclic antidepressants, and major tranquilizers. Several such deaths have been reported.

Buprenorphine has a high affinity for μ opioid receptors, and is not easily displaced by the antagonist naloxone. Naloxone doses of 10 to

35 mg/70 kg, which are 10 to 30 times the normal naloxone doses used to reverse heroin overdose, may be required to reverse the effects of buprenorphine toxicity.

Intoxicated presentations

Intoxicated patients should not be dosed with buprenorphine, and patients should be made aware of this prior to the commencement of treatment. These patients may attend again later the same day or the following day for dosing. The prescribing clinician must be notified prior to the next dose being administered. Patients with a history of repeated intoxicated presentations should be reviewed by the treating doctor and the treatment plan reviewed.

Incorrect dose administered

The risks associated are not as severe with an incorrect dose of buprenorphine as with other opioid medications. In the event of an incorrect dose being administered:

- The dispensing pharmacist or nursing staff should immediately notify the patient and medical officer of the error.
- The patient should be warned of the likely consequences such as increased sedation/drowsiness which may occur for several hours afterwards, and be warned against any additional drug use, and driving or operating machinery for the remainder of the day.
- The patient should be monitored for at least 6 hours after an incorrect dose by trained health professionals, or in the Accident & Emergency Department of a hospital if any of the following circumstances apply: the patient is sedated following the dose; the patient is in their first 2 weeks of maintenance treatment; the regular daily buprenorphine dose is ≤4 mg, and the patient was incorrectly administered a dose of ≥16 mg; a buprenorphine dose of ≥64 mg was incorrectly administered.

The patient should be reviewed by the prescribing medical officer prior to the next dose of buprenorphine. It may be that a lower dose or no dose at all is required the following day.

Diversion of buprenorphine

As buprenorphine is a sublingual tablet, it can easily be diverted by patients. They may try to avoid taking their buprenorphine as directed, at the pharmacy, for the following reasons: to take sublingually at a later time; to inject or snort the medication instead of the sublingual route of administration; or to give or sell to another person.

There are potential risks associated with these practices. Patients not taking their full dose of buprenorphine may be more likely to use heroin. Injection of buprenorphine is associated with risks of venous thrombosis, thrombophlebitis, and other local infections; and of systemic fungal or bacterial infections, particularly in circumstances where patients inject buprenorphine that has already been in their mouth.

Diversion of the medication to other people can result in overdose through combination with other sedating drugs or precipitation of withdrawal, such as when taken by a patient on a high dose of methadone.

To minimize the risks of diversion, a number of safeguards are recommended. Pharmacists should note carefully whether the full number of buprenorphine tablets have been taken sublingually by the patient. Patients should not be allowed to handle the tablets prior to dosing. Pharmacists or their assistants should supervise the patient closely until the tablets have dissolved, which generally takes about 3 to 7 minutes.

In circumstances where diversion of buprenorphine is a possibility, for example where there is inadequate time for supervision, the following strategies are recommended. The pharmacist and prescribing medical practitioner should warn the patient of the potential health risks associated with misuse of the medication. The pharmacist should crush the tablets, administering a fine powder sublingually to reduce the time required for absorption and the potential for medication to be removed from the patient's mouth. While the effect of crushing tablets on the bioavailability of the sublingual preparation has not been examined, it is thought to have little clinical impact.

Where there is ongoing misuse of the medication, patients should be warned that they may have to be transferred from buprenorphine treatment to methadone, which is easier to supervise.

Investigations

Urine tests reveal an individual's drug use in the preceding 48- to 72-hour period. This is an expensive investigation and should be conducted only if the results are likely to be important. At the time of writing, Australian pathology laboratories do not routinely test for buprenorphine in the urine, and it will not be detected as an opioid.

The only possible indications for buprenorphine urine screening are: to confirm whether a patient has taken the take-away doses and to see if a patient not in treatment is abusing buprenorphine.

Analgesia requirements for patients on buprenorphine

Patients maintained on buprenorphine will have a diminished response to opioids prescribed for analgesia. This is because of the 'blocking' effect of the buprenorphine on full opioid agonists. Consequently, patients on buprenorphine who suffer severe or chronic pain will require considerably higher doses of opioid analgesia than individuals not in buprenorphine treatment. Use non-opioid analgesics where possible, such as aspirin, NSAIDs and paracetamol.

Maintain buprenorphine dose if acute or subacute analgesia is required. A temporary increase in buprenorphine dose may provide additional analgesic cover. Patients who develop chronic pain which is not responding to buprenorphine, and who require ongoing additional analgesia, may require transfer to methadone treatment.

Where additional opioid analgesia is required, the dose of opioid should be clinically titrated according to clinical response. The dose of analgesic should be closely monitored if buprenorphine is reduced or stopped. The concern is that high morphine doses will be required while buprenorphine is exerting 'blockade' effects, but as the buprenorphine levels decrease there will be a corresponding reduction in the 'blocking' effects of buprenorphine which increases the potential for oversedation – or even overdose – from the high morphine doses. If buprenorphine treatment is stopped completely, the dose of opioid analgesic needs to be closely monitored every day for at least 4 to 5 days after the last buprenorphine dose. It will probably have to be reduced over time to avoid an overdose.

Pregnancy and lactation

Inadequate research has been conducted on the effects of buprenorphine during pregnancy and lactation in humans. For this reason, and because of certain adverse effects reported in animal trials, buprenorphine is contraindicated for both pregnant and lactating women.

Buprenorphine is a Category C drug in Australia, which has implications for pregnancy. The Australian Drug Evaluation Committee states that this group of drugs 'has caused, or may be suspected of causing, harmful effects on the human fetus or neonate without causing malformations. These effects may be reversible.' Opioid analgesics are capable of causing respiratory depression in the neonate, and withdrawal symptoms have been reported in cases of prolonged use. Any woman patient seeking maintenance treatment who might become pregnant should be counseled on the potential risks of buprenorphine during pregnancy, with this information being reinforced and presented to them in writing. Reliable forms of contraception must be recommended to women of child-bearing age.

The pregnant heroin user not in treatment

Heroin-dependent women who become pregnant should be advised to commence maintenance substitution treatment, with methadone the preferred option.

The patient who becomes pregnant while in buprenorphine treatment

If this happens, advice should be sought from a specialist multidisciplinary unit providing obstetric and pediatric services for chemically dependent women and their babies. Counseling should be provided regarding treatment options, and support offered when a choice of action is made.

Continuation of pregnancy and transfer to methadone maintenance treatment is the preferred option for the woman who wishes to continue with her pregnancy. The woman should be admitted to hospital for transfer to methadone, allowing for close observation of both the patient and the fetus for evidence of withdrawal or distress.

In rare circumstances, discontinuation of buprenorphine treatment may pose a greater risk to mother and baby than continuing with buprenorphine treatment. In particular, the woman who refuses to transfer to methadone should be given the option of continuing her buprenorphine treatment after the risks to the fetus and baby, and the concerns about breastfeeding whilst in buprenorphine treatment, have been explained to her. The woman must be capable of giving informed consent.

Women wishing to terminate the pregnancy should be referred to appropriate services.

Neonates of women exposed to buprenorphine should be monitored for neonatal abstinence syndrome or any other adverse events. This group of children should be followed up by pediatricians with experience in caring for children exposed in utero to drugs of dependence. Long-term follow-up will be required to monitor for developmental abnormalities.

The effect of buprenorphine on infants of nursing mothers has not been well studied. Thus, buprenorphine treatment is contraindicated for breastfeeding mothers.

Writing prescriptions and dispensing buprenorphine

Note that this section refers to the situation in Australia.

Buprenorphine is an opioid and is registered as an S8 medication. Special precautions should be taken by clinicians in the prescribing, handling, dispensing, and storage of the medication.

Writing prescriptions

Prescriptions for buprenorphine may be on a standard prescription form. A valid prescription must specify the following:

- the name and address of the prescribing doctor who has been issued with the permit to prescribe;
- the patient's name and address;
- the date of the prescription;
- the preparation to be dispensed – buprenorphine sublingual tablets;

- the dose of buprenorphine to be dispensed in mg, using both words and numbers;
- different dose schedules must be written separately, i.e. 24-hour doses, 2-day or 3-day doses, specifying the days of the week the patient is to be dosed;
- the beginning and end dates of the prescription.

It is strongly recommended that the name of the pharmacy be included on the prescription.

Protocols for administering buprenorphine

Procedures prior to dosing

Staff authorized to administer buprenorphine generally include a pharmacist, a medical practitioner, or two registered nurses.

Prior to administering the medication, staff must: establish the identity of the patient; confirm that the patient is not intoxicated; and check currency and amount of prescription. A patient cannot be dosed if a prescription is not current; check that the current day is a dose day on the patient's regimen; confirm the dose for the current day if it is an alternate-day or three times a week regimen; and record the dose in the Drug of Addiction recording system.

After recording dose details in the necessary Drug of Addiction recording system, the following procedures should be observed:

- Count and check the buprenorphine tablets into a dry dosing cup. Double check number and strength.
- For patients unfamiliar with buprenorphine dosing, issue the following instructions:
  - place the tablets under your tongue;
  - do not chew the tablets;
  - do not swallow saliva until tablets have dissolved. This should take 3 to 5 minutes on average;
  - do not chew or swallow the tablets;
  - once the tablets are given to you they are your responsibility and will not be replaced.

- Give the cup to the patient and ask the patient to tip the contents under the tongue. Discourage patients from handling tablets.
- Observe the patient for at least 2 minutes until you are satisfied tablets are not divertable. Ask to see 'how the tablets are dissolving' enough times for this to become an acceptable part of the patient's pick-up routine.
- Patients should sign that they have received their dose. Offer cordial or water to rinse the taste of the dissolved tablets from their mouth.
- The prescribing medical practitioner should be notified if the pharmacist or the health care professional dispensing the buprenorphine has concerns that the patient may be attempting to divert their medication.

References

1. Ajir K, Chiang N, Hiber A, Ling W. Pharmacokinetics of liquid versus tablet buprenorphine, 1999.
2. Dunlop A, Thornton D, Lintzeris N, Muhleisen P, Khoo K, Lew R. Coming off methadone. Melbourne: Turning Point Alcohol and Drug Centre, 1996.
3. Bell J, Kimber J, Mattick RP, et al. Use of naltrexone in relapse prevention for opioid dependence. Interim Clinical Guidelines. Canberra: Commonwealth Department of Health & Aged Care, 1999.
4. American Psychiatric Association. Diagnostic and statistical manual of mental disorders. 4th ed. Washington, DC: American Psychiatric Association, 1994.
5. Mattick RP, Hall W. Are detoxification programmes effective? Lancet 1996; 347: 97–100.
6. Hubbard RL, Marsden ME, Rachal JV, Harwood HJ, Cavanagh ER, Ginzburg HM. Drug abuse treatment: A national study of effectiveness. Chapel Hill, NC: University of North Carolina Press, 1989.
7. Vaillant GE. What can long-term follow-up teach us about relapse and prevention of relapse in addiction? Brit J Addict 1988; 83: 1147–57.
8. Simpson DD, Sells SB. Effectiveness of treatment for drug abuse: an overview of the DARP research program. Advan Alcohol Subst Ab 1982; 2(1): 7–29.
9. Cheskin LJ, Fudala PJ, Johnson RE. A controlled comparison of buprenorphine and clonidine for acute detoxification from opioids. Drug Alcohol Depen 1994; 36: 115–21.
10. Nigam A, Ray R, Tripathi B. Buprenorphine in opiate withdrawal: a comparison with clonidine. J Subst Abuse Treat 1993; 10(4): 391–4.
11. O'Connor PG, Carroll KM, Shi JM, Schottenfeld RS, Kosten TR, Rounsaville BJ. Three methods of opioid detoxification in a primary care setting: a randomized trial. Ann Intern Med 1997; 127(7): 526–30.
12. Bickel WK, Stitzer ML, Bigelow GE, Liebson IA, Jasinski DR, Johnson RE. A clinical trial of buprenorphine: comparison with methadone in the detoxification of heroin addicts. Clin Pharmacol Ther 1988; 43: 72–8.

13. Lintzeris N, Bell J, Bammer G, Jolley D, Rushworth L. A randomized controlled trial of buprenorphine in the management of short-term ambulatory heroin withdrawal. Addiction 2002; 97: 1395–404.
14. Gowing L, Ali R, White J. Buprenorphine for the management of opioid withdrawal. Cochrane Database Syst Rev 2004 (4).

chapter 13

Clinical guidelines and procedures for the use of naltrexone in the management of opioid dependence

James Bell, Jo Kimber, Nicholas Lintzeris, Jason White, Benny Monheit, Sue Henry-Edwards, Richard P Mattick, Robert Ali, Alison Ritter, and Allan Quigley

Introduction

Naltrexone was first used in the treatment of opioid dependence in the USA in the 1970s. However, because there was seen to be only a small demand for the drug, it was not initially registered for use in Australia. During the 1990s, there was an increase in the prevalence of opioid dependence, and increasing interest in using naltrexone. A number of medical practitioners began prescribing naltrexone under the Special Access Scheme which, under specific circumstances, allows the prescribing of unregistered drugs. Results of the first Australian clinical trial of naltrexone in the management of opioid dependence were published in 1998. In 1999, the drug was registered for use in Australia.

These clinical guidelines have been prepared to aid medical practitioners in the selection and management of patients seeking treatment with naltrexone hydrochloride for management of opioid dependence, and to assist medical practitioners to provide patients with accurate information concerning naltrexone.

These clinical guidelines cover the use of naltrexone in the management of opioid dependence – in both relapse prevention and withdrawal. The approach taken in developing these guidelines was to review published evidence, paying most weight to appropriately controlled trials. Strong research evidence is not available on many issues, and clinical consensus from a panel of experienced clinicians has been employed in developing these guidelines.

The guidelines were prepared under the auspices of the National Expert Advisory Committee on Illicit Drugs (NEACID) in collaboration with the National Evaluation of Pharmacotherapies for Opioid Dependence (NEPOD) project, the Royal Australian College of General Practitioners (RACGP), and the Australian Professional Society on Alcohol and Other Drugs (APSAD), and are funded by the Commonwealth Department of Health and Ageing.

These clinical guidelines are based on international research literature and clinical experience with the use of naltrexone in Australia. The material presented has undergone a rigorous process of review and has been formally endorsed by the RACGP and APSAD.

The contribution of various individuals and organizations in the drafting and review process is gratefully acknowledged. Commonwealth Government and State Government support for the National Evaluation of Pharmacotherapies for Opioid Dependence (NEPOD) project allowed extensive clinical and research experience of naltrexone, and underpins the development of these guidelines.

Regulation of naltrexone in Australia

Naltrexone hydrochloride (Revia®) is registered in Australia for use in relapse prevention for alcohol dependence and opioid dependence. Naltrexone is available on the Pharmaceutical Benefits Scheme (PBS) for only one indication, as an authority prescription for relapse prevention in the management of alcohol dependence. Several studies have demonstrated the efficacy of naltrexone in alcohol dependence,[1,2] although the effectiveness of naltrexone in alcohol dependence is reduced by poor compliance.[3] Naltrexone is available on private prescription for relapse prevention in opioid dependence.

This treatment is designed to assist a detoxified and opioid-free former heroin user to remain abstinent from heroin.

Naltrexone is not registered in Australia for use in opioid withdrawal, although it is occasionally used to accelerate the process of withdrawal from opioids. Rapid detoxification is the term given to a wide variety of techniques employing an opioid antagonist to accelerate the process of opioid withdrawal.[4] The use of naltrexone in rapid detoxification is an 'off label' use of the drug, which places additional responsibility on medical practitioners to ensure that prospective patients are fully informed of the potential risks and benefits of the use of naltrexone to accelerate withdrawal and alternate treatment approaches available. Prescribers must ensure that written informed consent for the procedure is obtained.

Clinical pharmacology of naltrexone

General information

What is naltrexone?

Naltrexone is a highly specific opioid antagonist which has a high affinity for opiate receptor sites. It competitively displaces opioid agonists if they are present, such as methadone, heroin, and slow-release morphine. Naltrexone has few intrinsic actions besides its opioid-blocking properties. It does produce miosis or pupillary constriction by an unknown mechanism. Naltrexone does not cause any physiologic tolerance or dependence. It is not known to block the effects of other classes of drug besides opioids, however, naltrexone appears to block some of the euphoriant actions of alcohol, presumably due to its blockade of opioid receptors.

What form does it come in?

Naltrexone hydrochloride is available in Australia as Revia®, and is presented as a scored, pale yellow coated capsule-shaped tablet. Revia is available as 50 mg tablets in bottles of 30 tablets. Because the major limitation of naltrexone is patient compliance with the daily regimen, there is considerable interest in the use of depot preparations of naltrexone, designed to slowly release naltrexone into the circulation over a period of weeks to months.

Medical practitioners in Australia and elsewhere have experimented with naltrexone implants designed to do this.

Naltrexone implants are not registered for use in Australia, and their use is experimental. Medical practitioners are advised not to use naltrexone implants, except in the context of clinical trials registered with the Australian Government regulatory organization, the Therapeutic Goods Administration.

Absorption, distribution, metabolism, and excretion

Naltrexone is rapidly absorbed, with peak blood levels achieved about 1 hour after oral administration.[5] Naltrexone has a relatively short plasma half-life of 4 hours. It is primarily metabolized in the liver to a metabolite, 6β-naltrexol, which has a plasma half-life of about 10 hours and is also an opioid antagonist. Approximately 20% of the active metabolite is bound to plasma protein, and is distributed widely, with relatively high amounts in the brain, fat, spleen, heart, testes, kidney, and urine.[5] Naltrexone and 6β-naltrexol undergo enterohepatic recycling and are excreted primarily by the kidney. Less than 1% of naltrexone is excreted unchanged.

Despite both compounds having relatively short half-lives, the duration of naltrexone blockade is much longer. An oral dose of 50 mg naltrexone has been shown to produce 80% inhibition of radiolabeled carfentanyl binding for 72 hours.[6]

Rationale for the use of naltrexone in opioid dependence

The rationale for using naltrexone in relapse prevention is that the patient knows that taking naltrexone blocks the effects of heroin. Detoxified heroin users have described naltrexone as being a form of 'insurance', a protection against a sudden temptation to use heroin. Clinical experience indicates that patients who take naltrexone in the hope that it will stop them wanting to use heroin, or will maintain their motivation to remain abstinent, tend to be disappointed. Naltrexone should be seen as a medication which may help motivated patients to remain abstinent, rather than a drug which reduces patients' desire to use heroin. Furthermore, it should be remembered that 'motivation' to remain drug-free can be very variable over time. It is common that people in crisis express a strong intention to become and remain drug-free, but within a relatively short time such determination disappears.

Indications

Naltrexone is indicated for opioid users seeking abstinence from opioids and who are capable of giving informed consent to treatment. Naltrexone treatment is only appropriate for opioid users committed to long-term abstinence.

Contraindications to naltrexone treatment

Contraindications to naltrexone treatment include current physiologic dependence on opioids. Those currently physiologically dependent should be offered detoxification or referred to specialist services. Those patients using opioids for chronic pain require specialist assessment. There needs to be a drug-free interval before commencing naltrexone and patients should not commence treatment in acute opioid withdrawal.

Treatment of patients with acute hepatitis or liver failure is contraindicated, as naltrexone can be hepatotoxic in high doses. The margin of separation between the apparently safe dose of naltrexone and the dose causing hepatic injury appears to be only 5-fold or less. Known adverse reaction or sensitivity to naltrexone is also a contraindication.

Precautions

Caution is advised in prescribing naltrexone to the following patients: women who are pregnant or breastfeeding, patients concurrently dependent on multiple drugs, patients with impaired renal function, patients with major psychiatric illness (including depression), children, and adolescents. In each of these cases, assessment by an alcohol and drug specialist is recommended.

Side-effects

Although major adverse events are very rare, side-effects of naltrexone are common, but tend to be transient, mild, and improve with time. Side-effects reported by more than 10% of patients include difficulty in sleeping, loss of energy, anxiety, abdominal pain, nausea and vomiting, joint and muscle pain, and headache.

Safety of naltrexone treatment

The greatest problem associated with naltrexone treatment is the increased risk of death from heroin overdose in patients who return to opioid use after being treated with naltrexone.

Increased risk of death for those patients who return to opioid use after naltrexone treatment is thought to be primarily due to loss of tolerance to opioids. An increase in the risk of death by overdose occurs in any recently detoxified group of formerly heroin-dependent patients, including people within 12 months of leaving methadone treatment.[7] After discontinuing naltrexone, a dose of heroin which the user had been accustomed to inject during their last period of addiction may now prove fatal.

Another factor contributing to the risk of death is that some people become depressed after discontinuing heroin, and may deliberately suicide. The experience with naltrexone indicates that there are few serious adverse reactions, other than the precipitated withdrawal, which occurs when the drug is administered to someone who is not opioid-free.

Although some years ago it was noted that high doses of naltrexone administered to morbidly obese subjects resulted in transaminase elevations, subsequent experience with use of naltrexone in alcohol dependence has found hepatotoxicity to be rare.[8]

Effectiveness of naltrexone treatment

The effectiveness of naltrexone treatment for relapse prevention is limited. Published literature on naltrexone in relapse prevention in general shows that only a small minority of opioid-dependent people seek naltrexone treatment, and among those entering treatment there is a very high rate of drop-out.

A significant proportion of people remaining in naltrexone treatment for periods of 3 months or longer remain abstinent from heroin. However, this represents only a small proportion of heroin users. Furthermore, most of these subjects appear to return to heroin use eventually. The only moderately long-term, published follow-up study of patients treated with naltrexone[9] reported that more than 90% of subjects became re-addicted to heroin at some time over the following 5 years. Patients in that study reported that they had found naltrexone helpful, as it had helped them to remain heroin-free for periods of time. This study concluded that naltrexone was not a 'cure' for heroin addiction, but was a useful medication in protecting patients from re-addiction for periods of time.

With more intensive supportive treatment, and with new methods of delivering naltrexone, it is thought that the effectiveness of treatment with this medication can be improved. However, at this time the available evidence suggests only very modest efficacy of naltrexone in relapse prevention for opioid dependence.

Entry into naltrexone treatment

Patient selection issues

Because of concerns over safety in the event of relapse, and the relatively low rates of abstinence achieved with naltrexone, naltrexone treatment is only appropriate for heroin users committed to long-term abstinence. It is preferable that such a commitment is assessed over time – at least a few days – rather than in a single interview.

Naltrexone is only one of a range of treatments for opioid dependence. Treatment options include detoxification, self-help groups, drug-free counseling, residential therapeutic communities, and maintenance treatment with methadone or buprenorphine. These treatment options are complementary, not competing, and many patients will access a variety of treatments over time, depending on their circumstances. The appropriateness of entry into one of these treatment options should be considered when assessing a patient for naltrexone treatment.

Clinicians should consider how prospective patients are to be inducted onto naltrexone. Induction onto naltrexone involves reversal of neuroadaptation to opioids, and usually produces considerable symptomatic distress for a few days.

Retention in drug dependence treatment programs is generally poor with the exception of agonist maintenance therapies.[10] Patients may be better suited to methadone or buprenorphine maintenance treatment if they are ambivalent about long-term abstinence, or if they are at high risk of relapse to heroin use. Such risk may be evidenced by virtue of a chaotic lifestyle, entrenched involvement with drug-using friends, and a lack of external supports to assist the patient to maintain abstinence.

Assessment for naltrexone treatment

Motivation and expectations

Motivation for treatment and expectations of treatment should be explored by clarification of reasons for presentation including immediate precipitants and clarification of the patient's goals such as long-term abstinence, respite, and attempt to regain control.

Many prospective patients see naltrexone as a 'wonder drug' which will stop them from wanting to use drugs. Naltrexone can be a useful adjunct in relapse prevention, but it does not motivate people to remain abstinent.

Drug use history

A drug use history comprises an assessment of current levels of drug use including quantity and frequency of use, duration of use, assessment of dependence including physiologic dependence, use of drugs other than the primary drug of dependence, and a history of treatment for drug problems. Careful drug use history taking is extremely important.

Patients may say they have been abstinent from heroin for a week, but may have been using street methadone and/or codeine or dextropropoxyphene preparations or compound analgesics such as Panadeine Forte®, or Digesic® and still be physiologically dependent on opioids. If a patient is on methadone or has recently been on methadone, or has been using street methadone, it is important to be particularly cautious when initiating naltrexone. If a patient's primary drug problem is amphetamine, cocaine, or cannabis use, it is very unlikely that naltrexone will be of use.

Evidence of drug use such as documenting the extent of vein damage, signs of liver disease, nutrition, and self-care should be sought. This may be of value in monitoring improvements during treatment, and providing patients with positive feedback about their progress.

Medical and psychiatric history

In general, patients with a history of medical conditions, which are acute or unstable, should undergo careful assessment prior to initiation of any new treatment. Consideration needs to be given to possible drug interactions in people taking prescribed medications.

Naltrexone treatment or, possibly, abstinence from heroin may exacerbate or unmask psychiatric problems, particularly depression, in susceptible subjects. Identification and monitoring of depressive symptoms is desirable, and if there is concern about a patient's mood, psychiatric assessment may be helpful. Mental state examination (mood, affect, attention, and concentration) is important to screen for depression or thought disorder, and to confirm that the patient is in a fit state to provide informed consent.

A psychosocial history should also be taken. A careful history should consider social circumstances including housing, relationships, children, employment, developmental history such as family of origin, schooling, occupational history, and forensic history including current charges.

Rapid detoxification causes considerable physiologic stress. Patients with history or signs of cardiac disease, particularly ischemic heart disease, arrhythmia, or hypertrophic cardiomyopathy, or respiratory disease should not undergo rapid detoxification. Patients with signs of acute or decompensated chronic liver disease (jaundice, encephalopathy) should not usually be commenced on naltrexone.

Investigations where clinically indicated

If a patient has a positive pregnancy test at assessment, do not perform a naloxone challenge, and reconsider naltrexone treatment. Patients should be advised of the potential risks of naltrexone during pregnancy.

Urinalysis can be undertaken as an adjunct to history taking and physical examination in confirming recent drug use. Opioids can be detected in urine for up to 48 hours. If a patient has an opioid-positive urine at assessment do not continue with the naloxone challenge test. Patients should be advised if random urine drug screens are used for monitoring purposes during treatment.

Injecting drug users are a high-risk group for parenterally transmitted diseases. It is therefore appropriate to screen new patients for hepatitis B and C, immunize against hepatitis B, and provide harm reduction information. Liver function tests (LFTs) and serology for blood-borne viruses are not mandatory prior to initiating treatment, and may better be undertaken during the first month of treatment.

In situations where patients report having completed detoxification, it is prudent to confirm that they are no longer physically dependent on opioids by performing a naloxone challenge test (see Appendix 1).

Treatment plan and informed consent

Informed consent for naltrexone treatment should include explaining treatment and providing written information. Patients should be appraised of the potential risks of treatment, particularly the overdose risks on discontinuing naltrexone. Contraindications for treatment should be discussed and excluded, and arrangements for induction onto naltrexone explained. The costs of treatment, frequency of appointments, and availability of support services should be explained and clarification sought as to whether the patient wants to enter into an arrangement in which his/her taking of naltrexone is supervised.

Supervision of naltrexone taking may improve compliance with treatment. Currently, several programs encourage patients to involve a significant other, carer, or friend to supervise the daily taking of naltrexone, and this may improve compliance and treatment outcomes. Research has demonstrated that treatment with naltrexone is more effective in highly supervised settings such as prisoners on probation,[11] or medical practitioners under the supervision of medical boards.[12] Whether these findings can be extended to having family members or friends as carers remains to be determined.

Finally, practitioners must document informed consent to naltrexone treatment and a medical warning card should be issued to patients in case analgesia is required in the event of sudden illness or injury.

Induction into treatment

The administration of naltrexone to people physiologically dependent on opioids will precipitate a severe withdrawal reaction. Precipitated withdrawal is much more severe than spontaneous withdrawal, and people undergoing precipitated withdrawal can become very ill. To avoid precipitating withdrawal, there are three approaches to induction onto naltrexone treatment.

The conventional approach is to undertake detoxification, and when patients have been free of short-acting opioids for 5 days, or free of methadone for 10 days, commence naltrexone treatment. As patient history can be unreliable, it is desirable to perform a naloxone challenge test prior to the first dose of naltrexone, to avoid inadvertently precipitating a withdrawal reaction. The procedure for undertaking a naloxone challenge is outlined in Appendix 1.

Antagonist accelerated induction or rapid detoxification involves administration of naltrexone or naloxone to opioid-dependent subjects, while providing symptomatic relief to make the ensuing precipitated withdrawal tolerable.

Buprenorphine-assisted detoxification can allow the introduction of naltrexone without severe precipitated withdrawal, either during buprenorphine treatment or within days of stopping buprenorphine.

Treatment with naltrexone

Dose and duration of treatment

The usual maintenance dose of naltrexone is 50 mg daily. However, 25 mg daily produces adequate blockade of opioid receptors, and may be a satisfactory dose in patients who experience side-effects from 50 mg/day.

The optimal duration for treatment with naltrexone is unknown. However, it is known that treatment for dependence is a long-term process, and there is still a substantial risk of relapse to heroin dependence for 2 to 3 years after last use of heroin. The optimal period of treatment will be different for different patients and advice about how long to take naltrexone should take into account lifestyle changes, environmental risk factors, and craving. Patients should generally be encouraged to take naltrexone for at least 6 months.

Supportive care for patients on naltrexone

Intensive follow-up is a critical component of optimizing the benefits of naltrexone treatment. The clinician performing induction onto naltrexone should review patients, or arrange for a suitably qualified health professional to review them, on two occasions during the first week after induction. Thereafter, clinical reviews should be conducted weekly during the first month of treatment.

There are many approaches to the delivery of supportive care. Medical monitoring involves a regular review with the prescribing doctor, with monitoring of compliance and review of drug use, sometimes with urine testing to confirm self-report. Regularly scheduled counseling sessions have frequently been used. Supervised dosing is where a family member or friend supervises the daily administration of naltrexone, sometimes administering the tablet crushed to minimize the risk of the patient spitting it out. Self-help groups may also be a valuable adjunct to people trying to maintain abstinence.

In the treatment of drug dependence, it is conventional to accept that it is only possible to help people change patterns of behavior if they themselves are motivated to make such changes. Motivation of treated heroin users to remain abstinent is generally transient,[13] and this is one reason why compliance with naltrexone treatment is generally poor, and a large proportion of subjects relapse. It is unclear how far practitioners should go towards trying to improve compliance with naltrexone treatment. In recent years, several practitioners have advocated a more aggressive approach to naltrexone treatment. Rather than accepting the ambivalence and shifting motivation to remain abstinent frequently demonstrated by patients, these practitioners have recommended: initiating treatment with rapid detoxification to minimize drop-outs prior to commencing naltrexone, supervised dosing by involvement of family or other carers who provide a high level of supervision ensuring patients continue to take their naltrexone, and aggressive re-induction after an episode of relapse.

There has been no systematic evaluation of this approach to treatment, certainly not one involving comparison groups or randomized design. Whether in the long term this approach leads to better, worse, or the same outcomes as conventional approaches to treatment remains to be determined.

It is important to remember that, while families are often keen to be involved in patient care on naltrexone, practitioners must obtain patient consent to involve family or discuss treatment with them. Remember that every family is different and that adverse family dynamics can contribute to a person's drug use. While most families try to support family members who stop heroin use, a person ceasing heroin can sometimes lead to considerable family tension. Sensitive handling of such changes could be important in reducing the risk of relapse.

Many people taking naltrexone are keen to engage in some form of counseling, and practitioners who do not feel they have the skills or time to spend in counseling patients should refer patients who express a wish for counseling.

Monitoring and review

Patients should be seen regularly while on naltrexone treatment. It is recommended that clinical reviews should be conducted weekly during the first month of treatment, then fortnightly or monthly as required.

Monitoring of compliance and progress should occur at each clinical review, including assessing: drug use for both heroin and other drugs, compliance with the naltrexone regimen, changes in social functioning and relationships, whether the patient is involved in counseling, and the presence of any side-effects, especially mood-related effects.

Relapse

At review, some patients will report that they have discontinued naltrexone use and returned to using heroin. Just as commonly, they may report that they are complying with treatment – yet have fresh injecting marks, a positive urine test for opioids, or other evidence of return to heroin use. Sometimes it is only the report of a significant other which may alert the doctor to the fact that the patient is not taking naltrexone, and has resumed heroin. Multiple missed appointments and the observations of the dispensing pharmacist can also be valuable indicators that something is wrong.

In these circumstances, the conventional approach is to re-assess the patient, clarifying their motivation. Patients should always be warned of the risks of overdose. Other treatment options should be considered. If the patient wishes to enter a residential treatment program, the program rules may allow them to remain on naltrexone. Some patients prefer to do this, so that they continue naltrexone after leaving residential treatment.

Re-induction onto naltrexone

Many patients who have relapsed will express a desire to resume naltrexone treatment. However, these patients need to be cautioned that reinstatement of dependence occurs rapidly within days of regular heroin use, and, therefore, somewhat unpredictably, resuming naltrexone can precipitate severe withdrawal.

If it is more than 5 days since the last dose of naltrexone, and the patient has used heroin each day since then, recommence on naltrexone as though a new patient requiring detoxification.

If it is within 5 days of the last naltrexone dose, restart naltrexone under medical supervision – patients may experience withdrawal, but this is usually not severe. Restart naltrexone in the morning, at least 24 hours after the last use of heroin, commencing with one quarter of a tablet (12.5 mg). Patients may need symptomatic medication.

Clinical experience to date has been that patients who relapse and return to naltrexone tend to remain in treatment a relatively short time. After multiple relapses, medical practitioners should seriously consider whether it is appropriate to continue naltrexone treatment, as it becomes increasingly likely that the patient will drop out, and it is preferable to actively manage cessation of treatment than for people to drop out and be receiving no treatment. Alternative approaches such as residential treatment or methadone or buprenorphine maintenance treatment should be discussed.

Transfer to maintenance substitution treatment

The patient may wish to transfer to maintenance substitution treatment with methadone or buprenorphine. This involves some risk, because when methadone is commenced too soon after the last dose of naltrexone, its actions will be blocked, and patients may appear to require a higher starting dose of methadone. This can give rise to a situation where people accumulate toxic levels of methadone, and the toxicity only becomes gradually apparent as the naltrexone blockade wears off. This risk needs to be balanced with the risk of people using heroin if the methadone dose is insufficient.

The first dose of methadone should ideally be delayed until 72 hours after the last dose of naltrexone. However, it may be possible to initiate treatment with 20 mg of methadone after only 48 hours, although patients should be warned of the possible residual receptor blockade. When methadone is initiated within 7 days of the last use of naltrexone, the starting dose should not exceed 20 mg daily for the first 3 days, as the patient may have low tolerance. When inducting onto buprenorphine, the initial dose should not exceed 4 mg, although rapid dose increases can occur following review by the prescribing doctor.

Management issues in naltrexone treatment

Intermittent naltrexone use

Some patients may wish to use naltrexone in an intermittent way. For example a patient may be abstinent, but when facing a high-risk situation will take one tablet, or a patient may want to avoid heroin use most days, but want to take heroin on weekends.

There are serious potential risks with these approaches, including overdose on opioids due to risk of misjudging level of tolerance and precipitated withdrawal due to resumption of naltrexone following reinstatement of opioid dependence. For these reasons, it is appropriate to caution people against irregular use of naltrexone. Also, in some situations it may be prudent to discontinue naltrexone treatment if the patient's level of risk taking outweighs any observed benefits of the treatment.

Diversion

Patients should be warned against giving or selling their naltrexone to other opioid users as it can precipitate acute withdrawal. Precipitated withdrawal is much more severe than spontaneous opioid withdrawal. Several patients have required hospitalization after taking naltrexone while still physiologically dependent on heroin. Guidelines for the management of precipitated withdrawal are included in Appendix 2.

Multiple drug use

Some heroin-dependent patients, when they cease heroin, commence or increase their use of other drugs, especially benzodiazepines, cannabis, amphetamines, and cocaine. Naltrexone does not block the effects of these drugs. Practitioners should caution patients against use of these drugs, and should monitor use of these drugs at each appointment. The risks and benefits of continuing naltrexone treatment should be assessed when patients are abusing or dependent upon other drugs.

Adjunct pharmacotherapies

To date, there is no evidence to support the routine use of drugs such as antipsychotics, benzodiazepines, and anticonvulsants during naltrexone treatment.

Many heroin users experience dysphoria at treatment presentation, upon completion of withdrawal and during the induction phase of naltrexone. The dysphoria usually resolves within weeks.

Antidepressants are indicated if there is a diagnosis of depression on the basis of features more substantial than dysphoria, such as suicidal ideation, anhedonia, sleep disturbance, and weight change. Although it has been suggested that use of selective serotonin re-uptake inhibitors (SSRIs) improve outcomes in unselected naltrexone patients, the weight of evidence does not support routine use of SSRIs in conjunction with naltrexone.

One study has reported that naltrexone has fewer adverse effects on sleep than methadone,[14] but despite this many patients complain of insomnia, particularly on initiation of naltrexone treatment. Benzodiazepines can help, but their use should be time limited – a period of less than 2 weeks is recommended. Patients need to be advised of non-pharmacologic treatment options for sleep disturbance.

There may be a role for the use of symptomatic medications in the first few days of naltrexone treatment to address ongoing withdrawal symptoms. Recommended medications include metoclopramide for nausea and vomiting, hyoscine butylbromide for abdominal cramps, non-steroidal anti-inflammatory drugs (NSAIDs) for joint aches, benzodiazepines for agitation and insomnia, and the use of non-opioid antidiarrheals for diarrhea.

Pain management

For mild pain, non-opioid analgesics such as paracetamol and NSAIDs should be used. Patients taking naltrexone will not benefit from opioid-containing medicines such as cough, cold, and antidiarrheal preparations.

Naltrexone should be discontinued at least 72 hours before elective surgery, including dental surgery, if it is anticipated that opioid analgesia may be required. The treating clinician should be informed that the patient has been taking naltrexone. The patient should then be abstinent from any opioid for 3 to 5 days before resuming naltrexone treatment, depending on the duration of the opiate use and the half-life of the opiate. A more conservative approach is to wait 7 days. As an alternative, a naloxone challenge test can be administered.

In an emergency, pain management may consist of regional analgesia, conscious sedation with a benzodiazepine, non-opioid analgesics, or general anesthesia. Ketorolac is an NSAID available for parenteral use. In an emergency, pain management should be coordinated with an alcohol and drug specialist.

Pregnancy

Patients seeking to remain opioid-free during pregnancy should have additional monitoring and support, as pregnancy can be a time of considerable psychologic stress. While pregnancy is often a time when women become motivated to stop drug use, it is also a time when previously stable patients may relapse.

The safety of naltrexone in pregnancy is not established. It has been classified as pregnancy risk B3. If the pregnant woman believes she is at low risk of relapse, and the doctor concurs, it is appropriate to cease naltrexone and monitor the patient through pregnancy. If the patient is highly concerned about relapse, and wishes to continue naltrexone, it is important to inform the patient about the risks of staying on naltrexone, and obtain consent for ongoing treatment. If the patient wishes to cease naltrexone but then reports that she has started using heroin again, it may be appropriate to consider methadone treatment. Patients need to be fully informed of the risks involved in doing so, including the risk that the baby will go through withdrawal on delivery.

Rapid detoxification – the use of naltrexone in withdrawal

Rapid detoxification is the process of accelerating acute withdrawal from heroin (or other opioids) by administration of an opioid antagonist, while providing symptomatic relief to enable patients to tolerate the procedure.

It is not recommended that practitioners use rapid detoxification as a means of induction onto naltrexone, particularly not on an occasional basis. These guidelines are intended for those practitioners who have decided to perform rapid detoxification on a regular basis.

Opioid antagonist precipitated withdrawal

The administration of opioid antagonists (such as naloxone or naltrexone) to an individual who is currently physiologically dependent on opioids precipitates an immediate abstinence syndrome, often of considerable severity. This is the basis for the naloxone challenge test to diagnose opioid dependence (see Appendix 1).

The acute phase of precipitated withdrawal involves three major clusters of symptoms: gastrointestinal, psychologic, and physiologic symptoms. Gastrointestinal symptoms include vomiting and diarrhea, often with cramping abdominal pain, lasting many hours. Without supportive treatment patients may become dehydrated and develop electrolyte disturbances as a result of severe vomiting. Psychologic disturbances may include agitation, dysphoria, and delirium which can last for up to 12 hours. Significant physiologic disturbances may include a marked increase in circulating catecholamines.

The trade-off is that some aspects of antagonist-precipitated withdrawal appear to be of shorter duration than the process of spontaneous withdrawal. For example, in anesthetized patients given a bolus dose of naloxone or naltrexone, signs of physiologic withdrawal resolve in 4–6 hours. Once acute withdrawal signs have subsided, further administration of naloxone evokes no further withdrawal signs, and this has been taken as definitive evidence that acute withdrawal is complete.

However, while acute signs of withdrawal subside, many patients remain ill for considerably longer than this acute phase. The key step to minimizing the severity of acute precipitated withdrawal, and the severity of persisting symptoms over the next several days, is to delay the introduction of naltrexone until 48 hours after the last use of heroin, or 5 days after the last use of methadone. Administration of naltrexone without observing such a delay risks severe physiologic and psychologic reactions.

Approaches

The published literature on rapid detoxification is characterized by a marked variation in approaches used, reported outcomes, and reported severity of symptoms associated with detoxification and in medium-term outcomes. Broadly speaking, two approaches to rapid detoxification have evolved: rapid detoxification under anesthesia, and rapid detoxification using sedation.

Anesthesia-based approaches to rapid detoxification involve airway protection to minimize the risk of aspiration. However, many patients are persistently unwell after the procedure. Use of anesthesia-based approaches requires skilled personnel, and high-level medical settings such as an intensive care unit (ICU) or operating room for 4–6 hours, and is more expensive than procedures involving sedation. Australian studies suggest that patient outcomes post rapid detoxification under anesthesia are no better than outcomes post rapid detoxification using sedation.

What all approaches to rapid detoxification have in common is the administration of an antagonist to precipitate withdrawal, use of symptomatic treatment to alleviate the severe precipitated acute withdrawal, and use of symptomatic treatment to alleviate persisting dysphoria and gastrointestinal symptoms after acute withdrawal has subsided.

The key components of rapid detoxification include assessment and informed consent, an adequate interval between the patient's last dose of an opioid and introduction of naltrexone, provision of symptomatic medication, and provision of an appropriate setting for care.

Assessment and informed consent

Naltrexone is not registered in Australia for use in rapid detoxification. Clinicians offering this treatment have an obligation to fully and accurately inform patients of the risks and benefits of the procedure, and alternative treatment approaches, and to ensure that patients are able to give informed consent to the treatment. Adequate assessment is the key to obtaining informed consent and appropriate patient selection.

The provision of accurate information about the procedure and naltrexone treatment is critical. Patients and their support people (if consent is given for their involvement in care) should be informed of the documented effectiveness of naltrexone treatment. Consumer demand for rapid detoxification appeared to be guided by the belief that it offered quick, painless detoxification, which committed patients to abstinence. However, these perceptions were not well founded. Research has consistently demonstrated that rapid detoxification is neither quick nor painless, with persisting withdrawal symptoms and malaise for several days.

Rapid detoxification does improve short-term induction onto naltrexone, but thereafter attrition from treatment is high. Sixty percent or more of patients undergoing rapid detoxification relapse to heroin addiction within 6 months.

Poorly motivated patients, and those in unstable social circumstances, are poor candidates for naltrexone treatment. Patients who are homeless or in highly unstable social circumstances require a comprehensive plan to stabilize their circumstances prior to undergoing rapid detoxification. It is probably best to defer naltrexone treatment in those patients who are ambivalent about remaining abstinent from opioids.

The assessment documented in the medical record should include: drug use and treatment history, medical and psychiatric history, psychosocial history, physical and mental state examination, and assessment of motivation.

Contraindications include pregnancy, a history of cardiac disease, or evidence of heart disease on clinical examination, chronic renal impairment, decompensated liver disease including jaundice, ascites, and hepatic encephalopathy, current dependence on benzodiazepines, alcohol, or stimulants, and a history of psychosis.

Relative contraindications to rapid detoxification include moderate or severe depressive symptoms. Psychiatric assessment is recommended in these cases.

Prospective patients should be supplied with written and verbal information about the nature of the proposed treatment, risks involved, steps to minimize the risk of severe withdrawal, known benefits and risks of naltrexone treatment, costs of treatment and the services that will be provided, and the role of any support people.

All patients must be warned at the outset, and at follow-up visits, of the risks of opioid overdose on discontinuing naltrexone and recommencing opioid use. There have been cases where patients on methadone treatment have undergone rapid detoxification without informing their methadone prescriber or their methadone-dispensing pharmacist, and where resumption of methadone has resulted in fatal overdose.

Patients on methadone should be asked to consent to the notification of their methadone prescriber and dispensing pharmacist of their proposed rapid detoxification. Where patient consent is not given, it is not appropriate to proceed with rapid detoxification.

Interval between last opioid use and rapid detoxification

Delaying the administration of antagonists until there are very low levels of circulating opioid drugs minimizes the severity of acute withdrawal and greatly reduces the severity of protracted withdrawal in the first week of naltrexone treatment.

After conventional detoxification, naltrexone should only be introduced after 5 days free of heroin or 10 days after the last dose of methadone. Rapid detoxification reduces the delay in commencing naltrexone. Naltrexone may be introduced after at least 48 hours free of short-acting opioids such as heroin or morphine, or at least 5 days free of methadone.

After these intervals, most opioid-dependent patients will experience moderate precipitated withdrawal and will require symptomatic support and monitoring.

Opioids must be entirely avoided in the interval prior to rapid detoxification. During this opioid-free interval, patients can be treated with clonidine and other symptomatic medications as needed to minimize withdrawal distress.

Provision of symptomatic medication

Prior to induction to naltrexone, clonidine is used in doses up to 300 μg 8 hourly with 900 μg per day maximum dose. Clonidine helps control agitation and restlessness. However, the dose which can be employed is limited by side-effects – most patients will become somewhat hypotensive, and should be warned of this risk.

It is generally safest to start with a dose of 150 μg every 6 hours, monitoring the symptomatic response and the patient's blood pressure. Clonidine should be withheld if the systolic blood pressure falls below 90 mmHg or patients complain of light headedness. Doses as low as 75 μg 4 to 6 hourly can help relieve withdrawal distress.

Clonidine should be commenced at around the time the patient begins to experience withdrawal symptoms, generally about 8 hours after the last use of heroin or 24 hours after their last dose of methadone. Clonidine should be continued until the patient has commenced naltrexone.

Other medications which may provide symptomatic relief in the period prior to induction onto naltrexone include: quinine sulfate 300 mg 2 times daily for muscle cramps, metoclopramide 10 mg 3 times daily for nausea and vomiting, and temazepam 20 mg at night for insomnia. Medications should not be given as a prescription, but should be dispensed daily to patients during the lead up to rapid detoxification.

On commencement of rapid detoxification, octreotide, a synthetic somatostatin analog, is the most effective agent for controlling gastrointestinal symptoms during precipitated withdrawal. Administer 100 µg subcutaneous octreotide prior to precipitating withdrawal.

Sedation is usually employed during the acute phase of precipitated withdrawal in non-anesthetized patients. Medications which depress consciousness, such as high-dose benzodiazepines, alleviate psychologic distress but increase the risk of aspiration as a result of depressed gag reflex. If patients have observed the appropriate opioid-free interval prior to commencement of naltrexone it is recommended that 5 mg diazepam be administered as premedication prior to precipitating withdrawal.

Precipitation of withdrawal

It is recommended that precipitated withdrawal be commenced with naloxone rather than naltrexone. Even with careful explanation to prospective patients, it is not always possible to be confident that people presenting for rapid detoxification will have observed the required opioid-free interval. For this reason it is recommended that precipitated withdrawal be initiated with naloxone rather than naltrexone.

Naloxone is a shorter-acting antagonist than naltrexone. If a patient has a severe withdrawal reaction to naloxone, the drug rapidly wears off, usually in less than an hour. In contrast, precipitated withdrawal from naltrexone lasts many hours and so it is highly desirable to initiate precipitated withdrawal with naloxone.

Administer 0.4 mg naloxone by intramuscular injection (im). If the reaction is too severe the procedure can be aborted. If the patient tolerates naloxone 0.4 mg im, naltrexone 25 mg can be administered orally.

All approaches to rapid detoxification involve balancing safety against tolerability. Clonidine can produce significant hypotension and bradycardia. In the context of dehydration, this can contribute to acute renal failure. Benzodiazepines can contribute to worsening of delirium, and to depression of consciousness, respiration, and gag reflex, and increased risk of aspiration. The more medications used to ameliorate symptoms, the greater the risks of drug interactions and potentiation of cardiovascular and respiratory toxicity. There have been several documented fatalities associated with rapid detoxification, mostly associated with the administration of multiple medications.

Setting for care

Anesthesia-based approaches to rapid detoxification require skilled personnel and high-level medical settings (ICU or operating room for 4–6 hours).

Rapid detoxification with sedation can be performed in settings with lower levels of care, and can be performed in ambulatory patients. However, as a precaution in the event of a severe precipitated withdrawal, rapid detoxification under sedation should only be performed where there is access to an adequate level of care, including: adequately trained nursing staff to deal with a severe reaction and possibly individualized nursing for 4 hours, medical staff on site for 4 hours from induction, and available on call for at least 24 hours after the first dose, access to medications, access to basic resuscitation equipment, and staff trained in the use of these devices.

Occasionally, even after great care in screening patients, a patient has a severe withdrawal reaction. During rapid detoxification, the first dose of naltrexone should always be administered in the morning to ensure that peak severity of precipitated withdrawal occurs at a time when medical support is most readily available.

Patients should be observed for a minimum of 3 hours after administration of naltrexone. If they are well, they can be discharged. On the evening after the first dose, temazepam 20 mg may be given, thereafter patients receive 50 mg naltrexone daily each morning.

Patients who are agitated or distressed at the end of 3 hours should remain under observation with regular monitoring and reassurance. Symptomatic relief is of some benefit: clonidine may be administered if the patient's pulse is above 55 and systolic blood pressure is above 90 mmHg systolic; buscopan is helpful for abdominal cramps, and quinine is helpful for muscle cramps.

Occasionally, the precipitated withdrawal may be of such severity that it is inappropriate to discharge the patient, thus arrangements should be in place to ensure a patient can receive inpatient care overnight if needed.

Patient information and warnings on naltrexone treatment

Patients should be supplied with take-home patient information and a medical warning card. Practitioners should cover the following points with patients:

- The patient (and carer if involved) must be made aware that naltrexone is not a 'miracle cure' for opioid dependence. Naltrexone does not influence the underlying reasons for opioid use and this is why appropriate counseling and support are integral to successful naltrexone treatment.
- Patients must be explicitly warned that attempting to overcome the naltrexone-induced opioid receptor blockade with large doses of opioids can result in fatal opioid overdose.
- Patients should also be warned that when they cease naltrexone treatment they will have an increased sensitivity or diminished tolerance to opioids, and that relatively small doses of heroin may result in fatal overdose. If the patient has decided to use heroin again they should consider themselves as a 'new user'.
- Patients should be advised that, on ceasing naltrexone, it takes very little use of heroin to develop physiologic dependence. After only a few days of daily heroin use, further ingestion of naltrexone may precipitate a withdrawal reaction. Patients should be cautioned about sharing their naltrexone with opioid-dependent friends or engaging in 'home detoxification'.
- Patients should be advised to carry a medical warning card or bracelet, which states they will not respond to opioid analgesia. Warning cards may be obtained from the sponsoring pharmaceutical company. The patient should also inform other relevant clinicians involved in their medical care that they are taking naltrexone so that appropriate pain management can be provided.
- Patients should be advised that they may experience increased sex drive and fertility compared to when they were taking opioids and to use reliable contraception to avoid pregnancy. Female patients in particular should be counseled about avoiding pregnancy while taking naltrexone as its safe use in pregnancy and while breastfeeding has not

been established. The decision to continue naltrexone treatment in pregnancy involves careful assessment of the relative risks to the fetus and the likelihood of relapse to heroin use.

- It is safe to drink alcohol while taking naltrexone. Naltrexone will not stop an individual becoming intoxicated. However, alcohol intoxication while taking naltrexone has been reported at times to be unpleasant.
- The potential for relapse after ceasing treatment is high. Clinical experience suggests that active attempts to contact people who discontinue treatment or miss appointments may improve the outcomes of naltrexone treatment. At the commencement of treatment, it is desirable to confirm with patients that they consent to attempts being made to contact them to reschedule appointments if they fail to attend.

References

1. Volpicelli JR, Alterman AI, Hayashida M, O'Brien CP. Naltrexone in the treatment of alcohol dependence. Arch Gen Psychiat 1992; 49: 876–80.
2. O'Malley SS. Opioid antagonists in the treatment of alcohol dependence: clinical efficacy and prevention of relapse. Alcohol Alcoholism 1996; 31(1): 77–81.
3. Volpicelli JR. Naltrexone and alcohol dependence: role of subject compliance. Arch Gen Psychiat 1997; 54(8): 737–42.
4. O'Connor P, Kosten T. Rapid and ultrarapid opioid detoxification techniques. JAMA 1998; 279: 229–34.
5. Gonzales JP, Brogden RN. Naltrexone: a review of its pharmacodynamic and pharmacokinetic properties and therapeutic efficacy in the management of opioid dependence. Drugs 1988; 35: 192–213.
6. Lee MC, Wagner HN, Tanada S, Frost JJ, Bice AN, Dannals RF. Duration of occupancy of opiate receptors by naltrexone. J Nucl Med 1988; 29(7): 1207–11.
7. Zanis DA, Woody GE. One-year mortality rates following methadone treatment discharge. Drug Alcohol Depen 1998; 52(3): 257–60.
8. Croop RS. The safety profile of naltrexone in the treatment of alcoholism: results from a multicenter usage study. Arch Gen Psychiat 1997; 54: 1130–5.
9. Rawson RA, Tennant FS Jr. Five-year follow-up of opiate addicts with naltrexone and behavior therapy. NIDA Res Monogr 1984; 49: 289–95.
10. Ward J, Mattick RP, Hall W, eds. Methadone maintenance treatment and other opioid replacement therapies. London: Harwood Press; 1998.
11. Brahen LS, Henderson RK, Capone T, Kordal N. Naltrexone treatment in a jail work-release program. J Clin Psychiat 1984; 45(9): 49–52.
12. Washton AM, Pottash AC, Gold MS. Naltrexone in addicted business executives and physicians. J Clin Psychiat 1984; 45: 4–6.

13. Ling W. The clinical investigator's dilemma. NIDA Res Monogr 1978; 19: 308–14.
14. Staedt J, Wassmuth F, Stoppe G, et al. Effects of chronic treatment with methadone and naltrexone on sleep in addicts. Eur Arch Psy Clin N 1996; 246(6): 305–9.

Appendix 1: Naloxone (Narcan®) challenge

It is strongly recommended that the Narcan® challenge test be undertaken when inducting patients onto naltrexone. There are however occasions where this may not be clinically indicated. Patients should be provided with information regarding the procedure, including the rationale behind the procedure.

Procedure

- Explain the test and the reason for performing it
- Intramuscular administration: 0.4 mg naloxone, repeat with another 0.4 mg in 10 minutes if no indication of withdrawal, or
- Intravenous administration: 0.2 mg naloxone and if no indication of withdrawal after 60 seconds, give a further 0.6 mg and observe for 5 minutes.

Withdrawal signs should peak within 10 minutes:

(a) piloerection – palpable and lasting more than 30 seconds;
(b) rhinorrhea, lacrimation, yawning (more than 3 times);
(c) sweating – wet rather than moist;
(d) vomiting.

Piloerection is the most decisive withdrawal sign. Restlessness is also a feature of a positive response to naloxone.

Interpretation

The naloxone challenge may be interpreted as positive (that is the patient is still physically dependent on opioids) if there is:

- a marked response with any one of the signs of withdrawal (a), (b), (c), or (d)
- a milder response with any two of the signs of withdrawal (a), (b), (c), or (d).

An alternative approach to interpreting the response to a naloxone challenge is to administer the Subjective and Objective Opiate Withdrawal Scales prior to administration of naloxone, and then repeat the administration of the scales at 10 and 20 minutes post-naloxone challenge.

A mild response is indicated as an increase of up to 2 points on the objective scale, or an increase of less than 5 points on the subjective scale. A positive response to naloxone is an increase greater than 2 points on the objective scale or 5 or more points on the subjective scale.

Response

If there is a mild positive response to naloxone, delay induction onto naltrexone and plan to re-challenge with naloxone after at least 24 hours. Reassure the patient that discomfort will pass in 20 minutes. If there is a severe response intramuscular morphine 10 mg can be administered, and detoxification from opiates advised.

If there are no signs other than a subjective response to naloxone, ask the patient if they would be able to tolerate this state for the next 24 hours. If the patient feels able to do so, they can be administered naltrexone 12.5 mg and be reviewed later that day.

If there is no response to the naloxone challenge, naltrexone treatment may be initiated with a starting dose of 25 mg. If there are no signs of withdrawal or side-effects following this initial naltrexone dose, the patient can go home, with instructions to take naltrexone 50 mg daily thereafter. If the patient complains of significant withdrawal or side-effects, maintain the patient on naltrexone 25 mg until symptoms have resolved.

Appendix 2: Management of acute opioid withdrawal precipitated by naltrexone

Introduction

Naltrexone is an opioid antagonist registered for use in Australia. There have been a number of reports of opioid-dependent people self-administering naltrexone, precipitating a severe withdrawal reaction requiring hospital treatment. These guidelines are to assist medical and nursing staff to recognize and manage naltrexone-precipitated withdrawal.

Precipitated withdrawal

Onset of naltrexone-precipitated withdrawal occurs 20 to 60 minutes following ingestion. Gastrointestinal symptoms are usually predominant, severe vomiting and diarrhea may occur. Patients become agitated and distressed, and delirium with confusion is common. Signs of sympathetic overactivity, particularly profuse sweating and piloerection, may occur. If a patient has taken sedative drugs in conjunction with naltrexone, as commonly occurs, delirium is exacerbated but other signs may be less clear.

There are significant risks associated with precipitated withdrawal. Most deaths associated with precipitated withdrawal appear to have been the result of aspiration associated with high doses of sedative drugs. In people who have received high doses of sedating drugs, delayed respiratory depression emerging after acute withdrawal has subsided may have contributed to deaths. Fluid and electrolyte problems can be secondary to vomiting and diarrhea. During acute delirium, confused patients must be considered at risk and require medical care.

Diagnosis and assessment

History may be difficult to obtain from confused patients, particularly if they are defensive about being identified as heroin users. Suspect naltrexone-precipitated withdrawal in any patient presenting with signs of opioid withdrawal in conjunction with delirium or intractable vomiting. A history of opioid dependence should be gained from the patient or significant others, or by inspection of injection sites for recent track marks. An absence of track marks should not exclude this diagnosis. Careful assessment of the degree of sedation and of the patient's capacity to protect their airway is essential. The use of flumazenil to reverse sedation is not recommended due to the chance of the presenting patient having concurrent benzodiazepine dependence and the risk of inducing life-threatening seizures. Deeply sedated vomiting patients may require intubation and ICU management. It may be desirable to check electrolytes and arterial blood gases.

Management

Naltrexone-precipitated withdrawal is self-limiting, with delirium usually lasting only about 4 hours. Treatment is supportive and symptomatic.

Patients with vomiting may require fluid and electrolyte replacement. Although most patients will experience fluid loss to some degree, the insertion of iv cannulae and administration of fluids should be balanced against potential problems. Patients in delirium frequently remove iv lines. Most patients will be capable of tolerating oral fluids within 12 hours of ingestion of naltrexone.

During naltrexone-induced withdrawal delirium, most patients can be reoriented. This is critical in both obtaining a history and in managing the confused patient. The most important part of management is reassuring the patient that symptoms, although severe, will be short lived. Treating staff should be aware that the antagonist-induced withdrawal syndrome is extremely traumatic and that patients expressing fear of death, for example, should not be treated contemptuously, but given appropriate repeated reassurance.

The administration of opioid agonists is unlikely to be helpful. Patients should be warned that taking heroin will not alleviate symptoms. In managing vomiting and diarrhea, clinical experience indicates that conventional anti-emetics provide little relief. Octreotide 100 µg subcutaneously is the drug of choice in reducing vomiting and diarrhea. Agitation and sympathetic overactivity can be treated with clonidine 150 µg orally, or 100 µg intramuscular administration, repeated after 2 hours if agitation persists and hypotension is not a problem. Urgent sedation is imperative where patients are violent and confused, midazolam 5–10 mg intramuscular administration may be helpful. When abdominal cramps are a problem, a single dose of hyoscine-*N*-butylbromide 20 mg can help.

Additional management

Patients and families should be informed that residual symptoms may persist for up to 7 days. Patients need to be warned of the risk of overdose if they use heroin following naltrexone.

chapter 14

Choosing treatments: The role of economics in informing future decisions

Marian Shanahan and Richard P Mattick

The foregoing chapters have set out the evidence on the effects of opioid pharmacotherapies on dependent users' health and drug-seeking behavior. Others have reached similar conclusions, giving converging support for the broad conclusions set out herein. For example, Amato et al,[1] in an appraisal of five Cochrane reviews on substitution maintenance treatments for opioid dependence, found that methadone maintenance was more effective in treatment retention than methadone detoxification, buprenorphine, LAAM, and heroin methadone maintenance and that higher-dose methadone is more effective than lower doses. Limited data existed on heroin use, but methadone was found effective at suppressing heroin use.[1] These are the robust findings about the effects of these pharmacotherapies.

Given the evidence, it is likely that treatments for serious drug problems will become more broadly available internationally, as new awareness of public health takes precedence over government and community concerns about the nature of the treatments. However, these treatments are not without cost and resource implications. A challenge that will continue to face governments that attempt to reduce problems associated with opioid dependence through such treatment options is the costs that will accrue to the government and community as a consequence of management of opioid dependence. Being able to justify treatment from a clinical perspective is feasible in terms of public and patient health, but the questions of cost and effects and cost–benefit are also very important in determining the use of these medications. Choosing between treatment options is not easy, and the economic literature is still limited in its coverage of the issues. However, the literature on costs and effects/benefits that is available tells us that treatment almost certainly pays for itself but there are other issues to consider. This final chapter addresses some of these issues.

Allocation of limited resources

One of the few truths in life is that resources are limited – this truth, combined with unbridled demand, creates challenges in resource allocation. However, when it comes to health care, 'more is not always better, people in general *do not* want ineffective, or minimally effective care, especially when it is inconvenient, unpleasant or dangerous'.[2] This discord can create tensions in the field of substance abuse, a chronic remitting disease, where evidence demonstrates that treatment can work for those who remain in treatment, but where there is often a high drop-out rate with many clients as aware of the limitations and side-effects of treatment as clinicians who are recommending treatment. Additionally, the allocation of resources to assist with what is almost universally seen as a stigmatized and highly self-indulgent behavior often raises questions for governments and society. Government and the community often prefer a policing and criminal justice response to a treatment response, although the costs of such a law enforcement response occur at some significant financial cost and these responses often appear not to be as closely evaluated as new clinical treatments. This is despite the fact that there is good evidence that treatment for opioid dependence can be effective as a crime prevention measure.[3] These are issues which economics may be able to speak to.

When assessing a treatment there are a number of questions which are asked and answered: does it work and is it safe (efficacy), will it work in real-life clinical settings (effectiveness), is the treatment cost beneficial from a societal perspective, and finally given scarce resources, is one treatment more or less cost-effective than another in general, or for specific populations (for example, those with comorbid mental health problems, pregnant women, or adolescents)?

Economics, based on the principles of technical and allocative efficiency, can help with answering the last of these two questions, but even with these tools there are a number of challenges and, unlike clinical efficacy and effectiveness, findings may not be generalizable from one setting to another.[4] For example, what is an efficient use of resources in a highly urbanized developed country may not be suitable in a lesser-developed rural environment. The term *technical efficiency* refers to the relationship between resources used and outcomes achieved with the use of those resources. A technically efficient result occurs when the maximum possible improvement in outcome is obtained from a given set of resource inputs. If the output could have been produced with less of one or more inputs, this is referred to as technical inefficiency. The disparity in relative costs of resources in different locales may lead to alternative treatments being found to be technically efficient in some locales but not in others. *Allocative efficiency*, on the other hand, is used to assess the broader costs and consequences. For example, if society produced only goods which no-one wanted to purchase, but they did it cheaply, this would be allocative *inefficiency*. In the case of opioid dependence treatment, a technically efficient treatment that produces what is needed or wanted (allocative efficiency) is the best option.

Cost-effectiveness and benefit

Ultimately, economics is about producing the outcomes which society desires, in the most efficient manner, whether it is within or beyond the health care sector. However, there is still room to explore efficient resource use within a given sector such as health. Within economics there are two major techniques which can provide guidance; cost-effectiveness and cost–benefit analyses. Typically, cost-effectiveness analysis (CEA) is used to address questions such as whether one treatment (e.g., buprenorphine) is more cost-effective than another treatment (e.g., methadone) in achieving a given outcome (e.g. reducing heroin use or saving lives). Cost–benefit analysis (CBA), by way of contrast assigns monetary values to health and non-health outcomes, and it is used to assess questions such as which treatments are of value to society.[2,5]

Starting with the second of these, in the substance abuse area CBAs typically assess whether the cost of treatment has positive societal benefits in terms of decreasing crime rates, decreasing use of health care services, and other social gains such as decreasing the rates of HIV/AIDS and hepatitis C and increasing productivity. The strength of CBA, valuing outcomes in a single currency, is also one of its challenges. Mooney effectively articulated one of these challenges 'to be trained in medicine, nursing or one of the other "sharp end" disciplines and then be faced with some hard-nosed, cold-blooded economist placing money values on human life and suffering is anathema to many'.[6] There are a number of methods (contingent valuation, human capital approach, and revealed/stated preference) that are used to value human life and suffering in CBA but each comes with its own set of difficulties and assumptions which are well described elsewhere.[5] Whichever method is used, in order to inform decision making, it is important that the methods used to value human life, pain, and suffering are clearly articulated and all assumptions clearly stated. In substance abuse, a number of challenges arise when trying to assign monetary values to family burdens related to substance abuse, communities' fear of crime, change in drug use, and change in injecting behaviors. Failure to capture these changes often leads to valuing only those items which are easier to value, such as use of health services in and out of treatment and costs related to criminal activities (police, court, and jail).

Cost-effectiveness analysis is the other main form of economic analysis. CEA compares the incremental economic costs and the incremental benefits of two or more treatments and provides a cost per unit of outcome gain. In CEA, the outcome is measured in some natural unit such as reduction in days of heroin use, abstinence, lives saved, or quality-adjusted life years saved. Such methods are widely used to assess new medications and technologies and are often required as part of submissions to government regulatory bodies (such as the US Food and Drug Administration or the Australian Pharmaceutical Benefits Advisory Committee) for funding of new treatments or medications. The results from these studies are often appealing and intuitive for policy makers and clinicians, particularly in areas where there appears to be a clear single outcome measure. In substance abuse treatment, however, there are many relevant outcomes (changes in days of substance use, total abstinence, changes in crime rates, mental health status, and productivity to name a few), and it is unlikely that changes in these measures all move in the same direction and with the same magnitude.[7] This then leads to contradictory incremental cost-effectiveness ratios when different outcome measures are used, as was found by Sindelar et al.[8] These authors argue that cost-effectiveness should be rejected for CBA. However, as discussed above, CBA also has limitations. Another limitation of CEA is that it is client focused, as it does not capture any externalities (effects which spill over to other persons).

While CBA is useful, in many situations the actual type of analysis which should be used is a function of the question being asked, as CBAs are often large and resource-intensive undertakings. Dismuke et al[9] suggests that while improved health is an outcome of addiction treatment, most program administrators and policy makers are interested in the non-health-related outcomes such as lower crime rates, improved employment status, and decreased use of social services.[9] It is understandable that politicians and economists are interested in these wider outcomes but one could question whether it is rational for local program administrators, clinicians, and policy makers within health to be interested in outcomes beyond health unless they receive monetary transfers (as a function of these positive benefits) from other government departments. For example, if methadone is more cost-effective than buprenorphine from the agency or funder's perspective when a health outcome is used, but buprenorphine is more cost-effective when crime costs are included, it may be argued that methadone provision should be the first choice from a health perspective but buprenorphine the first choice from a whole of government approach.

Cost–benefit of treatment

Several reviews of the literature have determined treatment is cost-beneficial from a societal perspective, but often study designs were weak, and the lack of controls further lessens the validity of the studies.[7,10,11] Ratios of benefits to costs have ranged widely from 1.33:1 to 39.0:1, which means that for every dollar spent on treatment, a benefit from $1.33 to $39 was gained. It is hard to know what to make of such a range, except the cost–benefit ratios are uniformly positive showing that treatment more than pays for itself, and that most benefits are accrued from a decrease in crime.[7,11,12] Examination of the studies included in these reviews found that very few pertain specifically to treatment for opioid misuse, rather many evaluate substance abuse more broadly. Some further identify alcohol or illicit drug use, but not whether the primary drug was an opioid, cocaine, or other.[13] If the results from the generalized substance abuse studies hold true for opioid misuse, then treatment is likely cost-beneficial, but crucially the cost savings may not be directly realized by the health department let alone the treatment agencies that are providing treatment.[14]

A model developed to explore the lifetime costs and benefits of methadone compared to no treatment determined that if 60% of ever-heroin users sought treatment they would use heroin almost half as long as those who never sought treatment (6.58 years compared to 12.4); would be employed for more years (16.07 compared to 6.08), and live for longer after the age of 18 (27.13 compared to 16.9 additional years). The lifetime benefit–cost ratio was estimated at 37.7. If the number of ever-users entering treatment increases from 60% to 73.7%, the benefit–cost ratio increases to 76. While there were a number of simplifying assumptions made in this model, it demonstrates the lifetime cost–benefits from a social perspective of a widely available, well-used methadone program.[15]

Cost-effectiveness analyses

Turning to the cost-effectiveness literature, there are a limited number of cost-effectiveness studies which address opioid use specifically. Only those studies which evaluate treatment for opioid misuse or report results separately for opioid users are included here. Moreover, the literature is largely made up of one-off studies, with little real replication. A recent review of economic evaluations of methadone or buprenorphine located 28 papers, but concluded that only 11 were of sufficient quality to be included.[16] And furthermore, the authors concluded that none of these 11 studies contained all of the necessary data, outcomes, or comparators to make their results generalizable for the UK NHS, nor could direct comparisons between studies be made due to different approaches, time horizons, and preference weights.[16] Still another review finds few (two) studies adopting a societal perspective and using final outcomes such as QALYs.[11]

A Cochrane review conducted in 2005 concluded that there was insufficient research to make recommendations as to the effectiveness or cost-effectiveness of various methods of opioid detoxification.[17] Subsequently, a study which compared the costs and clinical outcomes for rapid opioid detoxification with and without anesthesia found similar clinical outcomes but significantly higher costs for the anesthesia group.[18]

An Australian study compared five methods of detoxification for heroin use.[19] In this study, a buprenorphine-based outpatient detoxification method was found to be the most cost-effective method overall when compared to conventional outpatient (clonidine-based), rapid opioid detoxification under anesthetic, rapid opioid detoxification under sedation, and conventional (clonidine-based) inpatient treatments. Two clinical outcome measures were used (abstinence and uptake of ongoing maintenance treatment) and buprenorphine was the most cost-effective option with both outcomes. When methadone maintenance was compared to a 180-day methadone detoxification in a randomized trial, methadone maintenance was found to be more effective than detoxification, and at a cost of $15,967 USD per life-year saved was assessed to be cost-effective.[20]

Barnett also estimated the incremental cost-effectiveness of methadone maintenance relative to a placebo, estimating lifetime costs and the impact on life expectancy. The cost per life-year gained was $5,915 (1996 USD), which Barnett argued compared favorably with other common medical treatments.[21] Barnett and colleagues also addressed the cost-effectiveness of buprenorphine compared to methadone using a dynamic modeling process.[22] Using a price per dose ranging from $5 to $15 (USD) for buprenorphine (as there was no price available at the time of the study), the researchers reported that even at the highest price, the cost per quality-adjusted life year (QALY) (USD) gained was less than $45,000 in most of the scenarios considered, thus falling under the oft used $50,000 threshold. They concluded both treatments were worth purchasing.

In two Australian randomized controlled trials comparing methadone and buprenorphine, it was determined that when the outcome measure was change in heroin use there was no statistical difference in cost-effectiveness,[23,24] but when the outcomes were measured in QALYs and the costs of crime were included, buprenorphine dominated methadone, i.e. it was less costly and achieved additional but not significantly more QALYs.[24] This leads to the conclusion that, from the health perspective, there is no difference in cost-effectiveness between methadone and buprenorphine. However, from a societal perspective, it may be that buprenorphine is more cost-effective than methadone, although this is based on a single study. This lack of replication in cost-effectiveness analysis is a significant problem affecting this area generally.

Other data supporting methadone's cost-effectiveness come from 5 heroin maintenance trials whose data were pooled to enable direct comparison of the cost-effectiveness of 4 maintenance pharmacotherapies in the Australian National Evaluation of Pharmacotherapies for Opioid Dependence (NEPOD). The results of the cost-effectiveness analysis suggest, for the primary outcome measure of change in heroin-free days, that LAAM and MMT are statistically equivalent in terms of cost-effectiveness while MMT (and LAAM) are dominant treatment options compared with BMT and naltrexone.[25,26] Following a systematic review of the clinical effectiveness and economic literature on the use of oral naltrexone in opioid-dependent people it was concluded that there was no statistically significant difference in relapse prevention between naltrexone and a placebo with or without counseling.[27] Having found no economic evaluations of naltrexone in the literature, a decision analytic Monte Carlo simulation was used to estimate the cost-effectiveness of naltrexone. The cost per QALY was found to be £42,500, but the cost-effectiveness curves did not ever go above 55% for any willingness to pay threshold due to the uncertainty of the estimates used in the model.[27] The authors subsequently concluded that naltrexone is not cost-effective from the perspective of the UK National Health System.

The situation can be further complicated by coprescribing another medication. For instance, a Dutch cost–utility study coprescribed heroin and methadone (patients received methadone once a day and heroin up to 3 times per day) compared to methadone maintenance only. They found the combined treatment was more cost-effective. The outcome measure was the EQ-5D, a measure of quality of life, and the costs included the cost of treatment, other health care use, and illegal activities. There was a significant improvement in QALYs in the coprescribed group but no change in QALY in the methadone group. The two groups used similar quantities of methadone, there was no difference in other health care use, but the experimental group engaged in fewer criminal activities as measured by self-report days of crime and arrests. The experimental group had significantly higher treatment costs at €17,634 per year versus €1,412 for the methadone group. However, when the costs of damage to victims from criminal activities were factored in, the experimental group was less expensive at €37,767 compared to €50,560, leading to the conclusion that the combined heroin/methadone treatment was more cost-effective than methadone alone in patients who had previously failed to respond to methadone.[28] Obviously, what one chooses to value (and cost) affects conclusions drawn (as noted earlier).

In summary, of the pharmaceutical treatments currently available, methadone maintenance appears to be the most effective at maintaining individuals in treatment.[1] and the least costly program to provide.[23,24,26] However, when costs of crime are included, both buprenorphine and heroin maintenance (with coprescribed methadone maintenance treatment) appear to be more cost-effective than methadone. The small number of studies and the lack of robust replicated findings, and the extent to which what is costed affects results, make these latter conclusions tentative at best.

The introduction of office-based buprenorphine with or without naltrexone in the US and France, in particular, has expanded the availability of opioid treatment.[29] However, to date there is no conclusive evidence on the cost-effectiveness of this treatment modality,[29] although an Australian clinic-based study demonstrated that the effectiveness of buprenorphine/naltrexone was no different for the group receiving daily dispensing compared to a group which received weekly dispensing; however the later group had significantly lower costs.[30]

Beyond CEA and CBA – opportunity costs

As noted earlier, there are two sets of decisions to be made concerning health care resource allocation for the management of opioid dependence. The first is at the societal level – that is what proportion of scarce resources is to be used in the treatment of opioid use? The second question is how are those resources to be allocated? Data from good cost–benefit analyses permit comparisons with other wider demands for resources and so may help with the first decision, but may not assist with the second decision. This is when we turn to cost-effectiveness analysis; however, even cost-effectiveness analysis with incremental cost-effectiveness ratios (ICERs) may not be sufficient information for policy makers. For example, if the most cost-effective treatment (the one with the lowest ICER) is to be provided, as is widely recommended, or alternatively any treatment with an ICER under a particular threshold (nominally USD $50,000), the issue of opportunity cost is ignored.[31] Particularly important when there are no additional funds available, is whether the benefits of the new treatment exceed the benefits forgone from the treatment that is no longer supported in order to fund the new treatment.[31]

Data on buprenorphine uptake in England provide an illustration of the complexity of the issue.[32] Examination of the rates of prescriptions found that buprenorphine prescriptions increased in absolute and proportional terms, with buprenorphine accounting for 23% of all opiate prescriptions (up from 12% over a 2-year period). However, buprenorphine accounted for 45% of opioid prescription costs (up from 20%), placing treatment budgets under pressure and restricting the delivery of other treatments without substantiated benefit.

The coprescribed heroin study provides another case in point if this program were to be introduced, *without* additional funding. For every one person on coprescribed heroin approximately 12 methadone places might not be funded. The question then arises as to whether a gain of 0.058 of a QALY for the coprescribed person is worth the loss to the 12 persons who would benefit from methadone? A second issue is that the decision of those researchers to include the crime costs and costs of damage to victims (70% of the difference in the heroin trials) provides an implicit suggestion to treatment agencies and drug treatment policy makers that they should fund coprescribed heroin. However, if the benefits go to the individual and to the justice system, treatment providers may never see the benefit of treatment, and the harms may be increasingly visible if there are insufficient treatment places.

Future directions

The range of pharmacotherapies (and indeed the range of therapies more generally) that are deemed helpful for the serious disorder we call opioid dependence is surprisingly small although the current epidemic of opioid use and dependence is 40 years in the making. It is likely that the next 40 years will see an expansion in responses to the epidemic and some widening of policy and treatment options internationally. This widening will bring with it the likelihood that new medication formulations will be introduced to reduce problems associated with the current formulations and to target subgroups of users more specifically. This broadening of the treatment response to opioid dependence will bring with it a need for better data on the specific effectiveness of the new approaches as well as a need for better cost analysis and health economic approaches, while recognizing that what might be cost-effective (or cost-beneficial) in one geographic locale or at one time may not be so in others.

Contingency management (CM), the provision of a monetary incentive to improve compliance with treatment, is re-emerging as a topic for debate and additional research. The effectiveness of CM as a method of improving treatment responses has been evaluated for over 20 years.[33] Not all clinicians agree on the merits of CM, however; a survey of Australian and American clinicians reported broad acceptance of the use of CM,[33,34] although many remain concerned about the use of monetary rewards. There is increasing evidence on both the effectiveness and the cost-effectiveness of the use of CM in the treatment of opioid dependence.[35,36] In addition, National Institute for Health and Clinical Excellence (NICE) guidelines suggest consideration of the use of CM as part of a treatment plan for drug misuse. To date, the size of the incentive, conditions for its use, and society's willingness to pay for these incentives have not yet been determined.[36]

At this time, the research is clear that we do have effective treatments for opioid dependence, and that these are cost-beneficial. They should be delivered faithfully and not marginalized within the health care system, as the adequate delivery of these treatments is central to preserving their effectiveness and cost-benefits. The need to assess allocative efficiency in choosing treatments, and technical efficiency in treatment delivery, requires the interested policy maker and the clinician to focus on determining whether to choose to fund opioid pharmacotherapy in the first place and then how best to provide it clinically. These may remain the major challenges, especially for resource-poor countries where the choices are more stark than in some of those countries that already have a viable treatment response for opioid dependence.

References

1. Amato L, Davoli M, Perucci C, et al. An overview of systematic reviews of the effectiveness of opiate maintenance therapies: available evidence to inform clinical practice and research. J Subst Abuse Treat 2005; 28: 321–9.
2. Evans R. Towards a Healthier Economics: Reflections on Ken Bassett's problem. In: Barer M, Getzen T, Stoddart G, eds. Health, health care, and health economics. Perspectives on distribution 1998; 465–500. Toronto, Wiley.

3. Lind B, Chen S, Weatherburn D, Mattick R. The Effectiveness Of Methadone Maintenance Treatment In Controlling Crime: An Aggregate-Level Analysis Crime and Justice Statistics. Sydney, NSW Bureau of Crime Statistics and Research, 2004.
4. Drummond M. Pang F. Transferability of economic evaluation results. In: Drummond M, McGuire A, eds. Economic Evaluation in Health Care. Oxford, Oxford University Press, 2001.
5. Drummond M, Sculpher M, Torrance G, O'Brien B. Stoddart G. Methods for the economic evaluation of health care programmes. Third Edition. Oxford, Oxford University Press, 2005.
6. Mooney G. The economics of health and medicine. Brighton, Wheatsheaf, 1992.
7. Belenko S, Patpis, N. French, M. Economic benefits of drug treatment: A critical review of the evidence for policy makers. Treatment Research Institute, University of Pennsylvania, 2005.
8. Sindelar J, Joffre-Bonet M, French M, McLellan A. Cost-effectiveness analysis of addication treatment: paradoxes of multiple outcomes. Drug Alcohol Depen 2004; 73: 41–50.
9. Dismuke C, French M, Salomé H, et al. Out of touch or on the money: do the clinical objectives of addiction treatment coincide with economic evaluation results? J Subst Abuse Treat 2004; 27: 253–63.
10. Doran CM. Economic evaluation of interventions to treat opiate dependence: a review of the evidence. Pharmacoeconomics 2008; 26: 371–93.
11. McCollister K, French M. The relative contribution of outcome domains in the total economic benefit of addiction intervention: a review of first findings. Addiction 2003; 98: 1647–59.
12. Salome H, French M, Scott C, Foss M, Dennis M. Investigating variation in the costs and benefits of addiction treatment: econometric analysis of the Chicago Target Cities Project. Eval Program Plan 2003; 26: 325–38.
13. Harwood H, Malhotra D, Villarivera C, et al. Cost effectiveness and cost benefit analysis of substance abuse treatment: a literature review. Rockville, MD Substance Abuse and Mental Health Services Administration. Centre for Substance Abuse Treatment, 2002.
14. Zarkin G, Dunlap L, Hicks K, Mamo D. Benefits and costs of methadone treatments: results from a lifetime simulation model. Health Economics 2005; 14: 1133–50.
15. Connock M, Juarez-Garcia A, Jowett S, et al. Methadone and buprenorphine for the management of opioid dependence: a systematic review and economic evaluation. Health Technology Assessment. NHS R&D HTA Programme, 2007.
16. Day E, Ison J, Strang J. Inpatient versus other settings for detoxification for opioid dependence (review). In: Cochrane Database of Systematic Reviews; 2005, Issue 2. Art No CD004580. DOI 10.1002/14651858.CD004580.pub2.
17. De Jong C, Laheij R Krabbe. General anaesthesia does not improve outcome in opioid antagonist detoxification treatment: a randomized controlled trial. Addiction 2005; 100: 206–15.

18. Shanahan M, Doran C, Digiusto E, et al. The use of pharmacotherapies to aid detoxification from heroin: a cost effectiveness analysis. Addict Behav 2006; 31: 371–87.
19. Masson C, Barnett P, Sees K, et al. Cost and cost effectiveness of standard methadone maintenance treatment compared to enriched 180-day methadone detoxification. Addiction 2004; 99: 718–26.
20. Barnett P. The cost-effectiveness of methadone maintenance as a health care intervention. Addiction 1999; 94: 479–88.
21. Barnett P, Zaric G, Brandeau M. The cost-effectiveness of buprenorphine maintenance therapy for opiate addiction in the United States. Addiction 2001; 96: 1267–78.
22. Doran CM, Shanahan M, Mattick R, et al. Buprenorphine versus methadone maintenance: a cost-effectiveness analysis. Drug Alcohol Depen 2003; 71: 295–302.
23. Harris A, Gospodarevskaya E, Ritter A. A randomised trial of the cost effectiveness of buprenorphine as an alternative to methadone maintenance treatment for heroin dependence in a primary care setting. Pharmacoeconomics 2005; 23: 77–91.
24. Mattick R, Digiusto E, Doran C, et al. National Evaluation of Pharmacotherapies for Opioid Dependence: Report of Results and Recommendations. Monograph Series 52. Canberra, Australian Department of Health and Aging, 2001.
25. Doran C, Shanahan M, Digiusto E, et al. A cost-effectiveness analysis of maintenance treatments for dependent heroin users in the Australian National Evaluation of Pharmacotherapies for Opioid Dependence. Exp Rev Pharmaco Outcomes Res 2006; 6: 437–46.
26. Adi Y, Juarez-Garcia A, Wang D, et al. Oral naltrexone as a treatment for relapse prevention in formerly opioid-dependent drug users: a systematic review and economic evaluation. Health Technology Assessment 2007; 11: 1–85.
27. Dijkgraaf MGW, van der Zanden B, de Borgie CAJM, et al. Cost utility analysis of co-prescribed heroin compared with methadone maintenance treatment in heroin addicts in two randomised trials. Brit Med J 2005; 330: 1297–302.
28. Gunderson E, Fiellin D. Office-based maintenance treatment of opioid dependence. How does it compare with traditional approaches? CNS Drugs 2008; 22: 99–111.
29. Bell J, Shanahan M, Mutch C, et al. A randomized trial of effectiveness and cost-effectiveness of observed versus unobserved administration of buprenorphine-naloxone for heroin dependence. Addiction 2007; 102(12): 1899–907.
30. Birch S, Gafni A. The 'NICE' approach to technology assessment: an economics perspective. Health Care Manage Sci 2004; 7: 35–41.
31. de Wet C, Reed L, Bearn J. The rise of buprenorphine prescribing in England: analysis of NHS regional data, 2001–03. Addiction 2005; 100: 495–9.
32. Cameron J, Ritter A. Contingency management: perspectives of Australian service providers. Drug Alcohol Rev 2007; 26: 183–9.
33. Ritter A, Cameron J. Australian clinician attitudes towards contingency management: comparing down under with America. Drug Alcohol Depen 2007; 87: 312–15.

34. Brooner R, Kidorf M, King V, et al. Comparing adaptive stepped care and monetary-based voucher interventions for opioid dependence. Drug Alcohol Depen 2007; 88S: S14–S23.
35. Sindelar J, Elbel G, Petry N. What do we get for our money? Cost-effectiveness of adding contingency management. Addiction 2007; 102: 309–16.
36. Pilling S, Strang J, Gerada C. On behalf of the guideline development groups. Psychosocial interventions and opioid detoxification for drug misuse: summary of NICE guidance. Brit Med J 2007; 335: 203–5.

Index

Note: Page numbers in *italics* indicate tables.

Printed in the United States
by Baker & Taylor Publisher Services